Lead Like a NURSE

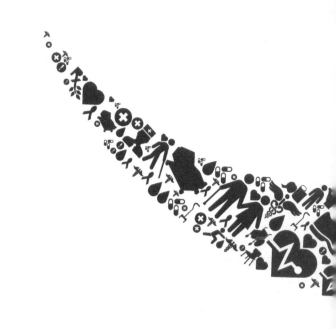

Lead Like a NURSE

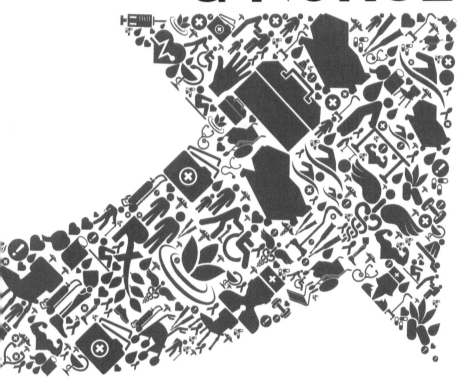

Jeffrey M. Adams, PhD, RN, NEA-BC, FAAN
Jennifer Mensik, PhD, RN, NEA-BC, FAAN
Patricia Reid Ponte, DNSc, RN, NEA-BC, FAAN
Jacqueline Somerville, PhD, RN, FAAN

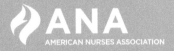

ANA
AMERICAN NURSES ASSOCIATION

Library of Congress Cataloging-in-Publication Data available upon request.

The American Nurses Association (ANA) is the only full-service professional organization representing the interests of the nation's 4 million registered nurses through its constituent/state nurses associations and its organizational affiliates. The ANA advances the nursing profession by fostering high standards of nursing practice, promoting the rights of nurses in the workplace, projecting a positive and realistic view of nursing, and by lobbying the Congress and regulatory agencies on healthcare issues affecting nurses and the public.

ISBN print 978-947800-25-0
ISBN ePDF 978-947800-26-7
ISBN ePub 978-947800-27-4
ISBN mobi 978-947800-28-1

First printing, October 2018

This book is dedicated to my family . . . Tieren, Kallen, Sabine, Ben, Susannah, Tony, Kathy, Todd, Aimee, Tyler, Camden, David, Taylor, Haley, Charlotte, and Pizza Monday . . . these concepts of "the importance of influence" and "positive environments foster better outcomes" have certainly borne truth in my life because of you. Thank you for the wonderful environment of life together.

I'd also like to acknowledge the many of scholarly nurse leaders who have both identified and lived the concepts contained within this book, most importantly "Leadership = Love." I am grateful to have had the gift to call many of you friends, teachers and mentors.

—Jeff

I dedicate this book to Jesse. Thank you for taking the time to know who I really am, for helping me to be more present each day, and for being my light.

—Jennifer

Love and gratitude to my family, friends, mentors, teachers, colleagues, and to those I have had the honor of caring for, teaching, or helping in some way. I gained more than I gave. To my mother, the first inspiring nurse in my life! To our sons, daughters-in law, and grandchildren with love and admiration. To my husband Bill, the foundation of all else.

—Pat

I dedicate this book to all who have taught me to live and lead from a place of wholeheartedness. To my husband Bob and my sons Connor and Jake, whose love is the foundation of my resilience. To the nurse executive team at Brigham and Women's Hospital whom I had the privilege to serve and who consistently pushed me to be my best. And lastly to my leadership coach Mary Connaughton whose wisdom and generosity of spirit is second to none. I love you all.

—Jackie

Brief Contents

Contents

Foreword

I was asked not long ago why I so readily agreed to participate in writing projects with the potential to compete with my own work. For me, the answer is always simple. One of my fundamental beliefs is that the more diverse the lens of life we look through, the richer and fuller is our own thinking and insight. This is no less true with the vital subject of leadership. I spent the last 40 years of my career, both in scholarship and practice, pursuing a deeper understanding of the meaning and action of leadership related to both individuals and the practice community. It has been a challenging pursuit but one that is mostly filled with the energy, excitement, and joy of learning and expanding my own insight on this topic. I mention this here because this text adds considerably to our understanding regarding effective leadership, especially that grounded in evidence-based knowledge and explicated through the discipline of personal experience and scholarly study and research.

The overriding driver for this book is ultimately to make a strong connection between leadership and the many ways it serves as a vehicle for expressing "agape," the experience, demonstration and expression of love between people. The effort to strengthen the connection between leadership and love is a logical initiative if at the end of the process human relationships are enhanced, effective interactions are advanced, and the quality of our lives is measurably improved. The connection between leadership and love demonstrates a concerted human effort to both enumerate and ultimately express that deep bond at the core of our humanity exemplifies our fundamental and primordial interdependence.

This relationship reflects collateral, equitable interaction between committed people to operate at our many human intersections in a way that demonstrates our capacity to embrace this fundamental interdependence and our willingness to use that energy together to advance our human condition. In a very powerful way, creating the conditions and methods that make this process possible and sustain it is the cornerstone of effective leadership.

Another important consideration bound into the fabric of this book is a deep understanding of the requisites of knowledge and truth that underpin leadership effectiveness and sustainability. There are a lot of popular articles, books, digital media, and the like that speak to leadership. However, the vast majority of these works are grounded in perceptions, beliefs, experiences, and notions of leadership that are not guided or disciplined by the rigors of science. As a result, a host of interesting yet periodic and incremental approaches to leadership are undertaken without any clear evidence that they are either rational or viable over the long term. Leadership reflects more than simply situational ideas, notions and experiences. While all of these can be included in the mosaic of reflections on sustainable leadership, unless they are bound to the evidentiary dynamic and validated by science, they remain simply ideas and notions. This demand becomes more critical as our human community enters more fully into the digital age and confronts the challenges of a new context for human relationships and the emergence of new media through which those relationships now evolve. Increasingly, the principles of complexity and the mechanisms of complex adaptive/responsive systems more strongly influence the context of our human expressions and relationships, creating new demands on our reflections and scholarship related to leadership and its unfolding expressions.

The breadth of topical chapters in this book reflects the bandwidth of leadership insights, experiences, and expressions in the wide variety of contexts and scenarios where leadership competence is critical. Clearly the context and mechanisms for leadership in an environment where the predominant frame for service is a geriatric population differs significantly from the places where the prevailing population is providers across the health system landscape. The leadership capacity and expression of the senior executive reflects a different palette of skills from those experienced at the point of service. Leadership in clinical partnerships across the disciplines requires a different alignment of equity and value and, thus, a different focus of leadership expression. All of these subtle yet unambiguous leadership expressions are reflected in each and all the chapters of this book in a way that calls the reader to more explicitly and intentionally comprehend the capacity to lead and exercise the requisite and appropriate skill sets.

There is much to engage both the novice and experienced leader in this text. The array of authors and chapters provide a wide range of insights and challenges to leadership that applies to leaders in a broad variety of settings and roles. Yet all are grounded in the inexorable connection between leadership and love and in the behaviors that demonstrate the energy of that interface at work in our communities of practice and in the human community. Reading this work through that lens will prove how important this leadership text is in adding to the armamentarium for evidence-based and relevant leadership for all of us going forward.

—Tim Porter-O'Grady, DM, EdD, APRN, FAAN, FACCWS

Introduction

*Even though there is now a vast body of
work on leadership, I find it far more enlight-
ening to consult our personal histories.*

—Margaret Wheatley

Margaret Wheatley states that in creating your own definition of good
leadership, you should reflect upon the leaders you were happy to serve
under. What were their behaviors? How did they make you feel? What
kind of worker where you? There is no one right way: no leadership
theory, behavior, or person that you can read about that will solve all your
leadership issues. Every situation, organization, team, and individual is
different in their own way. However one common element among all is
that we are all human and we thrive when love is part of the equation. In
our estimation, leadership in its highest form is love.

Our goal for this book is to provide you with the perspective of many
different nursing leaders and what worked for them. Read, and take from
the chapters what makes sense for you.

In this book there are 16 chapters. Each chapter builds upon leadership
in some aspect. Whether you are a staff nurse learning how you are a

leader or whether you are the most seasoned nurse executive and board member, there are many takeaways to learn from others so that you can create your own definition of good, if not exemplary, leadership.

Within each chapter there are various models, vignettes, case studies, and reflective questions to assist you in immediately applying the chapter learning into practice.

Chapter 1: This chapter describes a set of personal commitments that you can integrate into your behaviors in order to lead effectively.

Chapter 2: This chapter presents several essays on some of the most pressing issues that leadership in nursing is facing today. To address any issue, those in the profession must know where we have been, what is known today, and where we are going. Here you will read about leadership impact on patient outcomes, compassion fatigue, the professional practice environment, the value of nursing, influencing theories, and where we stand regarding evaluating leadership.

Chapter 3: So how do you determine if formal leadership is the career track you would like to pursue? What kind of questions should you be asking yourself? What kinds of experiences should you involve yourself in to help you with this important career choice? This chapter provides many case studies and reflective questions to help you determine these answers.

Chapter 4: As the largest workforce segment of healthcare delivery, nurses should lead in shaping future healthcare policies, regulation, workforce expectations, and the healthcare delivery model. This chapter discusses nursing's leadership role in supporting the Quadruple Aim.

Chapter 5: This chapter highlights the historical challenges and current points of strength for the profession of nursing. We discuss an evidence-based approach to enhancing nursing's influence in practice, research, education, policy, theory, media, and industry.

Chapter 6: We wrote this chapter with an eagerness that you would read it with interest in exploring what leading interprofessionally means to you, personally and professionally, and why being interprofessional and leading interprofessionally are aspirational, if not essential, nurse-leader attributes for you to model in your leadership for yourself and others.

Chapter 7: Complex technologies within complex healthcare organizations can no longer be relegated to one department for decision-making through the systems development life cycle. In this chapter you will learn how the chief nursing informatics officer, chief nursing officer, and nursing management leaders together are essential for the success of the planning, analysis, decision, implementation, and maintenance of healthcare technologies.

Chapter 8: This chapter has several goals: first, to provide an overview and background of diversity and health disparities; second, to examine leadership practice at the bedside, middle-management, and executive levels; third, to showcase leaders through exemplars who have leveraged their influence both personally and professionally to drive successful clinical and organizational outcomes, to create change, and to establish a legacy for the future; and fourth, to provide a plan of action to advance diversity at all leadership levels.

Chapter 9: This chapter provides an overview of innovation by defining it and then describing leaders of innovation in the context of a research study the authors conducted on the characteristics of innovative nursing leaders.

Chapter 10: This chapter explores the attributes of nursing leadership that lead to successful programs or initiatives that impact the health and wellness of patients and caregivers by utilizing healthcare-focused evaluation, quality improvement, and research. We focus on settings outside of those where nurses are typically well represented such as hospitals, healthcare organizations, academic medical centers, and academia.

Chapter 11: This chapter presents stories of how three Boston-based nurse leaders—one academic dean and two chief nursing officers—transformed what have been traditionally acknowledged as academic practice partnerships to address the recommendations made in 2010 in *The Future of Nursing: Leading Change, Advancing Health* report.

Chapter 12: In this chapter the authors reflect on their extraordinary ability to develop the gerontological nursing workforce and program within one hospital.

Chapter 13: This chapter explores the intersections of mindfulness and leadership from a pragmatic view that can be applied immediately.

Chapter 14: This chapter explores the impact of a relational care approach from the unique perspective of patients. Theory-infused practice that grounds nurses in this unique, holistic perspective ensures that nurses remain connected to the meaning and purpose of their work and supports their engagement in the current healthcare environment, whose focus may not always be consistent with nursing's worldview.

Chapter 15: This chapter challenges you to reflect upon and articulate what it is you are leading. In truth, unless you are leading the practice environment to facilitate nursing practice, you are not necessary. So how do you know you are meeting the expectations of your role?

Chapter 16: This chapter covers the need to prioritize health policy as a domain of nursing practice and discusses the role of nurse leaders in creating space for health-policy efforts in practice and research settings. Nurse leaders must be deliberate in devoting time and efforts to inform discussions at all levels of policy.

Our intention for this book is to generate a platform for advancing evidence through health services research and descriptions of action learning and empirical experiences about how best to prepare nurses to lead with love and effectiveness. Does leadership development matter? Do effective leaders influence patient, workforce and organizational outcomes? This book begins to answer these questions and stimulate people's thinking about them.

Chapter 1

Leadership Commitments That Drive Excellence

Patricia Reid Ponte, DNSc, RN, NEA-BC, FAAN
Jacqueline Somerville, PhD, RN, FAAN
Jeffrey M. Adams, PhD, RN, NEA-BC, FAAN

Effective leadership matters. It is essential for delivering and achieving high-quality healthcare. It is essential within colleges and universities to ensure positive learning experiences and outcomes. It is essential within research labs and programs to ensure highly productive and innovative teams, knowledge development, and knowledge dissemination.

The Obligation to Lead Well

Those educated and prepared as professionals have a societal obligation to lead effectively in all realms of their work, personal, and community lives whether holding a formal leadership role within an organization or not.

To support the commitment of professionals to lead effectively, in this chapter we describe a set of personal commitments that when integrated into one's behaviors increase one's capacity to lead effectively. We also provide vignettes illustrating the practical application of these commitments and share information about current approaches to analyzing the relationship between effective leadership and clinical, workforce, and organizational outcomes.

It's Complicated

It rings true for most people that good leadership makes a difference in the pursuit of any collective activity. There are numerous theories, models, and approaches that address the attributes of a good leader, how to learn to be a good leader, and how to enact good leadership. There is less known about whether good leadership impacts the outcomes of a given collective activity.

Analyzing the relationship between leadership effectiveness and outcomes is complex for many reasons: standardizing leaders' behaviors is very challenging, so measuring it becomes tricky; situations that require leadership action are complex and multifaceted; contextual issues vary greatly from organization to organization or situation to situation; human interactions and relationships are unique and situational; and standardizing behaviors based on a particular formula may not be desirable given the diversity and the unique needs of people. How, when, and why leadership is exerted varies greatly along with the context in which it occurs. And leadership is conceptualized in many ways: a set of personal attributes and attitudes; a knowledge base or set of experiences that prepare someone to lead; a technical, evidence-based skill set that can be applied; a commitment to using a set of competencies, principles, or practices that guide an individual's behavior; or an organizational role that gives an individual the power and authority to lead. These factors and more present healthcare-services researchers with a daunting set of attributes used to create models to define and measure leadership effectiveness and its impact on outcomes. That said, discovering ways to demonstrate how a leader's (or a group of leaders') actions and style impact the outcomes of a healthcare or academic organization would be useful for many reasons. One important reason is to help guide organizations and leaders to spend precious dollars on leadership development. But what's more important is that leaders in healthcare today—whether in practice, education, or research—are faced with some of the most daunting challenges and problems. The actions and decisions that leaders make to solve or improve situations is of great importance.

A common example of such a challenging situation is described in the following vignette.

> The clinic assistant was afraid of what the response might be. It was early and the physician she was working with that morning was running late—behind schedule already. But she knew that she needed to inform the physician about the pain-assessment level of her patient. She couldn't find the physician, so she paged her and just as the physician answered the page, the clinic assistant saw the physician rounding the corner with her cell phone to her ear. The physician said "I'm on my way to clinic now" and hung up. Minutes later the physician showed up and, upon seeing the clinic assistant, didn't stop and went directly into the exam room. The clinic assistant sought out the help of the nurse manager to ensure that the physician would become aware of the patient's pain and that it would be swiftly addressed.
>
> The other thing on the mind of the clinic assistant was that she felt ignored and disrespected by the physician, and she believed that should be addressed as well; after all, a team training refresher had just been conducted for this clinic. Both the clinical assistant and the nurse manager (and presumably the physician) knew what they should expect from the physician in terms of response time and interaction norms. The nurse manager knew that she would need to speak to the physician about the lack of follow-through on both counts but first talk with her to be sure there weren't other factors at play.

Essential Leadership Commitments

This vignette illustrates a common phenomenon in healthcare delivery occurring at the intersection of patient care and the interaction of staff who provide the care. At this intersection there are countless opportunities for effective leadership; how leaders engage, act, behave, and make decisions are all serious matters. More effective leadership in these spaces improves patient care processes and outcomes.

Guiding leaders to be most effective in their work and life can take many forms. The definition and promulgation of leadership competencies is one such approach, such as degree-granting programs in health administration. Leadership-development programs that promulgate and share evidence-based models and frameworks of leadership competencies are another example. A third approach is presented in this chapter.

We describe of a set of commitments based on our own leadership experience. These commitments are action oriented and, if applied consistently in life and work, may improve one's capacity to live and lead effectively. This is particularly true when applied within a context of self-reflection, self-evaluation, self-improvement, and a desire for feedback from others exemplified by asking the question, "Do actions I take and decisions I make appear to be congruent with these commitments?"

Sharing these commitments with others or using them to guide a leadership team could be useful. Novice and expert leaders alike can continue to grow and learn how to best integrate these commitments into their behaviors. As new knowledge and experiences emerge over time, individuals may choose to add to this list of foundational commitments.

The following section provides a set of commitments that are based on our experiences and in many cases are supported in literature about personal, interpersonal, and leadership effectiveness. These commitments are described to guide the thought process and behaviors of individual leaders as they live, lead, and learn.

There is a growing body of evidence suggesting that having a mindful attitude and incorporating mindful practices into one's personal and work life can improve one's sense of health and well-being and one's ability to be a more effective leader (Kabit-Zin, 2007; Marturano, 2015). The next vignette, *Be Mindful*, describes how an NP incorporated a mindful practice into her daily routine. Because of this, she was better equipped to make decisions based on evidence rather than emotion, to listen more intently, to have interactions that were more therapeutic than robotic, and to feel and emit compassion for herself and others. And as it turns out, the NP did coordinate an at-home intravenous

COMMITMENT ONE

Be Mindful and Encourage Others to Do So

The NP was ready to admit her 91-year-old patient to an acute care hospital bed, but something bothered her about proceeding. The patient's son had expressed concern about the decision and pleaded with the NP to come up with another alternative for the treatment of his mother's cellulites. "Isn't there some way to keep her in her apartment and treat her?" The NP knew this would be cumbersome to arrange and coordinate and would involve risks. But maybe the son was right; after all, the risks of admission to the hospital were probably greater for a woman this age. The NP was so busy and stressed now. She had five more patients to see before wrapping up her clinic session at 5:00 p.m., and it was currently 3:45 p.m. She needed to be at the daycare center to pick up her son—there was no choice in the matter since her wife was out of town on business. The NP decided to take five minutes to do some deep breathing before going back into the exam room. She sat in front of her computer, shut her eyes, got as comfortable as she could, began breathing, and focused her attention on her breath. Each time her mind moved to the situation at hand, to what she needed to prepare for dinner, to the likely high-traffic drive to the daycare center, to her patient and the son sitting in the exam room next door, she brought her mind back to her breathing. After about five minutes she got up from her seat, stretched, and proceeded with her care.

antibiotics treatment plan and she did also make it on time to her daycare provider. She felt that part of the reason both happened was because of her *finding the space to lead,* as titled in Marturano's (2015) book. Finding this space gives us more bandwidth—the ability to see, feel, hear, and reflect on what is in front of us and what is inside of us. "When we have that space, we can deal with even an urgent problem in a calm, creative and humane way, rather than have an expedient reaction to pressure." (p. x)

Marturano goes on to incorporate several practical approaches in everyday work and life. One is to take a "purposeful pause," which includes intentionally guiding your attention to the present moment by noticing and feeling your breath, hearing the sounds in your environment, and noticing the sensations in your body. Taking a purposeful pause allows you to bring focus and clarity to the situation at hand.

Finally, Marturano most importantly points out that mindfulness leadership practices enhance focus, control, creativity, and compassion.

There are other mindful practices that when incorporated into daily life and work can improve personal and interpersonal effectiveness, such as mindfully communicating, which involves listening deeply and speaking the truth. Edgar Schein (2013) coined the term "humble inquiry," which he defines as "the fine art of drawing someone out, of asking questions to which you do not already have the answer, of building a relationship based on curiosity and interest in the other person" (p. 2). This elegant and straightforward way of relating to others can transform a relationship.

A framework for building enduring trusting relationships among colleagues in work settings is described in Stephen Covey's book *The Speed of Trust* (2006). This framework includes what Covey calls the four cores of credibility, which he contends are elements that make one credible to oneself and others. The two cores of integrity and intent address character and the two cores of capabilities and results address competence.

Integrity involves integrating your inner values and beliefs with the courage to act them out. Intent involves your motives, agendas, and behaviors, and trust grows when these are mutually beneficial to yourself and others. Capabilities are your skills, attitudes, unique talents, knowledge, and style. They are the means used to produce results, which also involve execution and performance (Covey, 2006, pp. 54–55).

Covey goes on to describe a set of behaviors that establish and continuously grow trusting relationships over time as leaders consistently display them. These behaviors include talking straight, demonstrating respect, creating transparency, righting wrongs, showing loyalty, delivering results, getting better, confronting reality, clarifying expectations, practicing accountability, listening first, keeping commitments, and extending trust. Covey also offers an approach to restoring trust by using these behaviors after mistakes are made and trust falters.

The *Build Your Capacity to Create Trust* vignette introduces James, who came to understand upon reflection after the events discussed that he hadn't confronted reality and clarified expectations with his team of direct reports and so trust had diminished, particularly with

Commitment Two

Build Your Capacity to Create Trust in Your Relationships

James, a chief operating officer (COO) of a large community hospital, was called in to meet with his boss, Sue, the chief executive officer. She told James that several months earlier, the vice president (VP) of marketing, Dan, one of James's direct reports, asked to meet with Sue to let her know that he was being recruited to another job.

Sue told James that at the time she did not share this information with him but instead asked the human resources department to work with her to try to retain Dan through a variety of measures. And now, four months later, Dan had come back to Sue letting her know that the other hospital had increased the offer and he was hard pressed not to accept it.

Sue said that she felt she had no other recourse but to involve James at this time so that he could make a counteroffer that would include a significant bonus and salary increase to retain Dan. Several things about this bothered James: (1) there were performance issues with Dan that James had been working through with him; (2) Sue had engaged directly with James's direct report without his knowledge; (3) similarly, Dan had engaged in discussion with Sue—James's boss—without first conferring with James, which was a norm in this organization; and finally (4) for four months, James had no idea that his direct report was being recruited elsewhere. He likely would have recommended that Dan take the new job if he had known.

The trust that James had in both of his colleagues had diminished to the lowest level he could ever imagine. "Now what?" he said to himself. Six months later, Dan was appointed COO after Sue asked James to resign.

the VP. Because James hadn't behaved based on his own values (integrity) and hadn't set clear expectations with his direct reports regarding performance and communication, the VP was able to undermine and ultimately replace him. James learned that he had contributed to what happened by not setting expectations, not righting wrongs, and not confronting reality. Following this life lesson, James became a more effective person and leader as a result.

Angeles Arrien, noted anthropologist and author (1989, 2004) who studied indigenous cultures, related the importance of integrating an equanimous stance into our interactions with others. To do this well, she posited that people must have courage, show respect, and be honest, patient, and compassionate. So what is equanimity?

According to Mary Connaughton (2016), who worked closely over many years with Angeles Arrien, "Equanimity is the capacity to see something (self, others, circumstances) exactly as it is. It is a mindset, a choice to approach life in a calm, grounded and unflappable way" (p. 257). The equanimity framework that Connaughton uses in her coaching practice includes objectivity, the ability to see things for what they are and trust one's assessment of the situation; curiosity, always being open to seeing something in a new way; and emotional neutrality, having emotion but without reactivity. The model also includes steps to address problems:

1. Describe and acknowledge the situation.

2. Describe and acknowledge how you may be contributing to the problem.

3. Describe what you are learning as this problem has unfolded.

4. Describe what you will do the next time the problem arises.

Connaughton goes on to say that leaders who practice equanimity can reduce both their own stress and that of others, can diagnose and resolve problems more efficiently, and can better anticipate challenges or the negative behavior of others. Their calm nature enables them to see patterns and then alter their own reactions to the anticipated patterns and the behaviors of others to be more effective.

Connaughton and Hassinger (2007) describe compassion as a necessary leadership characteristic, defining it as the willingness to see the humanity in another person, to care deeply, and to express support without caretaking too much. Acknowledging the role of compassion in addressing the problematic behavior of another person is critical to leading effectively. Without compassion for the humanity of others, leaders can't truly effect change or improvement.

The researcher from the *Be Equanimous* vignette took the steps outlined above and returned to the next meeting with clarity and a resolve to find

COMMITMENT THREE

Be Equanimous and Compassionate

The researcher left the meeting feeling unsettled and angry. The meeting, which was held weekly, consisted of interprofessional team members who were leading a research project focused on patient progression and care coordination. As the only nurse scientist on the team, she felt like her contributions to the design of the study and the interventions that were central to it were unquestionable. But she often felt marginalized in discussions during the meetings. When she shared her perspectives or suggested alternative approaches or ideas, one of her colleagues would routinely dismiss her and talk over or disagree with her, and other colleagues tended to follow suit. This colleague also occupied a higher rung in the organization's hierarchy. As the researcher left the meeting she mused about how she could possibly ever get to a point where she could address this damaging and demoralizing interpersonal dynamic.

her voice and be respectful but assertive in responding to her colleague when she tried to squelch her ideas. She did so in the months and years ahead, coming from a place of compassion and equanimity and recognizing that whatever was driving her colleague's behavior likely had something to do her with own needs and desires and was not necessarily motivated by competition or negative emotions. The research project was a great success and the team who led it worked effectively and collaboratively.

Daniel Goleman is an expert in the field of emotional intelligence. He notes that

> *While our emotional intelligence determines our potential for learning the fundamentals of self-mastery and the like, our emotional competence shows how much of that potential we have mastered in ways that translate into on-the-job capabilities. To be adept at an emotional competence like customer service or teamwork requires an underlying ability in Emotional Intelligence fundamentals, specifically social awareness and relationship management.* (Goleman, 1996, p. xv)

COMMITMENT FOUR

Use and Promulgate Social Intelligence Skills

The newly elected chairman of the undergraduate school of nursing knew that his peers viewed him as technically competent to take on the account- ability and responsibilities of the role. He felt like his years of academic expe- rience positioned him well to be successful, but something was bothering him about the opportunities and challenges that lay ahead. He knew that some of his peers believed that his tendency to be domineering, controlling, and one sided in his views was a liability. Deep inside he believed that more than often than not his way of doing things was the best and right way; after all, he'd seen it all over the 22 years he had been at the college.

But he also knew that he could really turn people off, including students at times. He felt that this was true in his personal life as well. His grown chil- dren often didn't seek his advice because he tended to be overpowering and controlling, he thought. Considering his age, he wondered if there was anything he could possibly learn or do differently. He broached the subject with the dean that he reported to. They talked about it a few times, decided to look at the psychology and leadership literature, and came across the concepts of social and emotional intelligence. Through reading and with the help of a coach, the chair began to gain insight into his competency level regarding effectively relating with people. He knew he needed to build new behaviors and integrate a different mindset and style into how he developed and sustained relationships over time. The chair became very successful after a rocky start and continues to lead in this position today, eight years later.

He goes on to say that emotional competencies can be learned, but having these competencies doesn't mean that one is competent in the technical aspects of every scenario. He suggests that emotional self-awareness can be learned and improved over time. This awareness involves recognizing and naming the emotions we feel, understanding the causes of our feelings, and recognizing the difference between feel- ings and actions. He also advances the idea that managing our emotions is critical to effectively relating to others.

In his early work he posits four critical elements of emotional intelli- gence: self-awareness, self-management, social awareness, and relation- ship management. There are evidence-based approaches to improving one's capacity or competence in each of these domains. His later work advances the phenomena of "social intelligence" (Goleman, 2006) and its centrality to effective leadership in all aspects of life and across all industries. In his landmark book *Social Intelligence: The New Science of Human Relationships* he defines social awareness as the capacity to instantaneously sense the inner state of another person, including their thoughts and feelings. Elements of this interpersonal process include primal empathy, attunement, empathic accuracy, and social cognition.

The second domain of social intelligence is what Goleman terms social facility. He suggests that social awareness isn't sufficient for fruitful or effective interactions with others but rather sets the stage for the possibility. The social-facility capabilities include synchrony, interacting smoothly on a nonverbal level; self-presentation, presenting oneself effectively; influence, shaping the outcome of a social interaction; and concern, caring about others' needs and acting accordingly (Goleman, 2006, p. 84).

In the *Social intelligence Skills* vignette, the new chairman was able to identify through self-reflection the need to improve his capability to interact more effectively with other people so he could successfully enact his role. He was insightful enough to engage a coach to help him with this important personal-growth work. He demonstrated high competence in social intelligence because of this work, and the organization benefitted greatly as a result.

In the next vignette, *Drive Innovation*, a CNO leads a major departmental change that generated innovative ideas using a standardized framework for facilitating idea generation and creativity. Transformation doesn't happen on its own. This example illustrates that if things had been left to sort themselves out, the department may never have found the time to make a shared-governance model work.

Leaders need to know about and use tools for driving innovation, change, and improvement that are proven and evidence based. There are many models, frameworks, methods, and approaches, such as lean thinking (Womack & Jones, 2003) or lean philosophy. This philosophy seeks to supply exactly what the customer wants when the customer wants it. The methods that are used in lean thinking begin with defining what "value" means to the customer, followed by value stream mapping and ending with a means to constantly pursue perfection. This philosophy is steeped in the quality improvement process, and although it is not often thought to go hand in hand with driving innovation, using lean philosophy to

COMMITMENT FIVE

Drive Innovation, Change, Improvement, and Lifelong Learning

The chief nursing officer (CNO) believed that if she could find a way to get a diverse group of clinicians and staff together for a block of time, ideas would emerge about how to improve the shared-governance model in her department. It had become so impossibly difficult to get staff off the unit to attend meetings for information sharing and decision-making. The local-level leaders and staff themselves were ready to give up. There were also some rumblings from union leaders that shared governance was a farce and a means of "controlling the troops."

This was the furthest thing from the CNO's mind, as she was committed to inclusivity and shared decision-making. She knew that those individuals closest to the care of patients and families—what she termed as "the knowledge workers," just as Deming had done decades before—were the most precious and valuable organizational resource. Tapping into their energy and knowledge would be the most effective means of assuring excellence and continuous improvement in care delivery. So she decided to call together a four-hour work session devoted to coming up with alternative approaches to the current shared-governance structure. She decided she would use exercises from the Change Acceleration Process or CAP that she had learned about in an organization-wide lean hospital engagement with General Electric Healthcare Consulting.

In this first session, she focused on things like obtaining stakeholder buy-in, shaping a vision, and identifying metrics through consensus. The work was amazing, and she received much positive feedback from those who attended and those who didn't but had heard about it. The CNO facilitated the session herself, which received a positive reaction because much of the staff believed they didn't need an external facilitator or consultant for everything the department did. The shared-governance meeting structure changed drastically and with great organizational support. Six years later there continue to be quarterly full-day meetings, voting processes for representation on the councils, and robust work products of the councils and committees. Nurses and others feel very satisfied with their ability to truly contribute to the policy- and decision-making in the organization, as evidenced by high employee engagement and satisfaction scores.

improve a process or outcome often provides the seedlings of the greatest and most compelling ideas and results. Organizations that innovate are more sensitive to the quality of their business environment. They are highly committed to adopting and disseminating new knowledge, to relentlessly using and monitoring metrics, and to evaluating how benchmarks can be used to compare results with external competitors and partners to drive excellence in structure, process, and outcomes.

The CNO's instinct was to improve the capability of clinicians to physically participate in departmental decision-making and policy formulation. This instinct, along with her knowledge of and competency in the use of the CAP model to ensure inclusivity in decision-making and change, had significant organizational results in the years ahead relative

COMMITMENT SIX

Ensure Clear Lines of Accountability in Life and Work Roles

The new associate dean at a large college in the northwest was puzzled. She was on her way to attend the monthly faculty assembly meeting when her assistant called her and said that the invite to the meeting was not on her calendar after all. It had been on there, but it had recently been removed. Now it made sense to the associate dean. The newly appointed chair of the graduate program had told her that she wasn't invited to the faculty assembly meeting routinely, only periodically, but the associate dean thought for sure she didn't have her facts straight. After all, why an associate dean wouldn't be invited to a meeting in which business of the school of nursing program was routinely conducted was puzzling. So despite the calendar invite, she decided that she would attend anyway.

As she walked into the room the chair of the undergraduate program approached her and quietly said to her, "I'm sorry that I need to tell you this, but this meeting is for faculty represented by the college's union only. I don't necessarily agree with this, but as an administrator, you really shouldn't be attending this meeting."

The associate dean held her ground and said, "I don't agree with it either, so I'm staying. The business conducted in this meeting is all about my role and what I'm accountable for—I'm collaborative and inclusive and, union or not, I can be helpful to the both the process and outcomes."

to employee engagement, patient satisfaction, and clinical and organizational outcomes.

The clearer the role expectations, the more effective a person can be and the better the outcomes. When applied to organizational roles and performance outcomes this simple but powerful mindset can drive excellence and a culture of accountability. The most efficient and effective healthcare organizations with the highest performance and best results get that way because of their most precious resources: people. When people (employees) are unquestionably clear about what is expected of them and they are competent to perform the duties that are delegated to them, they produce accurate results in the most effective and efficient way. In healthcare however, there are inherent complexities particularly around coordinating and delivering care. Roles often have overlapping responsibilities, employees are often trained to assume a variety of functions based on resource allocation and constraints, and multiple healthcare teams of varying disciplines have shared accountability for seamless care of patients and families.

Job structure analysis, which results in clarification of each functional role's accountability, is the process by which employees who interact directly or indirectly with a function within an organization convene to design and implement job descriptions that describe key areas of functional accountability for each role within a functional unit. This creates job descriptions in tandem with other job descriptions to ensure that all related functions, separate functions, and overlapping functions are addressed and clarified. This process is known as role and responsibility charting, or RACI (responsible, accountable, consulted, and informed). It is a technique used for identifying functional areas where there are process ambiguities, bringing the differences out in the open, and resolving them through a cross-functional collaborative effort. This collaborative process focuses on three major processes aimed at clarifying relationships pertaining to (1) communication or actions required to deliver care (or a product in a sector outside of healthcare), (2) functional roles or department positions, and (3) participation expectations assigned to roles by decisions or actions. This process yields clarity in three areas: role conception, what a person thinks their job is; role expectation, what others in the organization think the role is responsible for; and role behavior, what the person does in carrying out the job. Through role and responsibility charting, or the RACI model, people assign certain roles to be

R—responsible for a specific or set of actions,

A—accountable or answerable for the activity or decision,

C—consulted prior to a final decision or action (often subject matter experts), and

I—informed after a decision or action has been taken.

(Value Based Management.net, 2016)

In *Accountability* vignette, the associate dean, the department chairs, and the dean would ideally participate in a responsibility charting exercise to generate clarity about functional accountability of each key role including faculty in the school of nursing. When organizations or departments are amid a major organizational change or leadership transition, it is critically important to take the time to conduct this process.

Committing to the process of ensuring role accountability drives staff and leadership engagement, satisfaction, and productivity. It leads to better patient- and family-centered care and outcomes. Jody Gittell (2009) in her landmark book *High Performance Healthcare* calls this process "designing jobs for focus" (p. 115). Using this approach, employees become better at coordinating with one another, have stronger relationships, and work toward shared goals. The same concepts apply to colleges and universities given the nature and importance of relationships and coordination between student and faculty experiences.

These commitments and related vignettes can provide a framework for living and leading effectively. There may be other commitments that guide your life, the decisions you make, and how you behave depending on your personal values and life's lessons. Having a framework like this positions you to lead from a place of consistency. Those whom you live and work with will experience you as a trustworthy, compassionate, and consistent presence.

Linking Leadership Effectiveness to Clinical, Workforce, and Organizational Outcomes

There is growing evidence that links certain structural elements of the healthcare work environment to positive clinical, workforce, and organizational outcomes (Aiken et al., 2002, 2011, 2014; Blegen et al., 2011; Cho et al., 2003; Duffield et al., 2001; Estabrooks et al., 2005; McHugh et al., 2016; Needleman et al., 2002). There is less evidence demonstrating that effective leadership positively affects clinical, workforce, and organizational outcomes.

It's natural to conclude that if evidence-based structural elements of a work environment are present—such as a shared-governance model that ensures inclusive decision making, effective interdisciplinary team work structures and processes, attention to employee and patient engagement, and a culture of safety and continuous learning—then the knowledge, skills, behaviors, and attitudes of leaders contribute to the goodness of the work environment. However, health services researchers have given this contention little attention primarily because it is very difficult to develop rigorous methods to evaluate it.

Despite this, organizations and individuals continue to seek out ways to make their leaders more effective. It's a natural inclination given the human-relationship element of healthcare practice and education. Leadership development and assessments of all types and approaches based on a variety of theoretical and philosophical foundations are abound. Which model to choose, how much to spend, how long a program should be, and who the audience should be are questions that are asked daily in organizations of all kinds. We hope this book will give you food for thought about how to answer those questions and will lead you to some good resources and evidence that will guide your improvement efforts.

Chapter Key Points

- Effective leadership matters.

- Leadership is conceptualized and operationalized in many ways.

- Leading in life and work can be more effective and consistent if a set of value-based commitments guide you.

References

Aiken, L. H., Clarke, S. P., Sloane, D. M., & International Hospital Outcomes Research, Consortium. (2002). Hospital staffing, organization, and quality of care: cross-national findings. *Int J Qual Health Care, 14*(1), 5–13.

Aiken, L. H., Clarke, S. P., Sloane, D. M., Sochalski, J., & Silber, J. H. (2002). Hospital nurse staffing and patient mortality, nurse burnout, and job dissatisfaction. *JAMA, 288*(16), 1987–1993.

Aiken, L. H., Sloane, D. M., Bruyneel, L., Van den Heede, K., Griffiths, P., Busse, R., . . . consortium, Rn Cast. (2014). Nurse staffing and education and hospital mortality in nine European countries: a retrospective observational study. *Lancet, 383*(9931), 1824–30. DOI: 10.1016/S0140-6736(13)62631-8

Aiken, L. H., Sloane, D. M., Clarke, S., Poghosyan, L., Cho, E., You, L., . . . Aungsuroch, Y. (2011). Importance of work environments on hospital outcomes in nine countries. *Int J Qual Health Care, 23*(4), 357–64. doi: 10.1093/intqhc/mzr022

Aiken, L., Rafferty, A. M., & Sermeus, W. (2014). Caring nurses hit by a quality storm. *Nurs Stand, 28*(35), 22–25. DOI: 10.7748/ns2014.04.28.35.22.s26

Blegen, M. A., Goode, C. J., Spetz, J., Vaughn, T., & Park, S. H. (2011). Nurse staffing effects on patient outcomes: safety-net and non-safety-net hospitals. *Med Care, 49*(4), 406–14. DOI: 10.1097/MLR.0b013e318202e129

Cho, S. H. (2003). Using multilevel analysis in patient and organizational outcomes research. *Nurs Res, 52*(1), 61–65.

Cho, S. H., Ketefian, S., Barkauskas, V. H., & Smith, D. G. (2003). The effects of nurse staffing on adverse events, morbidity, mortality, and medical costs. *Nurs Res, 52*(2), 71–79.

Connaughton, M. J. (2016). Equanimity: An essential leadership practice in challenging times. *Nurs Leader, 14*(4), 257–60.

Connaughton, M. J. & Hassinger, J. (2007). Leadership character: antidote to organizational fatigue. *J Nurs Adm, 37*(10), 464–70. DOI: 10.1097/01. NNA.0000285150.72365.b7

Covey, Stephen M. R. & Merrill, Rebecca R. (2006). *The speed of trust: The one thing that changes everything.* New York: Free Press.

Duffield, C. & Franks, H. (2001). The role and preparation of first-line nurse managers in Australia: where are we going and how do we get there? *J Nurs Manag, 9*(2), 87–91.

Duffield, C., Wood, L. M., Franks, H., & Brisley, P. (2001). The role of nursing unit managers in educating nurses. *Contemp Nurse, 10*(3-4), 244–50.

Estabrooks, C. A., Midodzi, W. K., Cummings, G. G., Ricker, K. L., & Giovannetti, P. (2005). The impact of hospital nursing characteristics on 30-day mortality. *Nurs Res, 54*(2), 74–84.

Gittell, J. H. (2009). *High performance healthcare: Using the power of relationships to achieve quality, efficiency and resilience.* New York, NY: McGraw-Hill Professional.

Goleman, D. (2006). *Social intelligence: The new science of human relationships.* New York, NY: Bantam Dell.

Kabat-Zinn, J. (2006). *Coming to our senses: Healing ourselves and the world through mindfulness.* New York: Hyperion.

Marturano, Janice. (2015). *Finding the space to lead: A practical guide to mindful leadership* (1st ed.). Bloomsbury Press.

McHugh, M. D., Aiken, L. H., Eckenhoff, M. E., & Burns, L. R. (2016). Achieving Kaiser Permanente quality. *Health Care Manage Rev, 41*(3), 178–88. DOI: 10.1097/HMR.0000000000000070

McHugh, M. D., Rochman, M. F., Sloane, D. M., Berg, R. A., Mancini, M. E., Nadkarni, V. M., . . . American Heart Association's Get With The Guidelines-Resuscitation, Investigators. (2016). Better Nurse Staffing and Nurse Work Environments Associated With Increased Survival of In-Hospital Cardiac Arrest Patients. *Med Care, 54*(1), 74–80. DOI: 10.1097/MLR.0000000000000456

Needleman, J., Buerhaus, P., Mattke, S., Stewart, M., & Zelevinsky, K. (2002). Nurse-staffing levels and the quality of care in hospitals. *N Engl J Med, 346*(22), 1715–22. DOI: 10.1056/NEJMsa012247

Schein, Edgar H. (2013). *Humble inquiry: The gentle art of asking instead of telling.* Oakland: Berrett-Koehler Publishers.

Value Based Management.net. (2016, January 6). RACI Model. Retrieved from http://valuebasedmanagement.net/methods_raci.html

Womack, James P. & Jones, Daniel T. (2003). *Lean thinking: Banish waste and create wealth in your corporation* (1st Free Press ed.). New York: Free Press.

Chapter 2

Today's Foundation for Nursing Leadership

This chapter presents several essays on some of the most pressing issues that leadership in nursing is facing today. To address any issue, the profession must know where we have been, what is known today, and where we are going. Here you will read about leadership impact on patient outcomes, compassion fatigue, the professional practice environment, the value of nursing, influencing theories, and where we stand regarding evaluating leadership.

Influence of Leadership on Patient Outcomes

Jennifer D. Eccles, MScN, MEd, RN, doctoral candidate

The goal of any nurse leader is to have positive patient outcomes, and this is also the goal of this book: to influence patient outcomes. However, the understanding of how best to accomplish this goal lacks definition due to the fluidity of the relationships involved.

Leadership and outcomes must be viewed as parts of a whole. Just as wellness does not occur in isolation from the entire being, positive patient outcomes are influenced by the whole system of care, including leadership and the work environment. Therefore, we must view leadership in a holistic manner, influencing and influenced both by the work environment and by patient outcomes (Adams & Natarajan, 2016).

Structure-Process-Outcomes Theory

Over 50 years ago, Avedis Donabedian (1966) began articulating this holistic viewpoint in his seminal work to assess quality in the healthcare environment. This framework (figure 2–1) evolved to include three major realms: structure, process, and outcomes. Structure refers to those aspects supporting the care of patients, such as facilities and equipment. Administrative structure and support also fall into this category, as this support is considered an underpinning of the ability of caregivers to provide quality care. Process refers to how care is achieved, and includes the providers who support care for the patients, how those providers offer care, their judgments, and their technical competencies among other factors. Outcomes are the results of the structure and processes of care delivery, such as patient outcomes including falls, morbidity, and mortality rates (Donabedian, 1988).

Many studies of quality healthcare have their basis in Donabedian's theory. In fact, in September 2017 an electronic search of articles citing Donabedian's 1966 work revealed over 5,500 citations in 51 years since the publication, with citations consistently occurring to the present day.

The Triple Aim

Another seminal work on quality in healthcare outcomes came out of the Institute for Healthcare Improvement (IHI), through Berwick, Nolan,

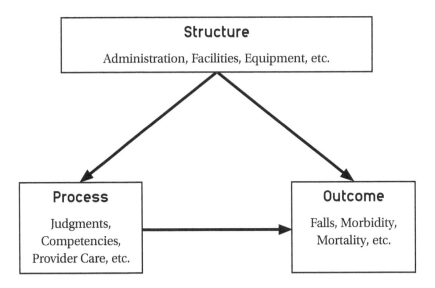

FIGURE 2–1. Donabedian's structure-process-outcome model of quality care

and Whittington's (2008) definition of the Triple Aim. This work took a different holistic view of quality improvement in healthcare, defining the Triple Aim as "improving the individual experience of care; improving the health of populations; and reducing the per capita costs of care for populations" (p. 760). Berwick, Nolan, and Whittington (2008) identified obstacles to healthcare improvement found within policy, healthcare culture, payment systems, and other political factors. These obstacles correspond to Donabedian's structure element, in turn affecting healthcare processes and outcomes to achieve the Triple Aim. It is important for the nursing leader to acknowledge all factors affecting quality healthcare in order to positively influence these factors.

The Quadruple Aim

The Triple Aim was expanded upon by Bodenheimer and Sinsky (2014) in proposing the Quadruple Aim, which includes the three aspects of the Triple Aim plus improving the work life of healthcare providers. The premise for this inclusion is that care team burnout leads to lower patient satisfaction, poorer patient outcomes, and higher healthcare costs, each of which affects accomplishment of the Triple Aim (Bodenheimer & Sinsky, 2014). Knowing that the work life of healthcare providers relates highly to patient outcomes, the nursing leader is then able to focus influence toward the professional practice work environment to improve patient outcomes.

Leadership Characteristics

Although nursing leadership characteristics and styles, such as relationship-based leadership and transformational leadership, have been studied in relation to how they affect perceptions of healthcare employees, these characteristics and styles and how they affect patient outcomes have been studied sparingly throughout the past two decades and seem to be increasing in importance. Wong and colleagues (2007, 2013) found that relational leadership styles, such as transformational or relationship-based leadership, were positively related to improved patient satisfaction, decreased adverse events, and decreased patient mortality. Task-oriented leadership styles, such as transactional leadership or styles focused on structures and processes, were related to increased patient satisfaction (Wong, Cummings, & Ducharme, 2013) but not significantly related to changes in mortality or adverse-event rates.

Conclusion

The concept of influence being a snapshot in time, requiring adaptation to feedback and differing issues (Adams & Natarajan, 2016), includes assumptions that nursing leaders can adapt and should respond differently depending on circumstances. Leadership teachings sometimes promote consistency in interactions and processes as a hallmark of great nursing leadership (Studer, 2009). Yet other leadership teachings hold individualization and strength-based leadership as key (Rath & Conche, 2009). Further, a leader using a different influential style or technique with one person as opposed to another may be viewed as inequitable. However, the interpersonal nature of influence appears to demand an individualized approach to different situations, holding fairness as an ethical imperative to improve equity.

Ultimately nursing leaders should have a holistic view toward the system of care and professional practice work environment, understanding the changing and fluid nature of all relationships involved, to positively affect patient outcomes.

Professional Practice Environment

Maria Ducharme, DNP, RN, NEA-BC

Having been a nurse leader in a Magnet organization for almost two decades, my primary focus has been the development and maintenance of a professional practice environment (PPE) that fosters autonomy and accountability for professional nurses. My goal is to create a structure of professional and shared governance that allows nurses the influence in development of the processes that result in optimal patient and nurse outcomes.

To ensure consistent success in achieving, sustaining, and growing a robust shared-governance structure, I wanted to examine and identify the impact of nurse-leader influence on the health of our professional environments. I struggled when our efforts were not always seen to fruition or our projects were abandoned midcycle. I had noticed that several projects that were not actualized involved processes that were considered sacred or sensitive or those in which financial resources were required, and improvement efforts circled the drain. I desired to further understand the barriers and assist in ensuring that the challenges to achieving success did not rest with a nurse leader's ability to be persuasive and influential.

You may note that the words impact and influence were used in the same sentence in the preceding paragraph, and many people may initially read that as redundant. It is not infrequently that the two words are used interchangeably. However, using the word influence as a passive word does not ascribe to it the criticality of the skill of influence. The American Organization of Nurse Executives (AONE) competencies (AONE, 2015) exemplify influencing behavior as a critical leader characteristic for communication and relationship building. The Institute of Medicine (IOM) report *The Future of Nursing* (2011) outlines the importance of nurses in influencing healthcare decision-making, and the IOM has called for the transformation of the profession through the development of influential leaders. A critical component of the American Nurses Credentialing Center (ANCC) Magnet 2014 standards focus on transformational leadership, ensuring that leaders develop a strategic vision and a professional practice philosophy and demonstrate advocacy for staff and patients. This is measured in part by the position of influence ascribed to the nurse executive to lead professionals and achieve leverage with other executive stakeholders (ANCC, 2014).

Professional Practice/Healthy Work Environments

Since the early research on Magnet hospitals, nurse leaders have been identified as integral in fostering and developing the structures necessary for a healthy and professional work environment (McClure, Poulin, Sovie, & Wandelt, 1983). Subsequently, three decades of evidence suggests that PPEs affect both nurse outcomes (Aiken, Clarke, Sloane, Lake, & Cheney, 2008; Friese & Himes-Ferris, 2013; Laschinger, Almost, & Tuer Hodes, 2003; McClure, Poulin, Sovie, & Wandelt, 1983; Upenieks, 2000) and patient outcomes (Aiken, Sloane, Lake, Solchaski, & Weber, 1999; Aiken, Clarke, Sloane, Lake, & Cheney, 2008; Armstrong, Laschinger, & Wong, 2009; Hall & Doran, 2004; Laschinger & Leiter, 2006; Mark, Slayer, & Wan, 2003; Tourangeau et al., 2007; Witkoski Stimpfel, Rosen & McHugh, 2014). The original Magnet hospitals were selected because they had evidence of the structures that resulted in positive nurse outcomes and because they retained qualified nurses who promote quality patient care. It was the further study of these hospitals that began to make the connection and inform those in healthcare as well as the public that nursing care delivered in an environment that fostered autonomy, interprofessional relationships, and lifelong learning resulted in enhanced patient outcomes as well. A landmark study noted a decreased mortality in these organizations (Aiken, Sloane, Lake, Solchaski, & Weber, 1999).

Following the introduction of the landmark Magnet hospital research, a tool was constructed to measure and evaluate the structural characteristics of PPEs (Kramer & Hafner, 1989). Later revisions sought to identify work processes essential to healthy work environments such as collegial nurse–physician relationships, autonomy, competent peers, perceived adequacy of staffing, and support for professional development; these revisions became known as the Essentials of Magnetism (EOM) instrument. The EOM instrument was based on clinical nurse–identified processes perceived as enabling quality patient care (Kramer & Schmalenberg, 2004; Schmalenberg & Kramer, 2008).

Nurse Leader Influence: State of the Science

If nurse leaders are instrumental in fostering these environments and the environments are critical to optimal nurse and patient outcomes, the logical question becomes, How is it that nurse leaders achieve successes in developing these professional ecosystems? In attempts to answer this question, many researchers have sought to define nurse executive or leadership competencies and characteristics that contribute to leader success and engagement. Some have even examined the impact of leadership characteristics on activities that empower clinical nurses to develop autonomy, to participate in continuous clinical inquiry, to form interprofessional relationships and overall to practice at high levels of professionalism (Adams & Ives Erickson, 2011; Bormann & Abrahamson, 2014; Friese & Himes-Ferris, 2013; Kramer & Schmalenberg, 2004; Kramer et al., 2007, 2008; Lankshear, Kerr, Spence-Lashinger, & Wong, 2013; Laschinger, Finegan, Wilk, 2009; Manojlovich, 2005; Patrick, Laschinger, Wong, & Finegan, 2011; Spence-Lashinger, Wong, Grau, Read, & Pineau Stam, 2011; Wong, Cummings, & Ducharme, 2013). However, fewer researchers have sought to measure or specifically define the attributes of leader influence and its impact on achieving success. Without measurement and a clear definition, how do nurse leaders cultivate the knowledge and self-assuredness to be influential, empowering, and transformational leaders?

While tools and measures of influence exist (Yukl & Falbe, 1990; Yukl, Falbe, & Youn, 1993; Yukl, & Tracey, 1992), their use is documented more extensively in non-healthcare-related fields. In nursing literature as early as 1977 Kanter explored the concept of organizational empowerment, and many researchers have used this theory to outline how nursing leaders can propel the health of the work environment through structures that enable staff empowerment (Laschinger, Almost, & Huer Hodes, 2003; Laschinger, Finnegan, Shamiam, & Wilk, 2001; Manjolovich, 2005; Upenieks, 2000). However, it is more difficult to directly ascribe these successes to the attributes of the leader.

More recently, researchers have begun to explore across the continuum of structure, process, and outcome utilizing more than one construct. For example, they have examined the combined presence of organizational empowerment and transformational leadership, hypothesizing that nurses' clinical leadership practices would be positively related to their nurse managers' use of the leadership practices. They found that nurse-manager leadership had a significant direct, positive effect on structural empowerment and a significant direct effect on clinical leadership (Patrick, Laschinger, Wong, & Finegan 2011). Kanter's theory of organizational power was also used with Yukl's (2006) influence tactics, as theoretical underpinnings, to examine a leader's organizational power and personal influence in creating a nursing PPE. Interestingly the leader role in this study had no direct line authority or budget responsibilities, and researchers hypothesized that the lack of organizational power ascribed to the role would impact the leader's ability to influence. The results indicated that there was a direct and positive relationship between the organizational power ascribed and role function as well as a direct and positive relationship between role function and nurses' perception of their practice environment.

However, leaders' lack of organizational support did not moderate their influence, role function, or the nurse's practice environment as was hypothesized. The influence tactics that the leader used achieved the necessary support and influence of key stakeholders, highlighting the importance of both organizational power and personal influence as factors that contribute to leaders' success and achievement of outcomes (Lankshear, Kerr, Laschinger, & Wong 2013). Other studies have examined the evidence on both the structure and processes that leaders employ to create and nurture PPEs and have measured and defined leader characteristics and relationships (Laschinger, Finegan, & Wilk, 2011; Laschinger, Purdy, & Almost, 2007; Lashinger, Read, Wilk, & Finegan, 2014); yet still, little research has specifically examined influence as a process and less has tied any specific influence characteristic to the health of the environment or to the outcomes.

Influence

I was interested in specifically focusing on influence as an active versus passive process with the goal to begin articulating how nurse leaders develop the competencies to be influential. One may ask why nurse-leader influence is different than that of another field and what additional benefit a tool specifically developed for nurse leaders provides.

While literature supports the notion that an influential nurse leader can create a positive environment, not only do nurse leaders describe a varying level of influence but the public also highlights similar discrepancies. In the Robert Wood Johnson Foundation (RWJF) Bedside to Boardroom survey (Hassmiller, 2011), 1,500 healthcare leaders viewed nurses as having less influence on healthcare than physicians, pharmaceutical executives, insurers, and patients. The same respondents articulated that nurses should hold a prominent level of influence in healthcare policy and planning. The dichotomy clearly outlines the gap recognized by these opinion leaders, with findings in alignment with nurse leaders' self-reports as well as clinical nurse reports that the chief nursing officer (CNO) was not equal in authority to other executives (Jones, Haven, & Thompson, 2009).

Influence as a Process

My desire was to conduct a study in which nurse-leader influence was purported as a process required for dissemination and enculturation of the structural elements necessary for a PPE: clinical and organizational autonomy, collaborative interprofessional relationships, and professional development. The Adams Influence Model provided the framework, where influence connects practice environments and outcomes, and we identified the Leadership Influence over Professional Practice Environment Scale (LIPPES) as the ideal tool to measure the components that collectively and specifically define nurse influence. Because of the abundance of literature suggesting that a PPE results in positive patient and nurse outcomes, research that focuses on how nurse leaders foster these environments and influence their optimization is important.

In proposing a study that examined influence as a process, the question was, Does a relationship exist between nurse leaders' perceived influence over the PPE and clinical nurses' reported engagement in essential professional nursing practice? The hypothesis was that the greater the influence nurse leaders perceive they have over the environment (measured by the LIPPES), the greater the clinical nurses' engagement will be in the essential professional practices. To measure the presence of work practices and relationships essential for a productive PPE and nurses' ability to engage in essential practices, we used the Essentials of Magnetism II (EOMII) tool.

Fast Forward: Findings of Study

The findings of our study were interesting. While the perceptions of leader influence were relatively high on a 1–4, never-to-always Likert scale, the ratings were variable. Authority was the highest score (3.7), suggesting leaders perceive that they have the right to act and that they are accountable and responsible. However, they perceived themselves as least influential in adequately procuring human, physical, information and financial resources (3.0). We anticipated relationships between several like concepts on the tools; however, we found the most significant relationships almost solely in the clinical nurses' domain of adequacy of resources (EOMII). Clinical nurses reported more positive perceptions (on the EOMII) regarding adequacy of resources when nurse leaders perceived themselves to be more influential (on the LIPPES) in collegial administrative approach, authority, access to resources, and leadership expectations of staff, where all were statistically significant. It is compelling that the area in which nurse leaders found themselves least influential was where the most-significant findings existed. The findings also suggest that the extent to which nurse leaders perceive they influence the decisions regarding resources is predictive of nurses' assessed ability to provide essential patient care (p = 0.022), which can be predictive of patient outcomes (McHugh & Stimpfel, 2012). Additionally, we found that clinical nurses' rating of the adequacy of staffing (EOMII) was significantly related to their perception of the quality of care (also EOMII) they deliver in the organization (Ducharme, Bernhardt, Padula, & Adams, 2017).

Implications for Practice

A nurse leader's influence in acquiring access to resources is undeniably a fundamental requirement in providing nurses the tools to deliver essential care. In the context of the IHI Triple Aim (Berwick, Nolan, & Whittington, 2008), in a healthcare environment where cost reduction is an imperative, the findings related to access and adequacy of resources are critical to achieving the balance required to improve the patient experience of care and the health of populations while decreasing costs (Dearmon, Roussel, & Buckner, 2013; Mensik, 2013) . Nurse leaders need to be versed and confident in providing persuasive evidence of the contributions of nursing care to patient outcomes. While the current climate challenges nurse leaders in achieving this balance, we have tools. Newer payment models that reward quality present the opportunity to educate key stakeholders about the value of nursing care; if these stakeholders don't fully understand the value, they may effect detrimental reductions in resources. Nurse leaders need to advocate for resources that support professional environments, the importance of which has been highlighted by the Quadruple Aim's adding the goal of healthy work environments to the Triple Aim (Bodenheimer & Sinsky, 2014; Sikka, Morath, & Leape, 2015). I have too often seen nurse leaders compromise on resources considered "softer resources," such as shared-governance initiatives and educational- and professional-development support, to ensure there is an adequate number of nurses caring for patients.

Staffing resources are at the forefront of every nurse leader's mind, as procurement of such constitutes a large part of a leader's role. However, the importance of the "softer resources" cannot be underestimated and cannot be excluded from the adequacy-of-resources discussion. As considerable debate exists within the profession regarding staffing resources and more specifically the concept of staffing ratios, it becomes paramount to consider all resources and ensure their presence. While most nurse leaders argue that there is no one-size-fits-all equation regarding ratios for nurse-to-patient care, all agree that adequate resources result in better patient care—under the right circumstances.

Conclusions

Mentoring nurse leaders to develop competencies and confidence in creating a shared vision, educating interprofessional and executive stakeholders on the financial implications of patient care decisions, and constructing and presenting a business case for adequate nursing resources that support nursing are all critical in today's healthcare landscape. Influential nurse leaders advocate for resources utilizing evidence-based research and work to create an environment where success is measured by patient outcomes versus cost reduction. Expert-mentored guidance as well as self-reflection can expand influencing behaviors, provide measure to assist in evaluating the impact of influence, and position the nurse leader to inspire a professional practice environment that supports exemplary outcomes.

Nurse-Manager Practice Environment: Conceptual and Empirical Origins

Nora Warshawksy, PhD, RN, NEA-BC, CNE, FAAN

Professional practice environments are critical to high-quality nurse and patient outcomes (Swiger, et al., 2017; Warshawsky & Havens, 2011). The practice environment has been largely defined as the sociocultural dimensions of the organizational context of hospitals that support or hinder the practice of professional nursing from a clinical nurse perspective (Kramer & Schmalenberg, 2002; Kramer, Schmalenberg, & Maguire, 2010). Nurses have consistently reported that quality nursing leadership at all organizational levels is a critical dimension of the practice environment.

Other dimensions of PPEs include professional development, collaborative interprofessional practice, evidence-based practice, empowered decision-making, adequate staffing, and a patient-centered organizational culture. Nursing leadership, in particular nurse-manager leadership, has been consistently reported as the most significant predictor of nurses' job satisfaction and retention (Cowden, Cummings, & Profetto-McGrath, 2011). The impact of nursing leadership on patient outcomes has been more difficult to establish (Wong & Cummings, 2007; Wong, Cummings, & Ducharme, 2013).

Given that hospitals are bureaucratic organizational structures, the hierarchical nature of organizations must be taken into consideration when studying the effects of nursing leadership (Uhl-Bien & Marion, 2009). Most hospitals have at least three distinct layers of nurse leaders: the senior-executive level, the midlevel director, and the frontline nurse manager. All levels of an organization employ decision-making, with the executive level having the broadest reach. As decisions disseminate throughout an organization, the director and nurse manager may filter information and implement variations of the original decisions. In their unit-level position in the organization, nurse managers may in fact buffer the decision-making of the directors and nurse executives. Clinical staff do not always perceive the flow of information from the executive levels to the front line and may attribute all decisions to the nurse manager—regardless of how well the decisions are received. Thus to better understand the dynamic nature of organizational leadership, the practice environment was defined from the perspective of nurse managers.

Assessing the Practice Environment

Researchers and nurse leaders require valid and reliable instruments to assess their organizational context, identify the relative strength of the environment, and diagnose opportunities to direct interventions. Several instruments exist to assess the practice environment from the perspective of clinical nurses with the most commonly used tool being the Practice Environment Scale of Nursing Work Index, or PES-NWI (Lake, 2002). In order to account for the hierarchical nature of organizations, Warshawsky, Rayens, Lake, and Havens (2013) developed the Nurse Manager Practice Environment Scale (NMPES) to assess the organizational context from the perspective of nurse managers. The initial dimensions of the practice environment of nurse managers were primarily derived from the qualitative work of Shirey (Shirey, 2009; Shirey, Fisher, McDaniel, Doebbeling, & Ebright, 2010) and Mackoff (2010). The conceptual domains include three cultural aspects—a culture of patient safety created by administrative leaders and cultures of generativity and meaning (Warshawsky, Lake, & Brandford, 2013). Three priority nurse-manager relationships emerged: those with their directors, their unit staff, and their physicians. The final two domains were having adequate resources and fair and balanced workloads. Table 2–1 provides a summary of the NMPES.

The NMPES has been used to determine the impact of the practice environment, job design, and nurse-manager characteristics on their job satisfaction and intent to leave their positions (Warshawsky, Rayens, et al., 2013; Warshawsky, Wiggins, & Rayens, 2016). Findings suggest that nurse managers value working in organizations committed to patient safety, having time to coach and mentor clinical staff, having positive relationships with their director, and having a fair and manageable workload.

TABLE 2–1. Domains, definitions, and sample items of the Nurse Manager Practice Environment Scale

Subscales	Items	Definition
Empowering administrative leaders create a culture of patient safety	The actions of the executive leaders are consistent with the stated mission, vision, and values.	The administrative leadership team creates a culture of patient safety. Nurse managers are empowered to develop creative solutions to problems. Organizational decisions are consistent with the organization's mission, vision, and values.
	My executive nurse administrators encourage innovative solutions to problems.	
	The executive leaders value my ideas.	
	The executive leaders in this organization make decisions that reflect the mission, vision, and values.	
	I am empowered to do my job.	
	The executive nurse administrators keep me informed of important information.	
	I am a valued member of the leadership team.	
	The executive leaders put patient safety first.	
	Maintaining a reputation for excellence is important to my organization's leaders.	
	Organizational leaders work with me to find solutions to problems rather than assign blame.	
	I can try new processes in my patient care area(s) without fear of negative repercussions.	
	Educational opportunities are accessible to help me develop as a leader and manager.	
	I have flexibility in my work schedule.	
	The executive leaders respect the work of nurses.	
	I have a plan to further develop my leadership and management skills.	
Culture of generativity	I have time to collaborate with frontline staff to develop solutions to the challenges we are experiencing.	Nurse managers have adequate time to coach and develop their frontline staff.
	I have time to coach others.	
	I have time to advise my staff about their professional development.	
	I am able to coach my frontline staff.	
	I have time to reflect on my work performance.	
	Clinical staff are developed to assume higher levels of professional responsibility.	

Subscales	Items	Definition
Culture of meaning	I am able to translate the organization's mission and goals to the frontline staff.	Nurse managers align the care provided in their patient care areas with the organization's strategic plan.
	I routinely assess the quality of nursing care provided in my patient care area(s).*	
	I know how my department supports the hospital's strategic plan.	
	The behavioral standards are evident in the organizational culture.	
Constructive nurse manager–director relationships	I receive feedback from my director (immediate supervisor) that helps me develop my leadership skills.	Directors establish trust through clear communication and constructive performance feedback.
	My director (immediate supervisor) provides me with constructive feedback on my performance.	
	My director (immediate supervisor) clearly communicates their expectations.	
	My director (immediate supervisor) partners with me to improve patient outcomes.	
	My director (immediate supervisor) trusts my judgment when I make operational decisions.	
	I have a mentor who is trustworthy.	
Effective nurse manager-unit staff relationships	My unit staff partners with me to improve patient outcomes.	Nurse managers partner with their frontline staff to achieve quality patient outcomes.
	My unit staff works with me to resolve patient care issues.	
	My unit staff keeps me informed of important issues.	
Collegial relationships between nurse managers and physicians	Physicians understand my role as nurse manager.	Nurse managers and physicians partner to achieve quality patient outcomes.
	Physicians value my input to resolve patient care issues.	
	I have a physician partner who works with me to improve patient outcomes.	

(continued)

Subscales	Items	Definition
Adequate budgeted resources	The budget allocations for my patient care area(s) are adequate.	Allocations for human and material resources meet the needs of the unit. The process for obtaining additional resources is effective.
	I have enough budgeted staff to meet operational demands.	
	The process to obtain additional resources is effective.	
	Financial resources are available for professional development.	
Fair and manageable workload	The number of people that report to me is manageable.	Nurse managers' scope of responsibility and accountability are manageable and equitable.
	The number of patient care areas that I am responsible for is manageable.	
	My workload is equitable in comparison to my peers.	

* The NMPES has been used to determine the impact of the practice environment, job design, and nurse-manager characteristics on their job satisfaction and intent to leave their positions (Warshawsky, Rayens, et al., 2013; Warshawsky, Wiggins, & Rayens, 2016). Findings suggest that nurse managers value working in organizations committed to patient safety, having time to coach and mentor clinical staff, having positive relationships with their director, and having a fair and manageable workload.

Value: What We Know and What We Need To Study and Learn

Sharon Pappas, PhD, RN, NEA-BC, FAAN

Beginning with the belief that good leadership leads to stronger teams, better work engagement, lower turnover, better patient outcomes, and lower costs, this discussion establishes the connection between exemplary leadership and healthcare value. It was well established in the original research describing Magnet hospitals that nurse leaders are instrumental in fostering PPEs. Such environments are important because of the role they play both in vibrant nursing practice and in preventing harm and improving other outcomes such as patient experience. Improving the quality of patient care has always been a goal of hospitals, first to support their community image as a good hospital and later to reduce the financial burden of poor-quality care, because patient adverse events increase length of stay and because other costs now added financial risk. The association of cost and quality into a relationship describes value. In addition, the Affordable Care Act and Medicare's path to risk created financial incentives to improve quality. The idea of improving patient outcomes while also decreasing costs elevated the concept of value to a desirable and achievable outcome that is grounded in many aspects of nursing practice (Pappas & Welton, 2015).

The Concept of Value

The concept of value was explained best by Michael Porter when he defined value as health outcomes achieved per dollar spent. He went on to say that value should describe how healthcare improvement is measured and should be defined around the patient (Porter, 2010). In an acute care hospital, both quality and cost are quantified. Healthcare organizations deploy financial systems that report budget performance and measure direct costs. These patient care cost-measurement tools, the cost accounting systems, are grounded in concepts of activity-based costing. Federal and commercial payers also measure the cost to Medicare— charges billed to the payer for all services used by a patient both inpatient and outpatient including pharmaceuticals. Reporting the clinical and financial impact on the same outcome expresses value.

There are other organizational outcomes that describe the value of cultural health. One is employee turnover rates, which are associated with an average cost per RN turnover usually based on published research. In addition, as a measure of quality of work environment and often a predictor of turnover, employee engagement rates are measured to understand employee perceptions of specific workplace characteristics. Cultural engagement is a proxy for work environment quality and the cost of turnover is the related financial metric that describes value for the employee and ultimately the patient. These leader-influenced outcomes quantify exemplary leadership.

What We Know

Leaders shape and influence cultures. Saint and colleagues (2010) studied the importance of leadership in preventing infections. They found that successful leaders cultivated a culture when the leader focused on overcoming challenges and inspiring their team as a behavioral foundation to improving patient outcomes.

Hospitals can measure the cost of infections. Using data from the cost accounting system and isolating patients with and without specific infections, one can report the direct cost impact of a central line–associated bloodstream infection (CLABSI) or catheter-associated urinary tract infection. An example of this is a large academic health system that calculated the direct cost and determined that the cost of a CLABSI averaged $14,000 per case or infection. The cost avoidance by improving quality (preventing CLABSIs) allowed this organization to invest in important elements of direct patient care that sustained the elimination of the infection. The leaders here respected the wisdom of the care teams regarding improving care and supported the actions the teams recommended. By doing so they shaped a culture that supports patient value.

The characteristics of leaders also influence teams. Cummings, Midodzi, Wong, and Estabrooks (2010) conducted important research to understand the role that leader characteristics play in patient outcomes at the unit level. Findings showed that nursing leadership style explained some of the variance in patient mortality and that highly resonant leadership was significantly related to lower mortality. Resonant leadership, founded on emotional intelligence, was the basis for influencing outcomes and was defined by 13 leadership characteristics including conflict management, empathy, innovation, integrity, recognition, teamwork, developing others, sharing power and influence, and being achievement focused, empowering, participatory, relationship focused, and visionary/inspiring. This study operationalized the descriptions of emotionally intelligent leadership styles and drew a direct association between how the leader role influences and impacts patient outcomes.

There is also growing evidence on the cost of a continuum of care. The Centers for Medicare and Medicaid (CMS) Bundled Payment for Care Improvement Initiative (BPCI) bundled hospital payments for the multiple services beneficiaries received during an episode of care in an effort to control costs (CMS, 2018). This pre-acute, acute, and post-acute care was a measure of team effectiveness with a reliance on effective communication and collaboration as patients transitioned across multiple settings of care. Communication contributed to preventing the duplication or overuse of services. It also served to coordinate care toward an outcome. Rarely does a team magically accomplish this type of team effectiveness without the influence of leadership. Early BPCI results in some settings show a significant decrease in cost to Medicare for a patient population (CMS, 2018). The reductions were achieved largely through effective team behaviors that optimized collaboration and communication about use of services to achieve good patient outcomes.

Where Do We Go from Here?

Cultures for Innovation

Healthcare systems require both innovation and evidence-based practice to create and sustain both the people that will support the future of care and their systems of work. Leaders poise a culture for innovation through developing the structures of care and through team behaviors within systems of care. The concept of innovation leadership came from the clear need to eliminate silos and instead leverage the collective knowledge of individuals within a larger organization or system. The seven characteristics that influence an organization's movement through changing conditions include boundary spanning, risk taking, visioning, leveraging opportunity, adapting, coordinating information flow, and facilitating (Weberg, 2017). One leader doesn't have to enact all these characteristics; it is a collection of multiple leader behaviors that supports innovation. Innovation leaders are positioned to stimulate advancement into new territory to influence important changes. With changing payment models and incentives, new ideas emerge that require studying to answer questions about patient outcomes and care effectiveness and to adapt to a reforming system. Further study of the seven characteristics would reveal how to assemble teams and how to leverage individual characteristics in leaders. Innovation leadership is required in multiple areas where there is clearly an ability to measure both clinical and financial impact of innovation, thus quantifying exemplary leadership. The pressing areas in need of innovation are research structures, models of primary care access, and professional joy.

Research Innovation

Innovation is needed in research. From the study that associated leadership style and patient mortality, consider the importance of knowing what other patient outcomes are impacted by highly resonant leaders. There could be other leadership characteristics that influence patient outcomes in addition to resonant leadership. Discovering these requires additional study to further quantify leadership impact on the clinical and financial outcomes of patients.

Consider also the innovation of big data. Imagine using unique nurse identifiers in large databases to aid research. The ability to study individual nurse practice beyond the walls of one practice setting or electronic health record is important. An example is the examination how well a nurse manages pain, responds to assessment, monitors blood glucose, and other outcomes. This allows for knowledge of individual nurse practice competency and could influence the development of academic program curricula by ensuring inclusion of big data (Welton, 2013).

In addition, the ability to report the direct cost of care from the same database that houses clinical data would enable users to correlate these data in real time, instead of retrospectively, when making daily decisions about resources to use in patient care. This would require a national standard for cost measurement so that results could be generalized across care systems and settings. Advancing these innovations requires taking significant risks and adapting traditional systems into one that serves broader goals. This requires a culture of innovation.

Practice Innovation

Innovation comes from cultures where leaders create a context open to change. A leader who casts vision, mitigates risk, and is willing to step outside traditional boundaries to study new models is essential. There are other pressing issues such as patient access to care and the cost of prevention outside the sickness model that includes RNs in primary care and school nursing. Effectively implementing solutions requires additional knowledge. Understanding the role of nurses in primary care and their impact on patient engagement, which facilitates adherence to care plans, is important. This period of shortage of primary care providers is an important time for advancing the RN role. Facilitating these dialogues falls to leaders.

School nurses have a window into the health of families, and there is limited knowledge on the value of school nursing and the role it plays in primary care. This is probably due to the variation in models of school nursing and the variation in record keeping of their impact. In one study, innovative leaders established electronic communication between healthcare and school nurses (Reeves et al., 2016). Significant boundary spanning accomplished this innovation. With support of the American Academy of Pediatrics (AAP) policy statement on school nursing, leaders now must advance this innovation to elevate school nursing as key in the country's population health strategy (AAP, 2016; Butcher, 2016). Eliminating the duplicate costs from multiple silos of care, augmented with improving outcomes of problems such as obesity and mental health, demonstrates the value of exemplary leadership.

Cultural Innovation That Supports Professional Joy and Team Effectiveness
Given the cost of turnover, it is essential to understand the individual and team impact on nurse engagement and professional joy. Consider the value of the nurse residency, the value of team development, and how these impact patient outcomes. We need refinements to current research like understanding what matters in leadership development to make important things better or knowing what specific manager actions mitigate sources of stress in the work environment and increase the possibility for professional joy. As cost pressures increase, we must document the value of many of our programs such as leadership development and nurse residencies or we risk program elimination.

Summary
We understand the value of good nursing practice in both acute and post-acute care settings. We need to know specific leadership qualities that build effective, thriving teams and position a culture to innovate and change. Effective leadership creates strong cultures that yield exemplary clinical and financial performance. The benefactors of this value are patients, families, and our communities.

Compassionate Care in the Nurse Leader
Lesly Kelly, PhD, RN

In direct patient care roles, nurses can often identify the portion of their work life that they enjoy the most, whether it is the exhilarating rush of saving a life and feeling they have made a difference or the deep connection of conversations with patients. As a nurse leader, the ability to connect to your compassion, or the joy that you derive from your work, may be more elusive. Burnout occurs when the stressors of work life become a constant, chronic state and are detrimental to psychological and physical well-being. While stress is an inherent characteristic of a nurse leader's position, burnout has serious and detrimental consequences to the individual nurse, the organization—including the staff that the nurse leader directs—and the patients entrusted in the nurse's care. Even more concerning, burnout puts nurses at risk of leaving their position and the profession, creating increased stress on recruitment and retention.

There are ways to prevent, manage, and decrease burnout, with awareness and acknowledgment being one of the most powerful tools. Nurse leaders are one of the most critical components to helping create and sustain a healthy work environment for staff that promotes satisfaction and avoids burnouts. However, nurse leaders can often neglect their own risk for burnout. When an airplane loses altitude and oxygen masks drop from the ceiling, the directions are clear: you must place your own oxygen mask on first before you help others. The same analogy can be applied to the significance of addressing burnout in nurse leaders. As we recognize the need to address burnout in our nursing population, nurse leaders must first place their own oxygen mask so that they can then address the needs of their workforce.

The Burned-Out Nurse Leader

A nurse's work life can be visualized on a continuum of burnout to engagement, with three key dimensions influencing burnout: emotional exhaustion, cynicism toward work, and lack of personal accomplishment (Leiter & Maslach, 2009). Nurses who work in direct patient care roles may be able to recognize the physical and emotional signs of burnout, as examples are easily derived from caregiving, family interactions, overburdened workloads, or poor interactions with physicians (Han et al., 2015; Stimpfel, Sloane, & Aiken, 2012; Welp, Meier, & Manser, 2015). However, nurse leaders often do not recognize the risk for burnout or the stress, overwhelming experiences, and emotional burden associated with those roles. Furthermore, nurse leaders are in the same high-risk environment for burnout and are exposed to factors associated with it (i.e., caring for grieving families, handling patient complaints, managing employee welfare). Leaders can often develop an unhealthy relationship with stress, believing that they must always take on the burdens of their departments, never declining projects or requests and appearing to be constantly working hard for their departments. Rather than help their department, this behavior reflects poor role modeling to their staff and could be contributing to a trickle-down or contagion effect among staff (Bolger, et al., 1989).

The Compassionate Nurse Leader

Ideally we all strive to increase our joy in our professional lives or to move the equilibrium away from burnout and more toward engagement. Compassion satisfaction, or the joy we derive from our work (Stamm, 2017) often appears easier to understand in direct patient care, whether by finding connections with patients and families or having a sense of satisfaction with work in the clinical setting. As a nurse leader, the path to compassion satisfaction may look different and come from different sources; however, there are clearly many opportunities for the nurse leader to garner satisfaction with their role (Kelly & Adams, 2018). To minimize your organizational stress, be mindful of your practices, unplug or limit your technology, and utilize the technology (e.g., do-not-disturb features) to enhance your work. Find a way to connect with your nurses that is meaningful for you. While some leaders choose to participate in clinical activities (e.g., Walk in my Shoes programs), other leaders may choose to mentor nurses at conferences or start a journal club. Unequivocally, leaders must find time to restore their emotional and physical health outside of the workplace in order to be well-balanced and able to care for their staff and patients in their workplace.

Whether you've been a nurse leader for a year or three decades, burnout can be a consequence of the high demands of the role and work environment. Nurse leaders that can find their compassion satisfaction and connect to the joy or satisfaction in their work are more likely to decrease stress and prevent burnout.

Chloe Littzen, MSN, RN, CPN, AE-C

As an emerging nurse leader, I entered the nurse profession so enthusiastically that I burned out by the time I was 25 years old, exacerbating a chronic disease that prevented me from practicing in the field that I loved. While I may have had an underlying disease process, the exacerbation and associated effects resulted from overextending myself and constantly saying yes when asked by peers or managers for assistance. I worked nights, had a long drive to and from work, and would often find myself working long waves of shifts. In the hospital, I worked in a busy critical care environment while participating in staff meetings and organizing committees. Outside of the hospital, I was taking on leadership roles in nursing organizations, attending school full time for an advanced nursing degree, and attempting to maintain a work–life balance. Despite signs of burnout including exhaustion, illness, and safety concerns, I didn't acknowledge the severity of the situation and neither did my friends or family. It wasn't until the situation was so severe that I required medical attention, unable to function anymore from being so exhausted, that I was required to take time off from work and rebuild myself from the ground up while my health was evaluated. Prior to this, I believed what I was experiencing was a social norm. Nurses around me were doing the same things I was, and they had been for decades. I came into work with a smile on my face every day and I didn't think what I was experiencing was negative. Years later I still find myself recovering from this experience, with vivid memories that I never want to relive. This has driven me to make positive changes for my future, from changing my career trajectory within nursing to constantly reminding myself to put my health first; otherwise, I won't be able to be a nurse leader, take care of others, and practice in the field that I love.

Bob Dent, DNP, MBA, RN, NEA-BC, CENP, FACHE, FAAN

As an experienced nurse leader, I have learned that avoiding burnout is necessary for my own well-being and for creating a positive culture and environment for my staff. Personally I have experienced burnout and fatigue from working long shifts for days without adequate rest between when trying to meet the needs of our department and patients. As a nurse leader, it hasn't changed; I find myself at times getting overwhelmed with the amount of work to be done. To overcome the stress, I commit to eating healthier, exercising regularly (I love to play racquetball), and creating a back-yard vegetable garden. At work I do not schedule meetings on Fridays, calling this my Sharpening the Saw Day, a reference to one of Stephen Covey's habits of effective people. I also created a Leadership Team Pledge where we do not schedule meetings the full month of July or the last half of December to allow time to catch up on projects and prepare for upcoming ones. It is my responsibility for my own health, happiness, and success in my life. I must listen to my body and reflect on my leadership regularly. When I find that I'm not performing the way I need to be, I take a step back and take the necessary time to get back on track.

One of the greatest things I can do as a nurse leader is to recognize my nurses for the care and services they provide patients each day. We participate in the DAISY Award Program, a formal recognition program to acknowledge extraordinary nurses who provide compassionate care. To make it meaningful, the award is presented as a surprise and is often attended by the person writing the nomination. Many of these recognitions are streamed live through the internet so the DAISY nurse may share it, receiving thousands of views and comments from colleagues, family, and friends. In addition to acknowledging nurses' compassionate care, I strive to value nurses' education and long-term commitment to the profession. Each year, our hospital displays pictures of advanced degree graduates in the hospital lobby for staff and patients to see and holds an award ceremony with a tribute to Florence Nightingale. The award ceremony recognizes several hospital employees and nurses for various contributions to their profession and our organization, patients, and community.

As an executive leader, I realize that my nursing leadership team has a tremendous responsibility in meeting the demands of running operations inclusive of finance, IT, quality, patient safety, patient satisfaction, and workforce management. In taking care of myself, I can role model to them the value of preventing burnout and keeping the compassion in my leadership practice. Moreover, I have opportunities every day to meaningfully recognize my leaders and staff for their valuable contributions and create an environment for them to reduce burnout.

Leadership-Development Program Evaluation

Joshua Peltz, MSN, MBA, RN

The term *leadership development* has been described many ways, but to understand this we must first define what *leadership* is. Kouzes and Posner have stated that leadership is "not about personality; it's about behavior—an observable set of skills and abilities" (http://www. leadershipchallenge.com/about-section-our-approach.aspx). With specific reference to nursing, Watson has stated that "leadership style and engagement have a direct impact on the caring environment of the bedside nurse" (http://www.leadershipchallenge.com/resource/ caring-leadership-a-model-for-transformation.aspx). John Quincy Adams is attributed with stating "If your actions inspire others to dream more, learn more, do more and become more, you are a leader" As we combine these definitions into the term *leadership development*, we should note that "studying development involves mapping and understanding within-and between-person change patterns—as well as those involving groups, teams, and larger collectives—over time" (Day, Freenor, Atwater, Sturm, & McKee, 2014, p. 64).

Work environments for clinicians have a direct impact on patient outcomes; therefore leadership influence over the professional practice culture should be a top priority of any healthcare leader (Somerville, 2015). Healthcare executives must ensure that those who can positively influence care providers are in positions to help effectuate change that is needed to improve patient outcomes. These innovators of healthcare who are defining the future of care should maintain current knowledge as it relates to innovative leadership methods and responsibilities. The ability to assess the teaching and education of leadership development is vitally important to understanding how it has a direct impact on those who are learning.

As healthcare institutions of all sizes navigate the challenge of narrowing reimbursements, their priority has become operationalizing the delivery of care within a leaner environment while continually improving patient outcomes and care delivery in order to maintain financial stability and solvency. To maintain a presence and continue to be a top choice of consumers, healthcare organizations must ensure that they successfully match talent to role. Thereafter, institutions should define professional-development requirements on both an initial and ongoing basis to ensure that they are fully engaged and able to provide the management and leadership that is required.

It is therefore fundamentally imperative that a standardized mechanism exists to assess, evaluate, and provide feedback on leadership training and development throughout the health professions. It is necessary to evaluate the effectiveness of training and to benchmark its value to ensure that the future of healthcare has strong and knowledgeable resources.

The topic of evaluating leadership-development programs is significant because healthcare organizations often focus on acute issues to manage from day to day and do not necessarily have targeted succession planning in place. The future of any organization relies on identifying and developing a leadership pipeline. It is important not only to provide a method of talent development but also to ensure the content delivery is appropriate, effective, and serving the purpose identified by the organization and each individual in the program to advance his or her knowledge and skills. Individuals must have methods to measure their success, both within the program and afterward, by applying their knowledge.

Assessing leadership-development programs within the framework of a standardized model will help provide meaningful feedback to the faculty of the programs and to the participants and their sponsoring organizations. Understanding how to measure and sustain success through leadership development can help frame the future of healthcare leaders. By using this feedback and establishing leadership competencies, organizations can identify future leaders who are on track to excel within their careers. The following is a review of leadership-development program evaluation as it relates to the health professions.

We reviewed the following online databases for the period of 2007–2017: Cumulative Index of Nursing and Allied Health Literature (CINAHL) and Medline. A Google search was performed with specific search terms. Table 2–2 highlights the specific search criteria, including the databases, search terms, and number of articles located.

TABLE 2-2.   Search criteria

Database	Terms entered for search	Criteria	Number of articles
CINAHL	"Leadership development program evaluation" and "healthcare"	Peer reviewed English only	4
Medline	"Leadership development program evaluation" and "healthcare"	Peer reviewed English only	1
Google	"Leadership development program evaluation" and "healthcare"	Scholar section of Google	20,000

Findings

The CINAHL database returned four articles meeting the search criteria. Two of the articles highlight specifically evaluating a program as opposed to evaluation methods. One article describes current practices in leadership development for managers in Magnet and non-Magnet institutions. The fourth article was Throgmorton, C., Mitchell, T., Morley, T., & Synder, M. (2016).

This article reviews the first year of a Physician Leadership Academy that a Michigan healthcare system instituted. The article uses Kirkpatrick's model of evaluation as a theoretical framework to assess the outcomes of the education, stating, "Qualitative research methods, often lacking from learning evaluation design, uncover rich themes of impact" (p. 391).

The Medline database returned one article meeting the search criteria: by Pradarelli, J., Jaffe, G., Lemak, C., Mulholland, M., & Dimick, J. (2016).

This study discussed a leadership-development program that was established in 2012 and involved 21 surgeons voluntarily participating. The post-education results indicated reported improvements within multiple areas, including self-empowerment to lead, self-awareness, team-building skills, and knowledge in business and leadership. Perhaps most notable was that "surgeons felt 'more confident about stepping up as a leader' and 'more aware of how others view me and my interactions'" (p. 258).

A review of the literature identifies a gap in understanding how leadership-development programs are assessed, specifically for feedback on the value to the participant and, when applicable, the sponsoring organization. Within this space exists an opportunity to improve what is being presented to current and future healthcare leaders. This includes clinical and nonclinical professionals, many of whom are in positions of leadership because of their ability to drive change and positive results but some of whom have had no formalized education.

What Does This Mean?

Effective and meaningful leadership is essential in the current healthcare environment. An effective leader must be able to inspire trust and create and transform a vision into practice by removing barriers and engaging their team. Research continues to prove that overall patient care outcomes benefit greatly from staff that are engaged as the result of an effective nurse leader. Public reporting of consumer satisfaction scores and other outcome measures are creating a transparent environment in which patients are choosing where to seek their care based upon this information. Transparency through public reporting is a major contributor to compliance and improved outcomes.

The change that we need is a standard method to evaluate leadership education and curricula and the ability to associate learned knowledge with career progression. The objective within this is standardization and perhaps a longitudinal study to further understand the effects of various types of leadership education as a function of time through the length of one's career.

In considering this objective, we reviewed the Kirkpatrick Model, which is widely known as the "standard for evaluating the effectiveness of training" (Kirkpatrick Partners, 2017). However, the objective is to focus not necessarily on the sole effectiveness of the training itself but how it is incorporated into practice and implemented throughout the professional career of healthcare leaders.

There are numerous leadership-development programs throughout the country that are highly regarded for the education they provide to students. Considering that there is no standardized model of program evaluation and no longitudinal follow-through, these programs likely all complete their own type of survey, research, and continued follow-up after participant completion. Centralizing this information and having a repository would be extremely insightful to improving this type of ongoing education.

Research has demonstrated that work environments can directly impact and influence patient outcomes in a healthcare setting. For example, Durcharme, Bernhardt, Padula, and Adams (2017) state that "a healthy professional practice environment has been defined as an environment in which leaders create the structures and processes that allow nurses to practice safely and confidently and engage in relationships that results in quality patient outcomes" (p. 367).

It remains a challenge to find concise information relating to the assessment and evaluation of leadership programs for the health professions as a function over time and value to an organization and specific profession. This literature review was initiated to define what foundation is already in place as well as areas of further research opportunity. The findings, or lack of specificity thereof, indicate that this is an area ripe for a fresh perspective.

We must study the evaluation of leadership programs as it can provide a context of a learning-needs assessment and consequential outcomes data. Establishing a consistent minimum data set and subsequently developing a guiding framework to provide high-quality leadership programs is warranted.

Effective leadership improves culture, staff and patient satisfaction, and overall patient outcomes. It is therefore essential to develop a method to evaluate leadership programs in order to ensure that current and future leaders are destined to succeed within their respective roles. Gathering feedback, from the individual and organizational levels, will help us understand what information is useful to learners and how learners implement the information post-education to impact the care patients receive in the healthcare setting.

References

AAP Council on School Health. (2016). Role of the school nurse in providing school health services. *Pediatrics, 137*(6), e20160852. DOI: 10.1542/peds.2016-0852

Adams JM, Ives Erickson J. (2011) Applying the Adams Influence Model (AIM) in Nurse Executive Practice. *Journal of Nursing Administration 41*(4): 186–92.

Adams, J. M., Ives Erickson, J., Jones, D. A., & Paulo, L. (2009). An evidence-based structure for transformative nurse executive practice. *Nursing Administration Quarterly, 33*(4), 280-87. DOI: 10.1097/NAQ.0b013e3181b9dce3

Adams, J. M. & Natarajan, S. (2016). Understanding influence within the context of nursing: Development of the Adams Influence Model using practice, research and theory. *Advances in Nursing Science, 39*(3), E40-E56. DOI: 10.1097/ANS.0000000000000134

Agnew, C. & Flin R. (2014). Senior charge nurses' leadership behaviours in relation to hospital ward safety: A mixed method study. *International Journal of Nursing Studies, 51*, 768-80. DOI: 10.1016/j.ijnurstu.2013.10.001

Aiken, L., Clarke, S., Sloane, D., Lake, E., & Cheney, T. (2008) Effects of Hospital Care Environment on Patient Mortality and Nurse Outcome. *Journal of Nursing Administration, 38*, 223-29.

Aiken L.H., sloane D.M., & Lake E.T., Sochaski J., & Weber, A.L. (1999). Organization and outcomes of inpatient AIDS care. *Medical Care, 37*(8), 112-160.

Armstrong, K., Laschinger, H., & Wong, C. (2009). Workplace empowerment and magnet hospital characteristics as predictors of patient safety climate. *Journal of Nursing Care Quality, 24*, 1. Retrieved from http://dx.doi.org/10.1097/01.NNA.0000312773.42352.d7

American Nurses Credentialing Center. (2014). *2014 Magnet application manual.* Silver Spring, MD: American Nurses Credentialing Center.

American Organization of Nurse Executives. (2015). *AONE Nurse Executive Competencies.* Chicago, IL: Author. Retrieved from http://www.aone.org/resources/nurse-leader-competencies.shtml

Batchellor, J., Zimmermann, D., Pappas, S. H., & Adams, J. M. (2017). Nursing's leadership role in addressing the quadruple aim. *Nurse Leader, 15*(3). 203-6. DOI: 10.1016/j.mnl.2017.02.007

Berwick, D., Nolan, T., & Whittington, J. (2008). The triple aim: Care, health, and cost. *Health Affairs, 27*(3), 759-69. DOI: 10.1377/hlthaff.27.3.759

Bodenheimer, T., & Sinsky, C. (2014). From triple to quadruple aim: Care of the patient requires care of the provider. *Annals of Family Medicine, 12*(6), 573-76. DOI: 10.1370/afm.1713

Bolger N., DeLongis A., Kessler R.C., & Wethington E. (1989). The contagion of stress across multiple roles. *Journal of Marriage and the Family, 51*(1), 175-83. DOI: 10.2307/352378

Bormann, L. & Abrahamson, K. (2014). Do Staff Nurse Perceptions of Nurse Leadership Behaviors Influence Staff Nurse Job Satisfaction? The Case of a Hospital Applying for Magnet® Designation. *The Journal of nursing administration. 44*. 219-25. DOI: 10.1097/NNA.0000000000000053.

Butcher, L (2016, July 11). *Why the school nurse is key to a hospital's population health strategy.* Hospitals and Health Networks. Retrieved from http://www.hhnmag.com/articles/7351

Centers for Medicare & Medicaid Services. (2018, July 30). *Bundled Payments for Care Improvement (BPCI) Initiative: General information.* Retrieved from https://innovation.cms.gov/initiatives/bundled-payments/

Cowden, T., Cummings, G. G., & Profetto-McGrath, J. (2011). Leadership practices and staff nurses' intent to stay: A systematic review. *Journal of Nursing Management, 19*, 461–77. DOI: 10.1111/j.1365-2834.2011.01209.x

Cummings, G. G., Midodzi, W. K., Wong, C. A., & Estabrooks, C. A. (2010). The contribution of hospital nursing leadership styles to 30-day patient mortality. *Nursing Research, 59*(5): 331–39. DOI: 10.1097/NNR.0b013e3181ed74d5

Day, D., Fleenor, J., Atwater, L., Sturm, R., & McKee, R. (2014). Advances in leader and leadership development: A review of 25 years of research and theory. *The Leadership Quarterly, 25*(1), 63–82. DOI: 10.1016/j.leaqua.2013.11.004

Dearmon V., Roussel L., Buckner E. B., Mulekar M., Pomrenke B., Salas S., Mosley A., Brown S., & Brown A. (2013). Transforming care at the bedside (TCAB): Enhancing direct care and value-added care. *Journal of Nursing Management, 21*, 668–78.

Donabedian, A. (1966). Evaluating the quality of medical care. Milbank Memorial Fund Quarterly, 44(3 suppl.), 166–206. Reprinted in 2005 *Millbank Quarterly, 83*(4), 691–729. DOI: 10.1111/j.1468-0009.2005.00397.x

Donabedian, A. (1988). The quality of care: How can it be assessed? *Journal of the American Medical Association, 121*(11): 1145–50.

Ducharme, M. P., Bernhardt, J. M., Padula, C. A., & Adams, J. M. (2017). Leader influence, the professional practice environment and nurse engagement in essential nursing practice. *The Journal of Nursing Administration, 47*(7/8), 367–375. DOI: 10.1097/NNA.0000000000000497.

Fealy, G. M., McNamara, M. S., Casey, M., O'Connor, T., Patton, D., Doyle, L., & Quinlan, C. (2013). Service impact of a national clinical leadership development programme: Findings from a qualitative study. *Journal of Nursing Management, 23*, 324–32. DOI: 10.1111/jonm.12133

Friese, C. R. & Himes-Ferris, L. (2013). *Nursing practice environments and job outcomes in ambulatory oncology settings.* Lippincott Williams & Wilkins.

Frumenti, J. M., & Kurtz, A. (2014). Addressing hospital-acquired pressure ulcers: Patient care managers enhancing outcomes at the point of service. *The Journal of Nursing Administration, 44*(1), 30–36. DOI: 10.1097/NNA.0000000000000018

Hall, L.M. & Doran, D. (2004). Nurse staffing, care delivery model, and patient care quality. *Journal of Nursing Care Quality. 19*(1), 27–33.

Han, S. S., Han, J. W., An, Y. S., Lim, S. H. (2015). Effects of role stress on nurses' turnover intentions: The mediating effects of organizational commitment and burnout. Japan Journal of Nursing Science, 12(4), 287–96. DOI: 10.1111/jjns.12067

Hassmiller, S. B. (2011). Nursing Leadership from Bedside to Boardroom: Commentary. The *Journal of Nursing Administration. 41*(7/8), 306–8.

Institute of Medicine. (2011). *The future of nursing: Leading change, advancing health.* Washington, DC: National Academies Press.

Jones, C.B., Havens, D.S., Thompson, P.A. (2009). Chief nursing officer turnover and the crisis brewing: Views from the front line. *The Journal of Nursing Administration. 39*(6), 285–92.

Kanter, R. M. (1977). *Men and women of the corporation.* New York, NY: Basic Books.

Kelly, L. A., & Adams, J. M. (2018). Nurse leader burnout: How to find your joy. *Nurse Leader, 16*(1), 24–28. DOI: 10.1016/j.mnl.2017.10.006

King, I. (1981). *A Theory for Nursing: Systems, Concepts, Process.* New York, NY: John Wiley & Sons.

Kirkpatrick Partners. (2017). *The Kirkpatrick Model.* Retrieved from http://www.kirkpatrickpartners.com/Our-Philosophy/The-Kirkpatrick-Model

Kramer M. & Hafner L.P. (1989). Shared values: impact on staff nurse job satisfaction and perceived productivity. *Nursing Research, 38*(3), 172–77.

Kramer, M., & Schmalenberg, C. (2002). Staff nurses identify essentials of magnetism. In M. McClure & A. S. Hinshaw (Eds.), *Magnet hospitals revisited: Attraction and retention of professional nurses.* Silver Spring: American Nurse Association.

Kramer, M., & Schmalenberg, C. (2004). Development and evaluation of essentials of magnetism tool. *The Journal of Nursing Administration, 34*, 7–8.

Kramer, M., Schmalenberg, C., & Maguire, P. (2010). Nine structures and leadership practices for a magnetic (healthy) work environment. *Nursing Administration Quarterly, 34*(1), 4–17.

Kramer, M. Schmalenberg, C., Maguire, P., Brewer, B.B., Burke, R., Chmielewski, L., Cox, K., Kishner, J., Krugman, M., Meeks-Sjostrom, D., & Waldo, M. (2008). Structures and Practices Enabling Staff Nurses to Control Their Practice. Western *Journal of Nursing Research. 30*(5), 539–59.

Lake, E. (2002). Development of the Practice Environment Scale of the Nursing Work Index. *Research in Nursing & Health, 25*, 176–88. DOI: 10.1002/nur.10032

Lankshear, S., Kerr, M. S., Spence, L. H. K., & Wong, C. A. (2013). Professional practice leadership roles: The role of organizational power and personal influence in creating a professional practice environment for nurses. *Health Care Management Review, 38*, 4, 349–60.

Laschinger, H. K., Almost, J., & Tuer-Hodes, D. (2003). Workplace empowerment and magnet hospital characteristics: making the link. The *Journal of Nursing Administration, 33.*

Laschinger, H. K. S., Finegan, J., Shamian, J., & Wilk, P. (2004). A longitudinal analysis of the impact of workplace empowerment on work satisfaction. *Journal of Organizational Behavior, 25*(1), 527–45.

Laschinger, H.K.S, J Finegan J., & Wilk, P., (2009). New Graduate Burnout: the Impact of Professional Practice Environment, Workplace Civility, and Empowerment. *Nursing Economic$. 27*(6), 377–83

Laschinger, H.K., Purdy, N., & Almost, J. (2007). The Impact of Leader-Member Exchange Quality, Empowerment, and Core Self-Evaluation on Nurse Manager's Job Satisfaction. *The Journal of Nursing Administration. 37*(5), 221–29.

Laschinger, H. K. S., Read, E., Wilk, P., & Finegan, J. (2014). The Influence of Nursing Unit Empowerment and Social Capital on Unit Effectiveness and Nurse Perceptions of Patient Care Quality. *Journal of Nursing Administration, 44*(6), 347–52.

Leiter, M. P., Maslach, C. (2009). Nurse turnover: The mediating role of burnout. *Journal of Nursing Management, 17*(3), 331–39. DOI: 10.1111/j.1365-2834

Mackoff, B. (2010). *Nurse manager engagement.* Boston, MA: Jones and Bartlett.

Manojlovich, M. (2005). Linking the Practice Environment to Nurses' Job Satisfaction Through Nurse-Physician Communication. *Journal of Nursing Scholarship, 37*(4), 367–73.

Mark, B. A., Salyer, J., Wan, T. T. H. (2003). Professional nursing practice: Impact on organizational and patient outcomes. *Journal of Nursing Administration, 33*(4), 224–34.

McClure, M. L., Poulin, M. A., Sovie, M. D., & Wandelt, M. A. (1983). *Magnet hospitals: Attraction and retention of professional nurses.* Kansas City, MO: American Nurses Association.

McHugh, M. D, & Stimpfel, A.W. (2012). Nurse reported quality of care: A measure of hospital quality. *Research in Nursing & Health. 35*(6), 566–75.

Mensik, J. (2013). Nursing's role and staffing in accountable care. *Nursing Economic$ 31*(5):250–53.

Pappas, S., & Welton, J. (2015). Nursing: Essential to healthcare value. *Nurse Leader, 13*(3), 26–29, 38. DOI: 10.1016/j.mnl.2015.03.005

Parse, R. R. (2014). *The humanbecoming paradigm: A transformational worldview.* Pittsburgh, PA: Discovery International Publications.

Patrick, A., Laschinger, H., Wong, C., & Finegan, J. (2011). Developing and testing a new measure of staff nurse clinical leadership: the clinical leadership survey. *Journal of Nursing Management, 19*(4), 449–60.

Porter, M. (2010). What is value in health care? *New England Journal of Medicine, 363*(26), 2477–81. DOI: 10.1056/nejmp1011024

Pradarelli, J., Jaffe, G., Lemak, C., Mulholland, M., & Dimick, J. (2016). A leadership development program for surgeons: First-year participant evaluation. *Surgery, 160*(2), 255–63. DOI: 10.1016/j.surg.2016.03.011

Rath, T., & Conchie, B. (2009). *Strengths based leadership: great leaders, teams, and why people follow.* Washington, DC: Gallup Press.

Reeves, K. W., Taylor Y., Tapp, H., Ludden, T., Shade, L. E., Burton, B., Courtlandt, C., Dulin, M. (2016). Evaluation of a pilot asthma care program for electronic communication between school health and a healthcare system's electronic medical record. *Applied Clinical Informatics, 7*(4): 969–82. DOI: 10.4338/ACI-2016-02-RA-0022

Saint, S., Kowalski, C., Banaszak-Holl, J., Forman, J., Damschroder, L., & Krein, S. (2010). The importance of leadership in preventing healthcare associated infection: Results of a multisite qualitative study. *Infection Control and Hospital Epidemiology, 31*(9), 901–907. DOI: 10.1086/655459

Schmalenberg, C., & Kramer, M. (2008). Essentials of a productive nurse work environment. *Nursing Research, 57*(1), 2–13.

Shirey, M. (2009). Authentic leadership, organizational culture, and healthy work environments. *Critical Care Nursing Quarterly, 32*(3), 189–98. DOI: 10.1097/CNQ.0b013e3181ab91db

Shirey, M., Fisher, M., McDaniel, A., Doebbeling, B., & Ebright, P. (2010). Understanding nurse manager stress and work complexity: Factors that make a difference. *The Journal of Nursing Administration, 40*(2), 82–91. DOI: 10.1097/NNA.0b013e3181cb9f88

Sikka, R., Morath, J.M.,& Leape, L. (2015). The Quadruple Aim: Care, Health, Cost and Meaning in Work. *BMJ Quality & Safety. 24*(10), 608–10.

Somerville, J., Ponte, P., Pipe, T., & Adams, J. (2015). Innovation through a nursing academic practice research collaboration: Establishment of the Workforce Outcomes Research and Leadership Development Institute (WORLD-Institute). *Nurse Leader, 13*(6), 16–17. DOI: 10.1016/j.mnl.2015.10.002

Spence, L. H. K, Finegan, J., & Wilk, P. (2011). Situational and Dispositional Influences on Nurses' Workplace Well-Being: the Role of Empowering Unit Leadership. *Nursing Research. 60*(2), 124–31.

Spence, L. H. K., & Leiter, M. P. (January 01, 2006). The impact of nursing work environments on patient safety outcomes: the mediating role of burnout/engagement. *The Journal of Nursing Administration, 36*, 5, 259–67.

Spence, H. K. L, Wong, C. A., Grau, A. L., Read, E. A., & Pineau Stam, L. M. (2012). The influence of leadership practices and empowerment on Canadian nurse manager outcomes. *Journal of Nursing Management, 20*(7), 877–88.

Stimpfel, A.W., Rosen, J., & McHugh, M.D. (2014). Understanding the role of the professional practice environment on quality of care in Magnet® and non-magnet hospitals. *The Journal of Nursing Administration. 44*(1), 10–16.

Stimpfel, A. W., Sloane, D. M., & Aiken, L. H. (2012). The longer the shifts for hospital nurses, the higher the levels of burnout and patient dissatisfaction. *Health Affairs, 31*(11), 2501–9. DOI: 10.1377/hlthaff.2011.1377

Stamm, B. H. (n.d.). *Professional Quality of Life Scale: Compassion satisfaction and compassion fatigue*. Retrieved September 25, 2017, from http://www.proqol.org/

Studer, Q. (2009). *Straight A leadership: Alignment, action, accountability*. Gulf Breeze, FL: Fire Starter Publishing.

Swiger, P., Patrician, P., Miltner, R., Raju, D., Breckenridge-Sproat, S., & Loan, L. (2017). The practice environment scale of the nursing work index: An updated review and recommendations for use. *International Journal of Nursing Studies, 74*, 76–84. DOI: 10.1016/j.ijnurstu.2017.06.003

Tourangeau, A. E., McGillis Hall, L., Doran, D. M., & Petch, T. (2006). Measurement of nurse job satisfaction using the McCloskey Mueller Satisfaction Scale. *Nursing Research, 55*(2), 128–36.

Throgmorton, C., Mitchell, T., Morley, T., & Snyder, M. (2016). Evaluating a physician leadership development program: A mixed methods approach. *Journal of Health Organization and Management, 30*(3), 390–407. DOI: 10.1108/JHOM-11-2014-0187

Uhl-Bien, M., & Marion, R. (2009). Complexity leadership in bureaucratic forms of organizing: A meso model. *The Leadership Quarterly, 20*(4), 631–50. DOI: 10.1016/j.leaqua.2009.04.007

Upenieks, V. (2000). The relationship of nursing practice models and job satisfaction outcomes. *The Journal of Nursing Administration, 30*, 6, 330–35.

Warshawsky, N., & Havens, D. (2011). Global use of the Practice Environment Scale of the Nursing Work Index: A review of literature. *Nursing Research, 60*(1), 17–31. DOI: 10.1097/NNR.0b013e3181ffa79c

Warshawsky, N., Lake, S., & Brandford, A. (2013). Nurse managers describe their practice environments. *Nursing Administration Quarterly, 37*(4) 317–25. DOI: 10.1097/NAQ.0b013e3182a2f9c3

Warshawsky, N., Rayens, M. K., Lake, S., & Havens, D. (2013). The Nurse Manager Practice Environment Scale: Development and psychometric testing. *The Journal of Nursing Administration, 43*(5), 250–57. DOI: 10.1097/NNA.0b013e3182898e4e

Warshawsky, N., Wiggins, A., & Rayens, M. (2016). The influence of the practice environment on nurse managers' job satisfaction and intent to leave. *The Journal of Nursing Administration, 46*(10), 501–7. DOI: 10.1097/NNA.0000000000000393

Weberg, D. (2017). Innovation leadership behaviors: Starting the complexity journey. In S. Davidson, D. Weberg, T. Porter-O'Grady, & K. Malloch (Eds.), *Leadership for evidence-based innovation in nursing and health professions* (pp. 43–76). Boston, MA: Jones & Bartlett Learning.

Welp, A., Meier, L. L., Manser, T. (2015). Emotional exhaustion and workload predict clinician-rated and objective patient safety. *Frontiers in Psychology, 5*, 1573. DOI: 10.3389/fpsyg.2014.01573

Welton, J. (2013). *Nursing and the value proposition: How information can help transform the healthcare system.* Presented at Nursing Knowledge: Big Data Research for Transforming Health Care. Retrieved from https://www.researchgate.net/publication/265291987_Welton2013_08

Wong, C. A., & Cummings, G. G. (2007). The relationship between nursing leadership and patient outcomes: A systematic review. *Journal of Nursing Management, 15*(5), 508–21. DOI: 10.1111/j.1365-2834.2007.00723.x

Wong, C. A., Cummings, G. G., & Ducharme, L. (2013). The relationship between nursing leadership and patient outcomes: a systematic review update. *Journal of Nursing Management, 21*(5), 709–24. DOI: 10.1111/jonm.12116

Wong, C. A., & Giallonardo, L. M. (2013). Authentic leadership and nurse-assessed adverse patient outcomes. *Journal of Nursing Management, 21*(5), 740–52. DOI: 10.1111/jonm.12075

Yukl, G. (2006). *Leadership in organizations* (6th ed.). Upper Saddle River: Prentice-Hall

Yukl, G. & Falbe. C.M. (1990). Influence Tactics and Objectives in Upward, Downward, and Lateral Influence Attempts. *Journal of Applied Psychology. 75*(2), 132–40.

Yukl, G., Falbe, C.M., & Youn, J.Y. (1993). Patterns of Influence Behavior for Managers. *Group & Organization Management. 18*(1), 5–28.

Yukl, G., & Tracey, J. B. (1992). Consequences of influence tactics used with subordinates, peers, and the boss. *Journal of Applied Psychology, 77*(7).

Chapter 3

Preparing to Lead

Joyce Batcheller, DNP, RN, NEA-BC, FAAN

The first step to becoming an effective leader is being open to learning about yourself through feedback and a commitment to continuous learning.

Introduction: Purpose and Overview
Why Leadership?
Nurses are leaders at all levels in an organization. For example, leadership topics such as time management, delegation, and conflict management are reinforced in new RN residency programs. There is a lot of complexity in the RN role that requires all nurses to have at least a certain level of competency in key leadership areas. Being an RN also provides a good preview of the kind of knowledge and competencies that higher, more formal nursing-leadership positions require.

There is growing evidence in the literature linking the positive impact of a healthy work environment to key metrics such as staff satisfaction, retention, positive patient outcomes, and overall organizational performance (Sherman & Pross, 2010). Nurse leaders are pivotal in creating a professional practice environment that gives nurses the ability to deliver high-quality patient care. They are responsible for recruitment and retention, staffing, patient safety, patient satisfaction, and rewards and recognition. In addition, managers have a profound impact on the work life of the employees who report to them (Gray & Shirey, 2013).

Research shows that RN turnover and staff engagement scores are highly correlated to behaviors of unit/department leaders. Employees who rate their managers as excellent are more than four times as likely to be engaged as those who rate their managers as fair (Rothenberger, 2014).

The Discernment Process

So how do you determine if formal leadership is the career track you would like to pursue? What kind of questions should you be asking yourself? What kinds of experiences should you involve yourself in to help you with this important career choice?

Questions You Can Begin to Explore Are

- What do you enjoy doing the most?

- Do you know your strengths?

- What makes you feel energized?

- What makes you feel drained or bored?

- What is your vision of what your unit/department should look like?

- Do you like challenges?

- Are you comfortable having crucial conversations?

- Do you enjoy coaching and mentoring others?

Experiences to Explore

- Volunteer to be a charge nurse for your unit/department. This is a great way to gain exposure to what a higher leadership role involves. Directors and managers commonly select individuals they believe will be good role models and good reflections of their leadership styles.

- Become involved in or lead a performance-improvement project for your unit/department. Being exposed to effective meeting management, learning new skills and knowledge about performance improvement, and meeting and developing relationships with other key members or leaders in the organization help you gain a different perspective on how a leader truly gets the work done through others.

- Ask to attend key executive meetings with your leader to become exposed to the bigger picture of an organization and what is needed to continue to thrive.

- Become involved in a professional organization in your area to enhance your understanding of state or national challenges that you can become involved with. There are many leadership roles in these organizations and the work can be very impactful and rewarding.

CASE STUDY

Jane is currently working on a busy 46-bed cardiac care unit. She successfully completed her RN residency and now has a year and a half of experience. Jane is known for showing a high degree of compassion with her patients and for being committed to high-quality care standards.

Jane's unit director surprised her yesterday by telling her that she believes Jane is ready to become a charge nurse and that Jane will begin to assume this responsibility next week. Jane is not excited about this change and does not feel that she is ready to take on this role. One of the other nurses on the unit told Jane not to worry and that she feels confident Jane will do a great job. What should Jane do?

Questions

1. Does Jane's commitment to compassion and high-quality standards ensure she will be successful in this role?

2. Should someone with a year and half of experience be allowed to be a charge nurse?

3. Should Jane tell her unit leader she is not comfortable with this assignment?

4. Is there anything Jane can do to decrease her anxiety about being in charge?

5. What should the leader do to support Jane with this transition?

Discussion

1. Jane's success as a staff nurse does not alone ensure that she will be successful as a charge nurse or in some other leadership position. One of the biggest challenges first-time leaders face is changing their language from "it's about me" to "it's about you and me." The transition to managing people and displaying authority is a major change, and many new leaders may fail if they don't receive mentoring.

2. One's number of years as a nurse does not alone determine if someone will or will not be successful. This is particularly true since there are many nurses who enter nursing with a previous degree and who have years of life experiences and maturity. Successful leaders learn within three clusters of experience: coursework and training (10% of learning), developmental relationships (20% of learning), and challenging assignments (70% of learning; Rabin, 2010). Being a charge nurse is a great way for nurses to engage in challenging situations and to learn from these varied situations.

3. Jane should talk with her unit leader about why she is uncomfortable assuming this new role. She should also think about what kind of orientation and resources would be helpful. This approach demonstrates a willingness to assume this role and provides what the nurse believes would be helpful in ensuring a positive experience.

4. The unit leader should have an orientation process that includes mentoring for new charge nurses to assist with Jane's transition to this new role. This is an opportunity to begin growing the next generation of nursing leaders. Support and mentoring provide a person with a more accurate perception of what leadership is and why they may want to further their career in this specialty.

Are People Born to Be Leaders or Can Leadership Be Learned?

Fortunately the answer to this question is that leadership can be learned. However, an organization must be willing to provide certain kinds of investments and opportunities. In a recent survey, 50% of leaders responded that they plan to internally develop leaders through succession planning. However, two-thirds of those organizations did not have an existing program or a comprehensive program (Corhell & Noland, 2017). When succession-planning programs do exist they tend to be for the senior-executive level.

Since developing leadership skills is a journey, it is important to understand the most effective ways to help others learn these critical skills. For example, the number one way to learn leadership is through experience. There are five categories of key developmental experiences: challenging assignments, other people, hardships, coursework, and personal life experiences (Scisco, Biech, & Hallenbeck, 2017).

Challenging Assignments

Being asked to lead a new project, take on a great scope of responsibility, or turn around an area that is in trouble are examples that would cause someone to stretch beyond their current skill set. These kinds of opportunities have specific goals, timelines, and high visibility. They help teach someone how to cope with pressure, learn quickly, and deal with difficult situations. They provide a great deal of variety and represent what leaders must become comfortable doing. These kinds of experiences will likely push someone out of their comfort zone and enhance development.

Other People

One can learn a lot from working with and observing what both good and bad leaders do. Learning how to role model integrity and authenticity as well as learning what not to do are key.

Hardships

There is a lot that a leader can learn when they encounter a setback or failure of some sort. Spending time reflecting on what went wrong and what can be learned from such an experience can be very powerful. Most leaders, for example, have hired someone that they later realized was not an organizational fit. Spending time reflecting on this kind of experience can assist a leader in avoiding similar errors in the future. Unfortunately many leaders do not like to share what went wrong with others, but the opportunity for learning when they do talk about it is incredible.

Coursework

Many nurses are returning to school not only for their BSN but also for higher degrees. It is important for nurse leaders to know what they are learning so that it can be reinforced in the practice setting. In addition, there may be projects that student nurses need to complete for school, and an organization can enhance their investment by aligning what their nurses work on with their schoolwork.

There also is a great deal of online education available from organizations. In-person training, however, provides an opportunity for future leaders to learn from others and reinforces or builds their confidence by giving them a safe environment in which to practice what they've learned.

Personal Life Experiences

Off-the-job experiences can provide important leadership experience. Some nurses may be involved in local, state, or national nursing associations, which provide great experiences for learning and networking. Other examples include family, friend, or community experiences, which can also be both difficult and inspiring.

CASE STUDY

Jane has decided to schedule a meeting with her unit leader to discuss the charge nurse role that she will be assuming in a week. She initiated dialogue with some of the charge nurses to learn more about what is expected of someone in that role and what kind of training they received prior to moving into the role. Jane also found a few online modules that are offered at her organization. She is willing to complete these on her off time if she can be compensated for her time. Some of the charge nurses that Jane spoke with said they would be willing to act as a mentor if they were working and she had questions or concerns.

Questions

1. What do you like about what Jane is planning to do?

2. Do you have any concerns about what Jane is planning to do?

3. Is Jane being reasonable in what she plans to ask for?

Discussion

1. Jane is showing a lot of initiative and is being proactive in the approaches described above. She plans to meet with her unit leader to express her concerns and has some ideas on how to address them. By talking to some of the charge nurses she gained a better understanding of what the role entails. This knowledge along with that of the online modules seems like an appropriate approach to propose.

2. Jane may want to think about formalizing a relationship with an experienced charge nurse. She could suggest that she shadow a charge nurse for a day or two to gain more insights and experience prior to being on her own. Minimally she could ask that an experienced charge nurse be assigned to act as a mentor or resource person if her first idea is not accepted.

3. Jane seems to have reasonable requests. She may want to quantify the costs of the online education and two days of shadowing a charge nurse to help frame how much this investment really costs. Additionally she could commit to following up with the staff and charge nurses involved to evaluate how this process worked. She may end up helping establish a more consistent onboarding approach for other nurses transitioning to the charge nurse role in the future.

CASE STUDY

Jane receives support from her unit leader to be paid for the online modules as requested. In addition, Jane is scheduled to shadow a charge nurse for two days to orient to the role. The unit is busy with a lot of admissions, transfers, and discharges, which provides Jane with the opportunity to learn in a well-coordinated manner. Jane works with her unit leader and a few charge nurses to develop a consistent onboarding process to ensure that this is a smooth transition.

Self-Awareness and Self-Knowledge

Leaders need to be open to feedback and must commit to lifelong learning. For example, there are assessment tools that can help a leader gain insight into their leadership style, their strengths, and other key competencies. Many organizations utilize a 360-degree process, which provides a leader with feedback from their boss, their direct reports, and other key stakeholders. Mentors can also assist a leader in continuing to grow.

The kind of competencies that leaders have needed in the past will not necessarily be adequate to meet future challenges. Factors impacting this change are the pace of change, the movement to a culture of health, the need to manage a diverse workforce, and the impact that technology and artificial intelligence will continue to have in healthcare.

Key competencies that leaders will need include the ability to influence and lead change, inspire commitment, build effective collaborative relationships, think strategically, and shift to performance coaching and not performance management. Participative leadership has and will continue to be a key competency for all leaders.

Three new competencies for leaders, which are described in more detail later, include learning agility, self-awareness, and adaptability. Learning agility includes being able not only to learn more quickly but also to unlearn ways of doing things are no longer effective. There are many companies that now require their employees to complete the CliftonStrengths (formerly StrengthsFinder) assessment. Leveraging the strengths of employees and better matching work assignments enhances organizational effectiveness; employees view it as a more positive approach.

Leaders must learn to be more adaptable as the challenges they face continue to change rapidly. A leader's effectiveness also varies with how well they manage their self-care. Leaders need to remember that they were hired for their ability to think strategically and work effectively with others. Doing this is difficult when persons are tired or feel very stressed.

Leaders also must be adaptable and learn how to value the differences in the next generation of leaders. For example, this generation is very comfortable with technology and is used to connecting through different social networks. They tend to be creative and open to trying new ideas. Several exciting factors are that they have a sense of ethics, are service oriented, and want to make a difference. It is important to understand the link between the work they do daily and the overall success of the organization.

CASE STUDY

Jane has been very effective as a charge nurse and has also mentored other nurses in the role. Yesterday she learned that the manager on her unit had resigned. Several of the staff nurses are encouraging Jane to apply for the position. Jane is not sure whether she is ready or that she wants to move to a higher level of leadership. She really enjoys being able to spend time with patients and families.

Questions

1. Should Jane apply?

2. What questions could help her reflect and decide if this is something she should apply for?

3. What happens if Jane does apply and is not selected for the role?

4. What if Jane decides not to apply? Will she lose support of her peers? Will it mean she cannot apply for another leadership position in the future?

Discussion

1. Jane has an important decision to make. She may want to discuss her possible interest with the manager who is leaving. What kinds of insights could this person provide? Are there other managers she should talk to? Does she have a mentor who could help her think through her decision?

2. Jane seems hesitant to apply because she enjoys working with patients and families. Will she still be able to engage with patients and families in the manager role? Will her potential impact on the patients and families be greater if she is in this leadership role? How will her relationships change with the staff who are currently her friends?

Is she okay with this? What really gives her joy and meaning in the workplace?

3. If Jane applies but is not selected for the role, she will need to support the person who is selected. It may be a difficult experience, but she should use this as an opportunity to learn more about how to position herself for a similar role in the future. Jane also needs to demonstrate her support when the staff who want Jane to be their manager learn that she was not selected.

4. It is okay if Jane decides not to apply. She may be very happy as a great clinician and charge nurse. This is a personal decision that her team should accept. It also does not mean that Jane cannot apply for a leadership position in the future.

CASE STUDY

Jane applied and was selected as the new manager for her unit. As part of her orientation she plans to set up meetings with all the staff. Some of the staff have made comments like "Why do I need to do this?" "She already knows me," "I am not going to meet with her," and "This seems like a waste of time." She also overhears someone on her unit say, "Why does she need a mentor? I heard that she requested that one of the other managers be assigned to her as a mentor."

Questions

1. Is Jane's plan to meet with the staff on her unit a "waste of time"?

2. What is Jane trying to accomplish in these meetings?

3. What is the role of a mentor?

4. What are the common reasons new leaders fail?

Discussion

1. Jane's request to meet with the staff is an important part of her transition into the manager role. For example, it is important for Jane to learn more about each of the team members. By knowing the strengths and interests of each staff member she can begin to better match the staff's interests and passions with work that needs to be

done on the unit. It may also give her insights into work that they are already involved with so she can follow-up and recognize them when appropriate. It can also build trust within the team since Jane is open to hearing what is important to the staff.

Through the one-on-one meetings Jane can also begin to set expectations and establish herself as a leader on the unit. The shift from being a peer to a unit leader is especially important when someone is hired internally.

2. It is common for organizations to assign a mentor to assist a new or aspiring future leader. Having this kind of resource person to discuss challenges and general transition questions is invaluable. Mentors can provide hands-on support to assist a leader in being effective.

Many individuals have more than one mentor since they encounter various situations. Mentors may suggest other mentors or resource people that the leader may want to connect with. The power of this kind of networking is invaluable.

One of the most effective ways to develop a leader involves stretch assignments and making mistakes. The important part is to stop and think about why a situation went wrong—some of the most valuable lessons occur from this process. The key is to learn from mistakes to prevent making them again.

3. Leaders are usually selected based on how well they have been performing work that reflects their personal capabilities. Shifting one's language and thinking to be about *us* and not *me* is critical. The key competency centers on learning how to effectively lead team achievement and be comfortable putting others in the spotlight.

First-time managers also report having difficulty adjusting to displaying authority and becoming comfortable with managing people effectively. They need assistance on how to have difficult conversations and on conflict in general. It is not unusual for new leaders to be defensive when dealing with challenging employees. This is a great example where working with a mentor and role-playing through a difficult situation would be beneficial.

What Does a Leader Actually Do? What Are Other Key Competencies?

A major role that leaders play is in leading change. The one constant that exists in healthcare today is the fact that change is inevitable since healthcare is competitive and volatile. Ambiguity exists in the system due to changes in the reimbursement systems and due to the need for population management. Technological advances impact the industry and consumers expect more transparency of information, including pricing of healthcare procedures. Leaders must develop partnerships with key organizations in the community to be more visible and credible to outside agencies.

Another critical competency is learning agility, which is defined as the ability of leaders to move quickly and easily. Characteristics include being open to grow and adopting new ways of thinking. Agile leaders learn from experience and can apply this knowledge to a new challenge or situation (Eichinger, Lombardo, & Capretta, 2010). Others often describe these leaders as challenging the status quo, learning from difficult challenges, and resisting the tendency to be defensive in difficult situations. Research shows that most leaders learn from assignments in which they have failed or performed poorly (Eichinger et al., 2010). Leaders can share these lessons with their teams to role model behaviors that support an environment and culture of learning.

The focus on financial performance will continue to be a high priority. Nursing leaders must be able to speak to the value of nursing in their organizations. The nursing workforce directly impacts many of the outcomes for quality and safety, for example by preventing infections, pressure ulcers, patient falls with injuries, and readmissions (Aiken et al., 2008).

Another key competency is the ability to influence multiple stakeholders. For example, leaders are responsible for facilitating changes that have been identified through their work with quality and safety assurance. This kind of work often includes multiple stakeholders from different disciplines.

CASE STUDY

A unit leader is notified that a serious safety event has occurred in one of their units. A patient received an overdose of a pain medication that caused the patient to arrest and be taken to the ICU. The patient has been intubated and stabilized.

Questions

1. What does the unit leader need to do in a situation like this?

2. What resources are available to a leader if they have never been involved in a situation like this?

3. Who are the key stakeholders that the leader would need to involve?

4. What follow up should be done with the patient/family?

Discussion

1. The unit leader is responsible for investigating how this error was made. It is important that they discuss with the nurse who committed the error as well as the charge nurse of the unit. Questions may include the following: "Were there system errors that contributed to this error?" "Was this a skill, knowledge, or behavioral issue?" "What is the experience level of the nurse?" "What was the staffing on the unit and how were assignments made?" And to determine if fatigue was a factor, "How many hours had this nurse worked so far this week?"

2. Resources a leader can use include risk management, in-house legal services, quality leaders, and an experienced peer. The caregiver that committed the error is commonly referred to as the second victim. It is important for the leader to approach this individual in a caring and constructive manner. Offering employee-assistance and other support groups is also important to assist the individual in recovering from this incident.

3. Key stakeholders include the nurse, physician, pharmacist, charge nurse, risk manager, quality leader, the patient, and the patient's family.

4. The patient and family need to understand that an error has been made and also what has been done to correct the error. The leader may want to huddle the key stakeholders to develop a plan that outlines who will be responsible for talking to the patient and the family. It is also important for the family to feel comfortable allowing their loved one to return to the same nursing unit once a transfer from the ICU is needed. This kind of approach can help the unit staff and individual caregiver feel supported.

Does the Leader Really Make Difference?

What must an effective leader do to ensure the success of a unit/department? The health of the nurse work environment can be assessed by standardized, validated instruments such as the Practice Environment Scale of the Nursing Work Index (PES-NWI) and the Job Enjoyment and Job Satisfaction Scale-Revised (JSSR) (Warshawsky & Havens, 2011). Studies using these tools have shown that the outcomes are strongly correlated to nurse-manager effectiveness at a unit level. For instance, Press Ganey (2017) reported that while strong nursing leadership at all levels of an organization is important, the nurse managers at the unit level exert substantial influence on the work environment and on safety, quality, patient experience, and indicators of nurse engagement, such as nurse job satisfaction and retention.

The American Nurses Credentialing Center (ANCC) has recently made changes to the *2019 Magnet Application Manual.* The Magnet standards are strongly evidence based and span 20 years of research related to nursing care delivery, new nurse knowledge, and evidence-based clinical quality (ANCC, 2017). The role of the leader is evident throughout the standards and is best described as transformational leadership. These standards clearly demonstrate the impact that a nursing leader can have on a unit, department, or organization.

The Institute for Healthcare Improvement (IHI) Triple Aim, which includes improving the experience of care, improving the health of populations, and reducing per capita costs of healthcare, summarizes some key areas that a leader directly impacts in their unit/department and overall organization (Berwick, Nolan, & Whittington, 2008). Recently the IHI added a fourth area of focus, which a leader also directly impacts, and that is *joy in the workplace*, resulting in the Quadruple Aim. The goal is to create a work environment in which all caregivers can find joy and meaning in their work. In other words, leaders need to improve the experience of providing care so that staff can sense the importance of their daily work (Sikka, Morath, & Leape, 2015).

Additionally, focusing on joy allows leaders to think of the possibilities for improving the work environment and supports more open and innovative approaches. An engaged workforce tends to be more positive about their organization and more supportive of its mission and values. Increased engagement and joy correlate to improved patient experiences, outcomes, and safety, resulting in substantially lower costs (Burton, 2008).

The *IHI Framework for Improving Joy in Work* describes the essential areas leaders need to focus on to have happy, healthy, and productive people. These include real-time measurement, wellness and resilience, daily improvement, camaraderie and teamwork, physical and psychological safety, meaning and purpose, choice and autonomy, recognition and rewards, and participative management (Perlo et al., 2017). The framework, including its key change ideas for improving joy, describes a model that clearly illustrates the impact leaders can have.

Chapter Key Points

- Nurses are leaders at all levels in an organization.

- Talk with a few trusted leaders who can provide you more direct feedback about positions you may be interested in.

- Volunteer for a stretch assignment to help you grow and work with key leaders in the organization.

- Understand that leadership is a journey. No one starts with all the competencies they need to be successful; instead, leadership requires a commitment to lifelong learning.

- Being open to feedback and willing to work with a mentor demonstrates and models for others that you are creating a learning environment.

- It is also essential for leaders to network and involve themselves in professional organizations.

- Lastly, reflect on the depth and breadth of impact a leader can have and never lose sight of the goal: improving patient and staff outcomes.

References

Aiken, L., Clarke, S., Sloane, D., Lake, E. & Cheney, T. (2008) Effects of Hospital Care Environment on Patient Mortality and Nurse Outcome. *Journal of Nursing Administration, 38*, 223–29.

American Nurses Credentialing Center. (2017). *Transformational leadership: Criteria for nursing excellence.* Silver Spring, MD: American Nurses Credentialing Center.

Berwick, D. M., Nolan, T. & Whittington, J. (2008). The Triple Aim: Care, health, and cost. *Health Affairs, 27*(3), 759–69. DOI: 10.1377/hlthaff.27.3.759

Burton, J. (2008, July). *The business case for a healthy workplace* [white paper]. Retrieved from Industrial Accident Prevention Association: http://www.iapa.ca/pdf/fd_business_case_healthy_workplace.pdf

Corhell, P. & Noland, K. (2015, August 26). *Developing a leadership road map: the essential elements of succession planning* [white paper]. Retrieved from B.E. Smith: https://www.besmith.com/trends-and-insights/articles/developing-a-leadership-road map-the-essential-elements-of-succession-planning/

Eichinger, R. W., Lombardo, M. M., & Capretta, C. C. (2010). *FYI for learning agility*. Minneapolis, MN: Lominger International.

Gray, L. R. & Shirey, M. R. (2013). Nurse manager engagement: What it means to nurse managers and staff nurses. *Nursing Administration Quarterly, 37*(4), 337–45. DOI: 10.1097/NAQ.0b013e3182a2fa15

Perlo J., Balik, B., Swensen, S., Kabcenell, A., Landsman, J., & Feeley, D. (2017). *IHI framework for improving joy in work* [white paper]. Retrieved from Institute for Healthcare Improvement: http://www.ihi.org/resources/Pages/IHIWhitePapers/Framework-Improving-Joy-in-Work.aspx

Press Ganey. (2017). *2017 Press Ganey nursing special report: The influence of nurse manager leadership on patient and nurse outcomes and the mediating effects of the nurse work environment* [white paper]. Retrieved from: http://healthcare.pressganey.com/2017-Nursing-Special-Report

Rabin, R. (2010). *Blended learning for leadership: The CCL approach* [white paper]. Retrieved from Center for Creative Leadership: https://www.ccl.org/wp-content/uploads/2015/04/BlendedLearningLeadership.pdf

Rothenberger, S. (2014, January 13). How important is having an effective manager? Advisory Board Expert Insight. Retrieved from https://www.advisory.com/talent-development/employee-engagement-initiative/members/expert-insights/2011/how-important-is-having-an-effective-manager

Sikka, R., Morath, J. M., & Leape, L. (2015). The Quadruple Aim: Care, health, cost and meaning in work. *BMJ Quality & Safety, 24*(10), 608–10. DOI: 10.1136/bmjqs-2015-004160

Scisco, P., Biech, E. & Hallenbeck, G. (2017). *Compass: Your guide for leadership development and coaching*. Greensboro, NC: Center for Creative Leadership.

Sherman, R. & Pross, E. (2010). Growing future nurse leaders to build and sustain healthy work environments at the unit level. *The Online Journal of Issues in Nursing, 15*(1). DOI: 10.3912/OJIN.Vol15No01Man01

Warshawsky, N.E. & Havens, D.S. (2011). Global use of the Practice Environment Scale of the Nursing Work Index. *Nursing Research, 60*(1), 17–31.

Chapter 4

Addressing the Quadruple Aim

John Bowles, PhD, RN, CENP
Deb Zimmermann, DNP, RN, NEA-BC, FAAN

One in every 100 Americans is a registered nurse, and over 400,000 nurses serve in leadership positions that influence practice environments, the patient experience, cost per capita, and healthcare quality (Bowles et al., 2018). As the largest workforce segment of healthcare delivery, nurses should lead in shaping future healthcare policies, regulation, workforce expectations, and the healthcare delivery model. This chapter discusses nursing's leadership role in supporting the Quadruple Aim.

The Institute for Healthcare Improvement (IHI) Triple Aim framework focused on improving population health, improving the patient experience (including quality of care), and decreasing cost per capita. Hospitals and healthcare systems have adopted the Triple Aim to support and meet ACA requirements.

An example of the continued evolution of healthcare delivery includes the proposed Quadruple Aim. In 2014 medical leaders proposed a direct correlation between the achievement of patient outcomes and the resiliency and level of satisfaction of the care team. The physicians Bodenheimer and Sinsky (2014) boldly proposed that provider and staff satisfaction is a prerequisite for attaining optimum outcomes of the Triple Aim. For this reason they renamed the Triple Aim to the Quadruple Aim and outlined steps for addressing the fourth aim (Sikka, Morath, & Leape, 2015). Their recommendations have endured the test of time and are the foundation of the American Nurses Credentialing Center's Magnet standards (dams, Denham, & Neumeister, 2010), aligning with program's components of leadership, structural empowerment, professional practice, and innovation (McClure, Poulin, Sovie, & Wandelt, 1983).

Background

Future of Nursing Leadership

There is no single agreed-upon definition of leadership, much less nursing leadership. The literature is filled with different theories of nursing leadership and leadership from other disciplines to the extent of nearly 100 categories of leadership, nearly 300 definitions of leadership, and over 1,000 constructs relating to leadership (Gill, 2013). Leadership definitions and concepts vary among professional nursing organizations and may move others to conclude a simpler definition of leadership: "I know it when I see it."

The incongruences of defined nursing leadership among nursing organizations is one aspect that brought a group of nurse leaders together. The opportunity to explore the potential of a better future galvanized 16 scholarly nurse leaders from practice, academia, professional associations, and government agencies to come together for a weekend of dialogue focused on exploring nursing's leadership role in supporting each element of the Quadruple Aim. This chapter focuses on the findings of that discussion.

The theme of *all nurses are leaders* first emerged, and we discussed what competencies nurses need as leaders. These competencies include being a change agent and convener in the categories of advocacy, influence, and innovation. Figure 4–1 demonstrates the theme, with subcategories of data stewardship, role modeling, and engaging others that permeate through advocacy, influence, and innovation. Table 4-1 provides operational definitions of the concepts.

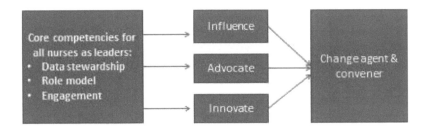

FIGURE 4–1. Nurse leader as convener and change agent to support Quadruple Aim model

TABLE 4–1.   Operational definitions: nurse leader as convener and change agent to support Quadruple Aim model

Concept	Definition	Source
Change agent	As an employee or consultant, the nurse can function as a catalyst and planner for change.	Kaplan, 1990
Convener	An individual or group responsible for bringing people together to address an issue, problem, or opportunity by using their influence and authority to call people to collaborate.	Adapted from CollaborativeLeadersNetwork.org, 2017; https://collaborativeleadersnetwork.org/leaders/the-role-of-the-convenor
Innovator	One who develops an idea, practice, or object that is perceived as new or who improves on something that already exists, individually or in collaboration, and produces a beneficial outcome.	Adapted from Porter-O'Grady & Malloch, 2010; Rogers, 2003;
Advocate	Examining options considering one's own value system using a personal interpretation of the scientific evidence with the aim of promoting a single policy option determined to be most desirable for society.	Barrows, 1994; Bogenschneider, Olson, Mills & Linney, 2006
Influence	The ability of an individual to sway or persuade another person or group based on authority, communication traits, knowledge-based competence, status, and use of time and timing.	Adams & Natarajan, 2016

Convener and Change Agent

All nurses are leaders who should be change agents (Kaplan, 1990) and conveners, holding responsibility for bringing people together to address an issue, problem, or opportunity (Wood & Gray, 1991). Considering the ever-changing healthcare delivery landscape, nurses must be agile and proficient change agents. If we are not able to drive change in our profession or professional environment, someone will do it for us and we will lose autonomy over how we as nurses deliver healthcare (Mensik, 2014).

Being a convener is not a new idea to nurses. Healthcare delivery is a collaborative process involving multiple participants including but not limited to patients, families, practitioners, and nurses. Nurses often act as conveners and coordinators of this process. We repeatedly discussed, with a variety of examples, convening groups to bring awareness and drive change, leading us to merge being a change agent and convener as one fluid action.

Influence

The importance of influence derived from participants describing a need for nurse data stewardship, role modeling, and engaging others; they used terms such as *influence, change, persuade, promote,* and *help others understand.* While chapter 2 describes the concept of influence at length, we defined influence as the ability to persuade others based on authority, communication traits, knowledge-based competencies, status, and timing (Adams & Natarajan, 2016).

Advocate

We defined the nurse-leader competency of advocacy as an examination of options using unbiased interpretation of scientific evidence to promote a policy option most desirable for society (Bogenschneider, Olson, Mills, & Linney, 2000; Tomajan, 2012). The term derived from participants' ideas of how nurse leaders advocate as data stewards and role models and facilitate engagement by promoting *calls to action* and *policy change.* Advocation is perhaps the most aligned, natural leadership competency all nurses demonstrate in their daily practice.

Innovate

The last category, innovation, derived from participants' descriptions of how nurse leaders act as data stewards and role models and facilitate engagement through developing and adopting evidence-based practice and research. As an innovator, the nurse as a leader improves or develops a new idea, practice, or object for adoption that results in a beneficial outcome (Malloch & Porter-O'Grady, 2010; Rogers, 2003).

Discussion

Nurses are regarded as one of the most trusted and ethical professions (Riffkin, 2014; Rutherford, 2014). With nurse competencies rooted in advocacy, influence, and innovation, all nurses can view themselves as conveners, change agents, and health leaders. It is necessary for all nurses to be good data stewards of financial and nursing-quality data, to role model the health behaviors we promote, and to facilitate the engagement of oneself and others with health promotion.

All Nurses as Leaders

Recognizing all nurses as leaders is not a new concept; however, not all nurses recognize that they are leaders or that they have a leadership role in the healthcare delivery framework. The terms *leader* and *manager* are often interchanged among nurses in the nursing profession but should not be.

A manager often holds an appointed hierarchical position of power over tasks and decision-making in an organization. A manager may or may not be a leader. A leader is in a position of power based on their ability to influence others through effective communication and relationships. A leader may not always be in an appointed position like a manager.

Nurses serve and influence patients, communities, and our profession daily through effective communication and relationships. This is evident as nursing continues to be voted the most trusted profession. As nursing moves forward in the current healthcare environment, we need to ask, How can we leverage our trusted-profession status to influence health promotion and support the Quadruple Aim?

Advocacy, influence, and innovation are core competencies to develop, implement, and evaluate health policy. We need to be purposeful and strategic in how we articulate nursing's leadership role in advancing each aspect of the Quadruple Aim through these competencies. As leaders and those most closely involved with aspects of the Quadruple Aim, we must support creating a practice environment to optimize improvements in the patient experience and population health and reductions in the cost per capita. We must encourage student nurses to develop these core competencies early to have greater impact at the point of care and reshape the healthcare delivery model.

Many of these concepts are included in various definitions of leadership in general and across professional nursing organizations. Training on these competencies is imperative to advance the profession, care delivery, the Quadruple Aim, and the health of everyone. We need to purse this purposefully. Our next steps may be to reconvene the nurse leaders from across the different professional nursing organizations, collecting their definitions and concepts of nursing leadership and comparing among one another and to the model described in this paper. Advancing through unification and moving from "I know it when I see it" to a unified definition of nursing leadership will support the Quadruple Aim.

Chapter Key Points

- There is no single agreed-upon definition of leadership.

- Nurses need to be agile and proficient change agents.

- The terms *leader* and *manager* are often interchanged among nurses in the nursing profession but should not be.

References

Adams, J. M., Denham, D., & Neumeister, I. R. (2010). Applying the Model of the Interrelationship of Leadership Environments and Outcomes for Nurse Executives: A community hospital's exemplar in developing staff nurse engagement through documentation improvement initiatives. *Nursing Administration Quarterly, 34*(3), 201–7. DOI: 10.1097/NAQ.0b013e3181e7026e

Adams, J. M. & Natarajan, S. (2016). Understanding influence within the context of nursing: Development of the Adams Influence Model using practice, research, and theory. *Advances in Nursing Science, 39*(3), E40–E56. DOI: 10.1097/ANS.0000000000000134

Barrows, H. S. (1994). *Practice-based learning: Problem-based learning applied to medical education.* Springfield, IL: Southern Illinois University.

Bodenheimer T. & Sinsky, C. (2014). From triple to quadruple aim: Care of the patient requires care of the provider. *Annals of Family Medicine, 12*(6), 573–76 DOI: 10.1370/afm.1713

Bogenchneider, K., Olson, J. R., Mills, J. & Linney, K. D. (2000). Connecting research and policymaking: Implications for theory and practice from the Family Impact Seminars. *Family Relations, 49*(3), 327–39. DOI: 10.1111/j.1741-3729.2000.00327.x

Bogenschneider, K. Olson, J. R., Mills, J., & Linney, K. D. (2006). How can we connect research with state policymaking? In K. Bogenschneider (Ed.), *Family policy matters: How policymaking affects families and what professionals can do* (2nd ed., pp. 245–76). Mahwah, NJ: Lawrence Erlbaum.

Bowles, J. R., Adams, J. M., Batcheller, J., Zimmermann, D., & Pappas, S. (2018). The Role of the Nurse Leader in Advancing the Quadruple Aim. Nurse Leader, 16(4), 244–48.

Gill, R. (2013). Theory and practice of leadership. London: Sage.

Kaplan, S. M. (1990). The nurse as change agent. *Pediatric Nursing, 16*(6), 603–5.

Malloch, K. & Porter-O'Grady, T. (2010). *Introduction to evidence-based practice in nursing and health care.* Burlington, MA: Jones & Bartlett Learning.

McClure, M. L., Poulin, M. A., Sovie, M. D., & Wandelt, M. A. (1983). *Magnet hospitals: Attraction and retention of professional nurses.* Kansas City, MO: American Nurses Association.

Mensik, J. (2014). *Lead, drive & thrive in the system.* Silver Spring, MD: American Nurses Association.

Porter-O'Grady, T. & Malloch, K. (2010). *Innovation leadership: Creating the landscape of healthcare.* Burlington, MA: Jones & Bartlett Learning.

Riffkin, R. (2014, December 18). Americans rate nurses highest on honesty, ethical standards. *Gallup.* Retrieved from https://news.gallup.com/poll/180260/americans-rate-nurses-highest-honesty-ethical-standards.aspx

Rogers, E. M., (2003). *Diffusion of innovations* (5th ed.). New York, NY: Free Press.

Rutherford, M. M. (2014). The value of trust to nursing. *Nursing Economics, 32*(6), 283–88.

Sikka, R., Morath, J. M., & Leape, L. (2015). The Quadruple Aim: Care, health, cost and meaning in work. *BMJ Quality & Safety, 24*(10), 608–10. DOI: 10.1136/bmjqs-2015-004160

Tomajan, K. (2012). Advocating for nurses and nursing. *Online Journal of Issues in Nursing, 17*(1), 4. DOI: 10.3912/OJIN.Vol17No01Man04

Wood, D. J. & Gray, B. (1991). Toward a comprehensive theory of collaboration. *The Journal of Applied Behavioral Science, 27*(2), 139–62.

Chapter 5

Advancing the Influence

Jeffrey M. Adams, PhD, RN, NEA-BC, FAAN
Debbie Chatman Bryant, DNP, RN, FAAN
Kirstin Manges, PhD, RN

Fight for the things that you care about, but do it in a way that will lead others to join you.

—Ruth Bader Ginsburg

Influence

As the largest, most trusted healthcare profession, nurses are regularly identified as major contributors to the quality, cost, and availability of high-performing healthcare (Adams et al., 2018). The nursing profession is well documented as having an enormous impact on patients' experiences—from birth through death, on each joyous, preventative, acute, and restorative stage throughout the lifespan. Evidence shows that nurses are key to keeping patients safe (Groves, Meisenbach, & Scott-Cawiezell, 2011), providing high-quality care (Aiken et al., 2012), and making care accessible (Salmond & Echevarria, 2017). Yet why are nurses not commonly thought of as leaders or influencers?

> Influence is best defined as the ability of an individual (agent) to sway or affect another person or group (target) based on authority, status, knowledge-based competence, communication traits, and use of time and timing (Adams, 2009; Adams & Natarajan, 2016).

This chapter highlights the historical challenges and current points of strength for the profession of nursing. We discuss an evidence-based approach to enhancing nursing's influence in practice, research, education, policy, and theory. Additionally, we discuss our team's work aimed at the question, How are nurses the largest and most trusted profession while also seemingly the least influential? At each stage we emphasize the key supportive relationships and access to resources that aided in advancing this trajectory, as these concepts have repeatedly been found to optimize influence (Diesing, 2016). Our exposure to the most influential nursing leaders (many of whom are highlighted within this chapter or contributed to this book) has helped form the foundation, or baseline, for the influence of nurses.

Strength in Numbers

With more than 4 million nurses in the United States, nurses constitute the largest professional group of healthcare providers (American Nurses Association, 2018). According to the US Department of Health and Human Services (2010), the number of nurses in the workforce is larger than 1 million more than the combined total of:

- Nutritionists (66,000),

- Occupational therapists (100,000),

- Pharmacists (300,000),

- Physical therapists (200,000),

- Physicians and surgeons (700,000), and

- Social workers (650,000).

Additionally, with more than 400,000 nurses (Bureau of Labor Statistics, 2017) in formal healthcare leadership roles, nurses constitute the largest segment of the leadership positions within the US healthcare workforce. Lastly, based on our estimations, nurses amount to more than 1% of the entire US population, and 2.4% of all women in the United States are part of the profession (U.S. Census Bureau, 2017, 2018). This is important to note as there is a current and needed groundswell focusing on the voice, advancement, equity, and equality of women across all sectors of work life in the United States and around the world.

While nurses are overwhelmingly the largest representatives of the healthcare workforce, and regularly recognized as the most trusted profession (Norman, 2016), the profession has been repeatedly recognized as "lacking influence." For example, a 2010 poll by the Robert Wood Johnson Foundation (RWJF) and Gallup found nurses to be the least influential compared to physicians, healthcare executives, insurance executives, government officials, pharmaceutical executives, and even patients when it comes to addressing health policy.

Additionally, an American Hospital Association–commissioned study identified that CEOs look to CNOs infrequently as part of their regular decision-making process (Health Research & Educational Trust, 2014). The findings were further supported by Adams and colleagues' research in which nurse-leader respondents self-identified as "less influential" than their nonnursing executive counterparts on a host of issues (Adams, Duffy, & Clifford, 2006; Adams et al., 2007). Further articulating that nurses lack influence is Modern Healthcare's "100 Most Influential People in Healthcare" (2018) list, which included only one nurse. These examples provide evidence that there is an understandable gap in understanding and actualizing influence of nurses.

The Nursing Influence Research Movement

The concept of influence has been significantly studied across many other disciplines such as psychology, marketing, communications, and anthropology. Psychologists French and Raven (1959) conducted the seminal studies of influence that focused on examining the interplay between social influence, leadership, and power. More recently, research about influence has examined influence behaviors, including influence upward (bosses), laterally (peers, vendors, or associates), and downward (subordinates) (Yukl & Chavez, 2002; Yukl, Chavez, & Seifert, 2005; Yukl & Falbe, 1990). Grenny et al. (2013) noted influence as a strategy for leading change management.

The Gap: Why Does the Largest and Most Trusted Healthcare Profession Lack Influence?

The remainder of the chapter discusses our beginning steps to understand and address this gap whereby the largest, most trusted profession is one that lacks influence. From the bedside to the boardroom and beyond, we provide a brief overview of historic and present challenges that have affected the influence of nursing, then we provide our team's work to date. While there is not a singular approach to optimizing nursing's influence, it is imperative to have a purposeful strategy across practice, research, education, policy, theory, media, and industry to improve healthcare for patients, organizations, and the workforce.

1996–2003: The Origins of the Influence Inquiry in Nursing

Experiences in Workforce, Work Environments, Nursing Informatics, and Language Standardization

Key Supportive Nursing Leadership Relationships: Linda Aiken, Sean Clarke, Donna Havens, Ada Sue Hinshaw, Gail Keenan, Roy Simpson, Julie Sochalski, and Ellen Marie Whelan

Access to Resources: Research supported through NINR T32 through the Center for Health Outcomes and Policy at the University of Pennsylvania

Starting in the early 1990s, The Center for Health Outcomes and Policy Research (CHOPR) at the University of Pennsylvania provided the foundation for understanding the importance of using research to influence practice and policy. The first author of this chapter was a research assistant on the CHOPR research team that published many seminal studies, including those linking the educational level of nurses to patient outcomes (Aiken et al., 2003) and demonstrating the relationship between quality work environments of nurses and patient, workforce, and organizational outcomes (Aiken, Sochalski, & Lake, 1997; Havens & Aiken, 1999; Scott, Sochalski, & Aiken, 1999; Aiken, Clarke, & Sloane, 2002). The leadership, expertise, and infrastructure at CHOPR provided immeasurable insight into the importance of being purposeful and assembling multiple factors to advance influence. Many of the influential nursing leaders and researchers (and authors in this book) have been a part of, or have learned from, experiences at CHOPR.

Building on these experiences, the first author of this chapter focused his early career around clinical informatics consulting including systems selection, implementation, design, upgrades, and staff education. As this career trajectory was near the advent of clinical informatics systems, most medical records systems were selected by a chief informatics officer, chief financial officer, chief executive officer, or even a chief medical officer. In the late 1990s, during his consulting career at more than 50 organizations, it was observed that chief nursing officers (CNOs) were not heavily involved (thus not influential) in most of the health system's clinical informatics decisions. Researchers and CNO groups identified nurses' lack of involvement in selection, design, and the like of clinical informatics systems as a troubling issue for many, as nurses were the largest user of these systems.

This lack of involvement and influence not only highlighted nursing's executive leadership challenges but also hampered documenting evidence of nurses' contributions, as vendor-driven clinical information systems didn't collect such professional information. Even if CNOs were influential in these decisions, the clinical systems left nurses without the ability to document good nursing practices or to generate quantifiable nursing evidence for the profession to influence across practice, research, education, policy, and theory.

From Exposure to Research

These exposures and experiences in the world-renowned CHOPR research lab and as a consultant across more than 50 health systems by the primary author have provided the foundation of this research, which has focused on the influence of nurse leaders. Specifically, our efforts are aimed at understanding influence within the approximately 5,500 CNOs

(American Hospital Association, 2017) and 400,000 nurses (Bureau of Labor Statistics, 2017) in formal management positions in clinical practice settings. Further, the nursing management population is unique because it is one of few populations where most leaders are women. Thus, the study of nursing leaders presents a unique opportunity to understand the implications of gender on influence.

2003–2008: Early Attempts to Understand and Research Nursing Influence

Examining Whether There Is an Influence Problem in Nursing

Key Supportive Nursing Leadership Relationships: Linda Aiken, Joyce Clifford, Mary Duffy, Jeanette Ives Erickson, and Dorothy Jones

Access to Resources: Projects sponsored by The Harvard Affiliated Hospital's Institute for Nursing Healthcare Leadership, Massachusetts General Hospital, Navin Haffty & Associates, Salinas Valley Memorial Healthcare System, and the Bogart Group, Inc.

The research journey into understanding nursing influence started with early discussions between researchers and practice leaders around the status of nursing's influence s a profession. Critical conversations with leaders in the field suggested that CNOs' limited influence over selecting clinical information systems was not an isolated issue and that in actuality nurses lacked influence in general.

Exploring the responsibilities of the rather small number of nursing senior leaders in contrast to the large volume of nurses gives additional clarity to the importance of nursing leadership and influence. For example, there is approximately one CNO for every one of the approximately 5,500 hospital/health systems (American Hospital Association, 2017) and one nursing school dean for each of the approximately 2,000 accredited schools of nursing (Accreditation Commission for Education in Nursing, 2016; Commission on Collegiate Nursing Education, 2018).

Therefore these 7,500 people lead a little more than half of the 4 million nurses. The problem of having a relatively few nurse leaders spans both clinical and educational settings. Thus, optimizing influential leadership is imperative for patients, organizations, and the profession. Over the next several years, our research team embarked on a series of studies focused on the knowledge, influence, and perceived success of nurse executives (Adams & Djukic, 2015).

2004–2008: Developing the Adams Influence Model (AIM)

Defining the Structure and Process of Influence

Key Supportive Nursing Leadership Relationships: Dorothy Jones, Jeanette Ives Erickson, Joyce Clifford, Callista Roy, Danny Willis, Ada Sue Hinshaw, and Gail Keenan

Access to Resources: Projects sponsored by Yvonne L. Munn Center Pre-Doctoral Fellowship Grant from Massachusetts General Hospital

Our earlier exploration and experiences left us with a confidence that expanding influence was an important concept to study for nursing, yet with such a broad topic, our team was faced with the question: Where to start? After identifying the critical gap in practices, we started by setting out on a multiyear journey to develop a theoretical model for the concept of influence. The resulting model, the **Adams Influence Model (AIM)**, is the result of extensive literature reviews, supportive targeted research, expert review, and validation-directed content analysis to define the components, structure, and process of influence (see figure 5–1).

The AIM design draws on an amalgam of theory, research, and practice knowledge that blends together concepts from Newman's Theory of Health as Expanding Consciousness (Newman, 2008), the Roy Adaptation Model (Roy, 2008) and King's Interacting Systems Framework and Theory of Goal Attainment (King, 1981).

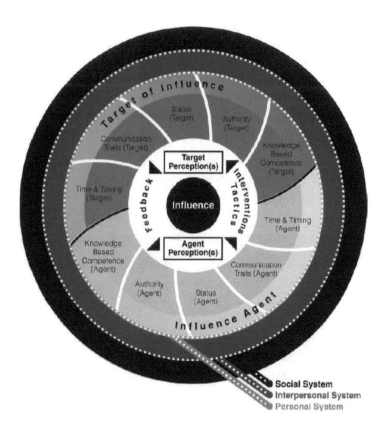

FIGURE 5–1. Adams Influence Model (AIM) (©Jeff Adams, LLC)

The AIM represents influence as occurring between an influence agent (i.e., one seeking to influence) and influence targets (i.e., those subject to influence) (Adams, 2009; Adams & Natarajan, 2016). The outer rings of the graphic (personal, interpersonal, and social systems) suggest that there are situational and relationship aspects (both within and outside our control) that impact the influence process. That structure of influence involves a mutual, two-way exchange (Adams, 2009; Adams & Natarajan, 2016) whereby both the influence agent and influence target possess influence factors (authority, communication traits, knowledge-based competence, status, and use of time and timing) and influence attributes (see table 5-1) in differing titrations that provide a foundation for the influence process.

TABLE 5-1.   Adams Influence Model influence factors and attributes

AIM Influence Factors	Definitions	AIM Influence Attributes	Definitions
Knowledge-based competence	The quality of being adequately or well-qualified intellectually so as to meet or exceed standards of performance	Empirical knowledge	The application of theories of science; factual knowledge of nursing, the scientific body of nursing knowledge
		Personal knowledge	Providing means to become more aware of culture, customs, beliefs, and emotions
		Aesthetic knowledge	Envisioning desired outcomes to respond with appropriate action; knowing how to be creative, open, empathetic, and holistic
		Ethical knowledge	The capacity to make choices regarding moral judgments within situations; expressed in codes, standards, and ethical frameworks
		Sociopolitical knowledge	Areas that affect the health of the population, such as class structure, poverty, sexism, and racism
Authority	The right to take actions or responsibility	Accountability	The state of being liable or answerable
		Responsibility	The social force that binds a person to the courses of action demanded by that force
		Access to resources	Ability to manage or oversee finances, information, or goods that are needed or valued by others
Status	Having high standing or prestige	Hierarchical position	An organized body of officials in successive ranks or orders
		Key supportive relationships	An emotional or other connection between people
		Reputation	A favorable and publicly recognized name or standing for merit, achievement, and reliability
		Informal position	An assumed or appointed role and the related pattern of expected interpersonal behaviors associated with the role
Communication traits	The proficiency or dexterity with which one person relates or interacts with other people	Message articulation	The shape or manner in which things come together and a connection is made
		Emotional involvement	To engage interests, emotions, or commitment
		Persistence	The act of persevering; continuing or repeating behavior
		Confidence	Belief in oneself and one's powers or abilities
		Physical appeal-self	The attractiveness of the individual
		Physical appeal-environment	An expected order to one's surroundings
		Presence	Being with another physically and psychologically
Use of time and timing	The understanding of both the interval in which action is available to be taken and the optimal judgment and delivery of when an action is taken	Amount of time to sell an issue	A limited period or interval, as between two successive events
		Timing to deliver the issue	The selecting of the best time or speed for doing something to achieve the desired or maximum result

Process of Influence

Further, at the center of the AIM is the process of influence, where an influence agent has a perception of him- or herself and the influence target. This perception then leads the influence agent to choose an influence tactic such as pressure, legitimizing, ingratiation, rational persuasion, coalition, exchange, personal appeals, inspirational appeals, consultation, collaboration, or apprising (Yukl & Falbe, 1990; Yukl & Chavez, 2002; Yukl, Chavez, & Seifert, 2005). The influence target also has a perception of him- or herself and the influence agent informed by the tactic chosen. The influence target then provides feedback as influence is achieved, or the process can start again with a new tactic if influence is not achieved.

The word or concept of *influence* is often used in informal conversation interchangeably with the word or concept of *power*. This is an incorrect equivalence. The AIM purposefully represents a camera shutter, signifying the AIM's focus and perspective on a moment in time and around a single issue. Within the context of the AIM, influence is different than the power that is a cumulative result of being influential over many issues.

2005–2007: Developing the Model of the Interrelationship of Leadership, Environments, and Outcomes for Nurse Executives (MILE ONE)

Determining What Nursing Is Trying to Influence

Key Supportive Nursing Leadership Relationships: Jeanette Ives Erickson, Joyce Clifford, Dorothy Jones, and Heather Laschinger

Access to Resources: Projects sponsored by an Yvonne L. Munn Center Pre-Doctoral Fellowship Grant from Massachusetts General Hospital.

A review of literature while developing the AIM revealed a unique conceptualization of three interrelated research and practice threads (Adams, Ives Erickson, Jones, & Paulo, 2009). These interrelated concepts led to a new framework, **The Model of the Interrelationship of Leadership, Environments, and Outcomes for Nurse Executives (MILE ONE)**, which provides a structure to articulate the work and role of nurse leaders and direct care nurses in improving patient, workforce, and organizational outcomes. The MILE ONE is distinct because the theory links existing evidence and identifies the continuous and dependent interrelationship among three content areas:

1. nurse leaders influencing professional practice/work environments (PPWE),

2. nurses' PPWEs influencing patient and organizational outcomes, and

3. patient and organizational outcomes influencing nurse leaders to try the next thing.

(Adams et al., 2009).

The MILE ONE (figure 5-2) additionally helps operationalize nurse-executive influence and define a measurement of CNO success. As represented in figure 5-3, nurse executives feel that their constituents place differing importance on their (the nurse executives') core competencies in context of the American Organization of Nurse Executives core competencies for nurse executives (Adams et al., 2008). The MILE ONE highlights a major role conflict that nurse executives face. While subordinates place an emphasis on a nurse executive's communication skills, superiors' expectations place emphasis on business skills. One hypothesis for the outcomes of this role conflict suggests that existing short average CNO tenures and high CNO turnover rates (Jones, Havens, & Thompson, 2008) are largely related to the lack of universally accepted performance measures or defined "success" by upward (bosses), lateral (peers), or downward (staff) constituencies (Adams & Djukic, 2015). The MILE ONE postulates that the nurse leader provides continuous influence to optimize the PPWE. Therefore, the optimization of the PPWE also meets the business-skills expectations of superiors and communication-skills expectations of subordinates. Thus, perhaps the MILE ONE could be used to articulate improving the PPWE as the *focus* and measure of nurse leader success as it is valued by each constituent group and their identified expectations.

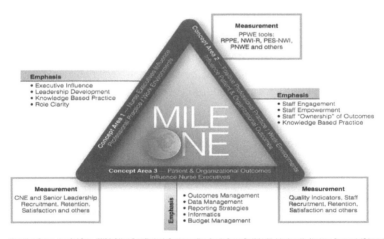

FIGURE 5–2. Model of the Interrelationship of Leadership, Environments, and Outcomes for Nurse Executives

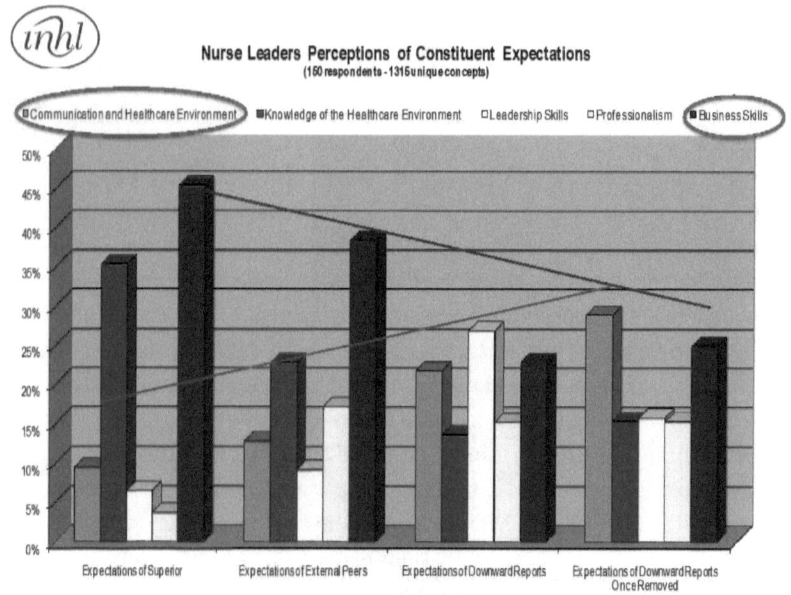

FIGURE 5–3. Nurse leaders' perceptions of constituent expectations

The MILE ONE provides a guide in support of the literature suggesting that the PPWE is an equalizing proxy measure for all constituencies (Adams & Djukic, 2015). The three components (concept areas) are interrelated and have a profound impact on each other. Concept area 1, the leadership's ability to impact the environment, has primarily been described and explored qualitatively and only more recently emphasized quantitatively (Batcheller et al., 2017; Diesing, 2017; Manges, Scott-Cawiezell, & Ward, 2017; Somerville et al., 2015; Wong, Cummings, & Ducharme, 2013). Concept area 2, the positive professional practice/work environments (PPWEs), has been qualitatively and quantitatively correlated to better patient, workforce, and organizational outcomes for nearly a quarter century (Aiken et al., 2008; Barnes, Rearden, & McHugh, 2016; Copanitsoanou, Fotos, & Brokalaki, 2017; Jayawardhana, Welton, & Lindrooth, 2014; Kutney-Lee et al., 2015; McHugh et al., 2013; Silber et al., 2016; Stimpfel et al., 2016). And concept area 3 suggests that as outcomes improve, nurse executives are encouraged to identify the next opportunity to improve the work environment in a continuous cycle to improve the PPWE.

2009–2012: Developing the Leadership Influence over Professional Practice Environment Scale (LIPPES)

Quantifying Leadership Influence

Key Supportive Nursing Leadership Relationships: Linda Aiken, Gaurdia Banister, Marianne Ditomassi, Jeanette Ives Erickson, and Dorothy Jones.

Access to Resources: Projects sponsored by an Yvonne L. Munn Center Post-Doctoral Fellowship Grant, Connell Research Scholar Grant and Connell Research Scholar Competitive Extension from Massachusetts General Hospital, American Organization of Nurse Executives Research Grant, and American Nurses Foundation—American Nurses Credentialing Center Research Grant

After developing the AIM, defining the structure and process of influence, and identifying the MILE ONE, conceptualizing the importance of nurse leaders' influence on enhancing the PPWE, we became aware of the necessity of measuring nurse leaders' ability to influence the work environment. We developed the **Leadership Influence over Professional Practice Environment Scale (LIPPES)** to address this need (Adams, Nikolaev, Ives Erickson, Ditomassi, & Jones, 2013). The LIPPES merges two evidence-based structures: the AIM (Adams, 2009) and the Revised Professional Practice Environment scale (Ives Erickson, Duffy, Ditomassi, & Jones, 2009). LIPPES uses the following definitions of influence and PPWE:

- Influence is the ability of an individual (agent) to sway or affect another person or group (target) based on authority, status, knowledge-based competence, communication traits, or use of time and timing (Adams, 2009; Adams & Natarajan, 2016).

- Professional practice/work environment is an organizational culture that advances the clinical practice of health professionals by ensuring unity of purpose and organizational alignment (Ives Erickson, 2012).

2015–2017: Developing the Leadership Influence Self-Assessment (LISA)

> ### *Preparing to Inventory Individual Influence*
>
> *Key Supportive Nursing Leadership Relationships:* Casey Shillam, Suzanne Miyamoto, Joy Deupree, Linda Cronenwett, Susan Hassmiller, and Mary Joan Ladden.
>
> *Access to Resources:* Projects sponsored by the Robert Wood Johnson Foundation

Further advancing the measurement of influence, and as part of the RWJF Executive Nurse Fellowship, an action-learning team used the AIM to develop an instrument toward understanding and thus enhancing leadership influence for leaders seeking to transform health and health-care across disciplines. What emerged was a valid and reliable 80-item instrument, the **Leadership Influence Self-Assessment (LISA)**, which is composed of four subscales—status, authority, strategy, and integrity— identified through a rigorous instrument-development process (Shillam et al., 2017). The LISA identifies gaps, strengths, and weaknesses of indi-viduals seeking to gain insights and knowledge, as well as to provide directions for enhancing leadership and influence. Nurse leaders can support themselves by understanding their individual needs and seeking targeted educational- and professional-development opportunities to optimize individual influence. Longitudinally, outcomes of studies using the LISA will help nurses cultivate, promote, and assert influence to ensure that their voices are respectfully acknowledged and valued as part of a healthcare leadership team.

Notably, the LIPPES and LISA were developed using the AIM. Although there are some similarities between them, the purpose of each instru-ment differs. LIPPES specifically explores the self-perceived influence of acute care nurse leaders and managers over practice environments, as well as the relationship of their influence to workforce and patient outcomes. LISA purposefully examines self-awareness of one's influence regardless of setting or role.

Next Steps to Enhance Nurse-Leader Influence

Beyond continuing to refine, use, and disseminate for research information about nurses' influence using the instruments and models described above, to move the field forward we must have a purposeful strategy for continuing to enhance the influence of nurses. Current plans for next steps in this effort are described below.

The Influence of Language (Used and Accepted)

First there are steps that every person can take to enhance the influence of nurses. The words we use, and how we use them, change both our perception and the public's perception of nursing's influence. For example, the phrase "I am just a nurse" has become an expression repeated all too often by nurses across every setting. One strategy is to correct this self-deprecation every time it is shared, and to encourage nurses to talk about their nursing expertise. Another language strategy is rephrasing the concept of "doctors and nurses" to "nurses and physicians." It is a minor change, but it is accurate when addressing the volume of the healthcare workforce (nurses can be doctors, too). Likewise, balking at the concept of "orders" as opposed to a team "care plan" is another important approach to moving the needle for personal and professional equality of importance. There are many other examples of the importance of language in enhancing or diminishing influence, from gender stereotypes to capturing the contribution of nurses in electronic medical records (Reid Ponte, Somerville, & Adams, 2016).

Articulating the Influence of Nurses on Healthcare Systems

From the bedside to the boardroom there is a continued need for research demonstrating the critical influence that nurses have on patient access, cost, and quality of care across the health-system continuum (Institute of Medicine, 2011). MILE ONE can help identify key under-examined areas of research that can better articulate the influence that nurses have on healthcare. There are ongoing efforts to more critically understand and advance nursing's influence, including the American Academy of Nursing's Expert Panel on Building Expert Health Systems 2016 retreat framed around the MILE ONE (Batcheller et al., 2017), the efforts to describe nursing leadership's role in addressing the Quadruple Aim (Adams et al., 2018; see also chapter 4), the efforts of the American

Organization of Nurse Executives (AONE) Foundation to focus specifically on nurse leader–related outcomes, and the *Nursing Special Report* (Press Ganey, 2017) using the MILE ONE to frame ongoing nursing research within the Press Ganey research infrastructure.

Individual and Team Influence Coaching

Nurses need leadership skills and competencies to influence and improve the delivery of care. The secondary author of this chapter (Bryant) with the support of the RWJF Executive Nurse Fellowship and the Center for Creative Leadership has developed an influence and coaching leadership program. This program focuses on the coach–client relationship with active listening and stresses the factors of the AIM, MILE ONE, LIPPES, and LISA as a mechanism toward enhancing a nurse leader's development over the course of their career. Within this context, there is an intentionality to optimizing and understanding influence within the minority nurse population to close the gap and advance diversity in the nursing-leadership workforce.

Galvanizing Nursing Organizations' Influence Strategy and Access to Resources

Additionally, the American Academy of Nursing's Expert Panel on Building Expert Health Systems has developed an influence initiative to address and enhance nursing influence within and across practice, research, education, policy, and theory. There is additional opportunity to further coordinate with the major supporters of nursing research and training programs such as the American Nurses Foundation, AONE Foundation, National Clinician Scholars Program, RWJF, and the Jonas Center for Nursing and Veterans Healthcare. The strategy for this initiative is still being finalized, but the planning and purposeful approach to enhancing influence through nursing's major organizations is underway.

Summary

To quantify nursing leadership, as this book strives to do, one must understand and enhance personal and professional influence. Nurses serve as the fulcrum of healthcare in our society, contributing to each point in the care delivery experience. Simply identifying nursing in a supportive role is neither accurate of the training nor correct in addressing the needs of the population. The models and instruments we used and developed as part of our nearly two decades' worth of substantive research focused on nursing influence and leadership are only a start to advancing this agenda. A purposeful approach to enhancing each nurse's influence within practice, research, education, policy, and theory can help address the health system's needs in access, cost, quality, and the clinician work environments.

Chapter Key Points

- Nurses have been the least influential in policy changes.

- The term influence should not be considered interchangeable with the term power.

- All nurses need leadership skills and competencies to influence the healthcare system.

References

100 most influential people in healthcare—2018. (2018) *Modern Healthcare*. Retrieved from http://www.modernhealthcare.com/community/100-most-influential/2018/

Accreditation Commission for Education in Nursing. (2016). *Accreditation Commission for Education in Nursing home page*. Retrieved from http://www.acenursing.org

Adams, J. M. (2009). *The Adams Influence Model (AIM): Understanding the factors, attributes, and process of achieving influence*. Saarbrüken, Germany: VDM Verlag.

Adams JM, Denham D, Neumeister I. Applying the Model of the Interrelationship of Leadership, Environments & Outcomes for Nurse Executives (MILE ONE): A community hospital's exemplar in developing staff nurse engagement through documentation improvement initiatives. *Nursing Administration Quarterly, 24*(3): 201–7.

Adams, J. M. & Djukic, M. (2015). Nurse leaders face incongruent measures of success by their upward reports, peers and downward reports. *Organization of Nurse Leaders MA, RI & NH Newsletter*. Retrieved from http://www.oonl.org/assets/docs/2015-2016/adams%20jm%20djukic%20m%202015%20-%20nurse%20leader%20success.pdf

Adams, J. M., Duffy, M. E., & Clifford, J. C. (2006). *Knowledge and influence of the nurse leader: A survey of participants from the 2005 conference*. Boston, MA: Institute for Nursing Healthcare Leadership.

Adams, J. M., Ives Erickson, J., Duffy, M. E., Jones, D. A., Aspell Adams, A., & Clifford, J. C. (2007). *Knowledge and influence of the nurse leader: A survey of participants from 2006*. Boston, MA: Institute for Nursing Healthcare Leadership.

Adams, J.M., Ives Erickson J, Jones D.A., & Paulo L. (2009). An evidence-based structure for transformative nurse executive practice: The model of the interrelationship of leadership, environments & outcomes for nurse executives (MILE ONE). *Nursing Administration Quarterly, 33*(4), 280–87.

Adams, J. M. & Natarajan, S. (2016). Understanding influence within the context of nursing: Development of the Adams Influence Model using practice, research, and theory. *Advances in Nursing Science, 39*(3), E40–E56. DOI: 10.1097/ANS.0000000000000134

Adams, J. M., Nikolaev, N., Ives Erickson, J., Ditomassi, M. A., & Jones, D. A. (2013). Identification of the psychometric properties of the leadership influence over professional practice environment scale. *The Journal of Nursing Administration, 43*(5), 258–65.

Adams JM, Paulo L, Meraz-Gottfried L, Aspell Adams A, Ives Erickson J, Jones, DA, & Clifford JC. (2008). *Success Measures for the Nurse Leader.* Boston, MA: Institute for Nursing Healthcare Leadership.

Adams, J. M., Zimmermann, D., Cipriano, P., Pappas, S., & Batcheller, J. (2018). Improving the work life of health care workers: Building on nursing's experience. *Medical Care, 56*(1), 1–3. DOI: 10.1097/MLR.0000000000000839

Aiken, L. H., Clarke, S. P., Cheung, R. B., Sloane, D. M., & Silber, J. H. (2003). Educational levels of hospital nurses and surgical patient mortality. *JAMA: The Journal of the American Medical Association, 290*(12), 1617–23.

Aiken, L. H., Clarke, S. P., & Sloane, D. M. (2002). Hospital staffing, organization, and quality of care: Cross-national findings. *Nursing Outlook, 50*(5), 187–94. DOI: 10.1067/mno.2002.126696

Aiken, L. H., Clarke, S. P., Sloane, D. M., Lake, E. T., & Cheney, T. (2008). Effects of hospital care environment on patient mortality and nurse outcomes. *The Journal of Nursing Administration, 38*(5), 223–29. DOI: 10.1097/01.NNA.0000312773.42352.d7

Aiken, L. H., Sermeus, W., Van den Heede, K., Sloane, D. M., Busse, R., McKee, M., . . . & Kutney-Lee, A. (2012). Patient safety, satisfaction, and quality of hospital care: Cross sectional surveys of nurses and patients in 12 countries in Europe and the United States. *The BMJ, 344*, e1717.

Aiken, L. H., Sochalski, J., Lake, E. (1997). Studying Outcomes of Organizational Change in Health Services. *Medical Care, 35*(11 suppl.), NS6–NS18.

American Hospital Association. (2017). *Fast facts on U.S. hospitals 2017.* Retrieved from http://www.aha.org/research/rc/stat-studies/fast-facts.shtml

American Nurses Association. (2017). *About ANA.* Retrieved from http://www.nursingworld.org/FunctionalMenuCategories/AboutANA

Barnes, H., Rearden, J., & McHugh, M. D. (2016). Magnet hospital recognition linked to lower central line associated bloodstream infection rates. *Research in Nursing & Health, 39*(2), 96–104. DOI: 10.1002/nur.21709

Batcheller, J., Zimmermann, D., Pappas, S, & Adams, J. M. (2017). Addressing nursing's leadership role in addressing the quadruple aim: An overview from the American Academy of Nursing's Expert Panel on Building Health Systems Excellence. *Nurse Leader, 15*(3), 203–7.

Bureau of Labor Statistics. (2017). *Healthcare occupations.* Retrieved from https://www.bls.gov/ooh/healthcare/home.htm

Commission on Collegiate Nursing Education. (2018, January 3). *Accredited baccalaureate & graduate nursing programs.* Retrieved from https://directory.ccnecommunity.org/reports/accprog.asp

Copanitsoanou, P., Fotos, N., & Brokalaki, H. (2017). Effects of work environment on patient and nurse outcomes. *British Journal of Nursing, 26*(3), 172–76. DOI: 10.12968/bjon.2017.26.3.172

Diesing, G. (2016, April 4). Nurse leaders' authority, access to resources play large role in patient outcomes, study finds. *Hospitals & Health Networks.* Retrieved from http://www.hhnmag.com/articles/7091-nurse-leaders-authority-access-to-resource-plays-large-role-in-patient-outcomes-study-finds

French, J. R. P. & Raven B. (1959). The bases of social power. In D. Cartwright & A. Zander (Eds.), *Group dynamics* (pp. 150–67). New York, NY: Harper & Row.

Grenny, J., Patterson, K., Maxfield, D., McMillan, R., & Switzler, A. (2013). *Influencer: The new science of leading change.* New York, NY: McGraw Hill Professional.

Groves, P. S., Meisenbach, R. J., & Scott-Cawiezell, J. (2011). Keeping patients safe in healthcare organizations: a structuration theory of safety culture. *Journal of Advanced Nursing, 67*(8), 1846–55. DOI: 10.1111/j.1365-2648.2011.05619.x

Havens, D. S., & Aiken, L. (1999). Shaping systems to promote desired outcomes: The magnet hospital model. *The Journal of Nursing Administration, 29*(2), 14–20.

Health Research & Educational Trust. (2014, April). *Building a leadership team for the health care organization of the future.* Chicago, IL: Health Research & Educational Trust.

Institute of Medicine. (2011). *The future of nursing: Leading change, advancing health.* Washington, DC: National Academies Press.

Ives Erickson, J. (2012). 200 Years of nursing: A chief nurse's reflections on practice, theory, policy, education, and research. *The Journal of Nursing Administration, 42*(1), 9–11.

Ives Erickson, J., Duffy, M., Ditomassi, M., & Jones, D. (2009). Psychometric evaluation of the Revised Professional Practice Environment (RPPE) scale. *The Journal of Nursing Administration, 39*(5), 236–43. DOI: 10.1097/NNA.0b013e3181a23d14

Jayawardhana, J., Welton J. M, & Lindrooth, R.C. (2014). Is there a business case for Magnet hospitals? Estimates of the cost and revenue implications of becoming a Magnet. *Medical Care, 52*(5), 400–406. DOI: 10.1097/MLR.0000000000000092

Jones, C. B., Havens, D. S., & Thompson, P. A. (2008). Chief nursing officer retention and turnover: A crisis brewing? Results of a national survey. *Journal of Healthcare Management, 53*(2), 89–105.

King, I. A. (1981). *Theory for nursing: Systems, concepts, process.* New York, NY: John Wiley & Sons.

Kutney-Lee, A., Stimpfel, A. W., Sloane, D. M., Cimiotti, J. P., Quinn, L. W., & Aiken, L. H. (2015). Changes in patient and nurse outcomes associated with Magnet hospital recognition. *Medical Care, 53*(6), 550–57. DOI: 10.1097/MLR.0000000000000355

Manges, K., Scott-Cawiezell, J., & Ward, M. M. (2017). Maximizing team performance: The critical role of the nurse leader. *Nursing Forum, 52*(1), 21–29. DOI: 10.1111/nuf.12161

McHugh, M. D., Kelly, L. A., Smith, H. L., Wu, E. S., Vanak, J., & Aiken, L. H. (2013). Lower mortality in Magnet hospitals. *Medical Care, 51*(5), 382–88. DOI: 10.1097/MLR.0b013e3182726cc5

Newman, M.A. (2008). *Transforming presence: The difference that nursing makes*. Philadelphia, PA: F.A. Davis Company.

Norman, J. (2016, December 19). Americans rate healthcare providers high on honesty, ethics. *Gallup News*. Retrieved from http://news.gallup.com/poll/200057/americans-rate-healthcare-providers-high-honesty-ethics.aspx

Press Ganey (2017) *Press Ganey nursing special report: The influence of nurse manager leadership on patient and nurse outcomes and the mediating effects of the nurse work environment*. Retrieved from http://healthcare.pressganey.com/2015-Nursing-SR_Influence_Work_Environment

Reid Ponte, P., Somerville, J., & Adams, J. M. (2016). Assuring the capture of standardized nursing data: A call to action for chief nursing officers. *International Journal of Nursing Knowledge, 27*(3), 127–28. DOI: 10.1111/2047-3095.12136

Robert Wood Johnson Foundation & Gallup. (2010). *Nursing leadership from bedside to boardroom: Opinion leaders' perceptions*. Retrieved from http://www.rwjf.org/en/library/research/2010/01/nursing-leadership-from-bedside-to-boardroom.html

Roy, C. (2008). *The Roy adaptation model* (3rd ed.). Upper Saddle River, NJ: Prentice Hall.

Salmond, S. W. & Echevarria, M. (2017). Healthcare transformation and changing roles for nursing. *Orthopedic Nursing, 36*(1), 12–25. DOI: 10.1097/NOR.000000000000030

Scott, J., Sochalski, J., & Aiken, L. (1999). Review of magnet hospital research: Findings and implications for professional nursing practice. *The Journal of Nursing Administration, 29*(1), 9–19.

Shillam, C., Adams, J. M., Bryant, D. C., Deupree, J. P., Miyamoto, S., & Gregas M. (2017). Development of the Leadership Influence Self-Assessment (LISA©) instrument. *Nursing Outlook, 66*(2), 130–37. DOI: 10.1016/j.outlook.2017.10.009

Silber, J. H., Rosenbaum, P. R., McHugh, M. D., Ludwig, J. M., Smith, H. L., Niknam, B. A., . . . Aiken, L. H. (2016). Comparison of the value of nursing work environments in hospitals across different levels of patient risk. *JAMA Surgery, 151*(6), 527–36. DOI: 10.1001/jamasurg.2015.4908

Somerville, J., Reid Ponte, P., Pipe, T., & Adams, J.M. (2015). Innovation through a nursing academic practice research collaboration: Establishment of the Workforce Outcomes Research and Leadership Development Institute (WORLD-Institute). *Nurse Leader, 13*(6), 16–17.

Stimpfel, A. W., Sloane, D. M., McHugh, M. D., & Aiken, L. H. (2016). Hospitals known for nursing excellence associated with better hospital experience for patients. *Health Services Research, 51*(3), 1120–34.

U.S. Census Bureau. (2017, March). *Annual Estimates of the Resident Population for Selected Age Groups by Sex for the United States, States, Counties and Puerto Rico Commonwealth and Municipios: April 1, 2010 to July 1, 2016.* Retrieved from https://factfinder.census. gov/faces/tableservices/jsf/pages/ productview.xhtml?src=bkmk

U.S. Census Bureau. (2018). *Population clock.* Retrieved from https://www. census.gov/popclock/

U.S. Department of Health and Human Services. (2010). *The registered nurse population: Findings from the 2008 National Sample Survey of Registered Nurses.* Retrieved from https://bhw. hrsa.gov/sites/default/files/bhw/ nchwa/rnsurveyfinal.pdf

Wong, C., Cummings, G.G., & Ducharme, L. (2013). The relationship between nursing leadership and patient outcomes: a systematic review update. *Journal of Nursing Management, 21,* 709–24

Yukl, G. & Chavez, C. (2002). Influence tactics and leader effectiveness. In L. Needier & C. Schriesheim (Eds.), *Leadership: Research in management* (vol. 2, pp. 139–65). Charlotte, NC: Information Age Publishing.

Yukl, G., Chavez, C., & Seifert, C. F. (2005). Assessing the construct validity and utility of two new influence tactics. *Journal of Organizational Behavior, 26*(6), 705–25. DOI: 0.1002/job.335

Yukl, G. & Falbe, C. M. (1990). Influence tactics and objectives in upward, downward, and lateral influence attempts. *Journal of Applied Psychology, 75*(2), 132–40.

Chapter 6

Leading Interprofessionally

Karen Saewert, PhD, RN, CPHQ, ANEF

The work of leaders is to create the conditions that will allow innovation and creativity to flourish. We do this by modeling the way: creating language and contexts that encourage all of us to be engaged and authentic.

—Davidson, 2016

Introduction

We wrote this chapter with an eagerness that you would read it with interest in exploring what leading interprofessionally means to you—personally and professionally—and why being interprofessional and leading interprofessionally are aspirational if not essential nurse-leader attributes for you to model in your leadership for yourself and for others. During these explorations, you will meet Dr. Gerri Lamb, an extraordinary nurse leader. Dr. Lamb exemplifies being interprofessional and leading interprofessionally as a nurse. This chapter offers glimpses into her perspectives, which are unquestionably powered by her passion for work as a nurse leader in the interprofessional space and distinctively shaped by her personal, educational, and practice-based experiences and trans-formative discoveries (her inward focus for outward application).

Exemplary Nurse and Interprofessional Leader Profile

Gerri Lamb, PhD, RN, FAAN

Dr. Gerri Lamb directs the Center for Advancing Interprofessional Practice, Education and Research at Arizona State University (ASU) and is a professor at the ASU College of Nursing and Health Innovation. She received her master's degree as an adult nurse practitioner from the University of Rochester and her PhD in clinical nursing research from the University of Arizona. Dr. Lamb began her nursing career as a visiting nurse in New York City and has had diverse senior administrative roles in both academic and clinical settings. She was introduced to interprofessional education at the University of Rochester by Dr. Madeline Schmitt, a nurse sociologist and international leader in teams and teamwork. Dr. Schmitt continues as her mentor and colleague to this day. Dr. Lamb also is known to the nursing community for her work in care coordination and case management, both of which are integral areas of nursing practice that she considers high-performance teamwork.

Consider engaging in this conversation—one important to the future of nursing—linked to nurses as interprofessional partners and leaders. We start by examining historical and current interprofessional imperatives for being and leading interprofessionally. As we reach for a shared yet emergent understanding of the meaning of leading interprofessionally, we offer opportunities to engage in thoughtful reflections geared to self-leadership and interprofessional leadership development. We also present strategies for examining and enhancing your knowledge, skills, and values associated with leading interprofessionally in the context of practical competencies—an inward focus for outward practice application. Driving questions for this chapter include:

- What are some of the historical and contemporary interprofessional imperatives?

- What does it mean to lead interprofessionally?

- What individual behaviors are evident and observable when one is leading interprofessionally (quantitative terms)? What subjective aspects are associated with leading interprofessionally (qualitative terms)?

- What does leading interprofessionally involve?

- Why should you care? What difference does this make to you?

Curious enough to get started? If not, or if you're undecided, please reconsider; those we provide care to and receive care from need all of us. If you're ready (or you have reconsidered!), let's begin by examining some of the historical and contemporary interprofessional imperatives.

Interprofessional Imperatives

The interprofessional dialogue has its roots in the past, its talons in the present, and its future being written in the here and now. Being professional includes being interprofessional, both now and in the future (Hammick, Freeth, Cooperman, & Goodsman, 2009, p. 37). The concept and structure of leadership is changing with the rise of team-based care bringing a democratization unparalleled in traditional leadership (Anonson et al., 2009, p. 19). The concept of interprofessional education and practice is a theme in the literature and other material from a variety of health professions, with almost every profession putting forth recommendations in favor of teamwork over the past three decades; it has become a mandate for most disciplines. Yet uncertainty about interprofessional practice remains disquieting and prompts nurses and other members of the health professions to voice concerns (Sommerfeldt, 2013, p. 520).

Historical

Understanding the history of interprofessional education and practice can reinforce its importance today (Hammick et al., 2009, p. 28). You may be questioning the relevance of knowing how it was in the past. The value of examining how we arrived at the present exists in not repeating mistakes of the past (Davidson, 2017, p. 450). So what important learnings can we derive from the past?

The landmark 2011 Institute of Medicine (now the National Academy of Medicine) report, *The Future of Nursing: Leading Change, Advancing Health,* focused on the rapid changes occurring in healthcare and on the critical role of nurses in developing policy, implementing changes, providing and coordinating care, and measuring healthcare improvements. After its release, the Robert Wood Johnson Foundation in collaboration with the Future of Nursing: Campaign for Action initiated efforts to help clarify and implement the report's recommendations. The Robert Wood Johnson Foundation also asked the Institute of Medicine to examine the changes and progress made since the release of the initial report. The Institute of Medicine's 2015 follow-up report subsequently documented significant progress and conveyed additional considerations for further study.

Together these reports called for a fundamental transformation of the nursing profession in practice, education, and leadership and highlighted the need for data on the healthcare workforce (Rutherford-Hemming & Lioce, 2018, p. 9). Both the 2011 and 2015 Institute of Medicine reports focused considerably on the importance of interprofessional collabora-tion and the valuable abilities of nurses to collaborate with patients, other clinicians, educators, and researchers. These reports targeted collaboration and leadership, recommending that great attention be paid to these areas (Moss, Seifert, & O'Sullivan, 2016, p. 6). The interprofessional approach to delivering health services contrasted strongly with the traditional ways of working in healthcare—characterized by long-standing, high-status professional groups—creating challenges within an interprofessional team (Hammick et al., 2009 p. 25). Reforms in western healthcare also resulted in increased interprofessional delivery of care. The early driving forces toward more collaborative models of care were initially economic, with few outcomes-related considerations (Sommerfeldt, 2013, p. 520).

Contemporary

Practitioners of health professions have always had to interact with others during their work. However, the consciousness and accountability for professional action in collaborative working initially lacked a sharp focus. This required us to increase our understanding of our interprofessional actions and duties and our ability to carry them out (Hammick et al., 2009, p. 60).

In the current complex healthcare environment, nurses in all roles and settings are called on to be leaders in advocating for a healthier future. The reform of healthcare, the rise of the evidence-based practice movement, and the proliferation of new educational options are among the forces opening opportunities as never before for nurses to expand their leadership capacity to an interprofessional level (Stiles, Horton-Deutsch, & Andrews, 2014, p. 487). However, for nursing to influence the evolving interprofessional world of healthcare, nurses in all roles and settings need to engage in that world and be prepared to articulate to others what nursing is and what it is not (Sommerfeldt, 2013, p. 519).

Nursing's focus on education and practice also must incorporate leadership in interprofessional education and demonstrate and encourage other health professionals as colleagues poised for change and ready to act (Clark & Hassmiller, 2013, p. 335). Nurse leaders can occupy a pivotal position in developing and promoting effective interprofessional collaboration and should be full partners with physicians and other healthcare professionals in leading change, advancing health, and redesigning healthcare in an evolving healthcare system (Hoying, 2017, p. 188; Pollard, Ross, & Means, 2005, p. 339). Even so, being interprofessional and working collaboratively needs some things besides the usual attributes ascribed to other teams: a different approach to leadership (Hammick et al., 2009, p. 60).

This leads us to ask, How can the profession of nursing contribute to and shape efforts to promote and achieve interprofessional collaboration in practice and education (Hoffart, Brown, & Farrell, 2015, p. 376)? How does the nursing profession respond to opportunities to demonstrate leadership in interprofessional education and practice—opportunities that can create systems of care that monitor the health needs of individuals, families, and populations in relation to complex evolving healthcare systems (Clark & Hassmiller, 2013, p. 335)? Do we know enough yet about who we are as nurses to know who we are or should be in the interprofessional space? Some of would respond to this question with a yes but others with a no or with uncertainty.

Identity Formation

> ### IDENTITY FORMATION
>
> *Interprofessional leadership challenges individuals to develop professional or disciplinary identities and master new ways to balance professional and interprofessional perspectives and priorities. It requires being secure and confident in your own professional identity so you don't have to wear it on your sleeve or fanfare it to everyone in the room. People I work with in the interprofessional space know I'm a nurse; they also know that I can think at a systems level and integrate my professional values and expertise in a much bigger context.*
>
> *Interprofessional leaders acknowledge that different professions are different—they respect this and know how to optimize bringing people together. They know that these differences are important as they seek to find common ground.*
>
> —Gerri Lamb, PhD, RN, FAAN (2017)

What does it mean to lead interprofessionally? Examining our own condition as leaders and digging deep for the courage and vulnerability needed to rehumanize healthcare starts within each of us and is the place to begin (Davidson, 2016, p. 97). As leaders, all nurses are—or should be—invested as collaborative interprofessional partners in creating outcomes of value for the patients, families, and communities they serve (Moss et al., 2016). Yet there is limited research on how well health professionals are socialized to work interprofessionally or prepared to build an interprofessional identity in interprofessional environments (Arndt et al., 2009, p. 18). It is important that nurses factor interprofessionalism into their practice to identify their distinctiveness as nurses and cultivate a culture within nursing that supports interprofessional identities (Sommerfeldt, 2013, p. 522). This conceptualization is fundamental to positively influencing collaboration of healthcare delivery and interprofessional practice and to creatively reshaping healthcare in innovative and noticeable ways. Articulating what makes nursing essential in interprofessional healthcare is complex and is a concern for nurses in practice, administration, and education.

Nursing emulates the evolving state of healthcare practice. It resides at a crossroads in which core nursing knowledge development meets practice theory and evidence-based ideology, and it faces an identity crisis both within itself and the larger healthcare community (Clark & Hassmiller, 2013, p. 335). Changing from a state of doing to one of collaborating becomes clouded when coupled with the domineering hierarchy of persisting health systems.

Collaborative leadership is a key competency that affects patient outcomes and team effectiveness, making its development critical in health-profession students and practitioners alike (Anonson et al., 2009, p. 17). Even so, interprofessional familiarization in both academic and practice settings is neither consistently espoused nor systematically embedded, and development of interprofessional competencies is neglected with a notable absence of socialization processes centered on how *we* work together (Arndt et al., 2009, p. 22). Future teaching of effective interprofessional care must include a focus on interprofessional socialization, formally and informally, in both academic and clinical settings. Today's health-profession students undertake the process of professional socialization alongside their learning to become part of an interprofessional community of practitioners. This can lead one to assume that professional values and beliefs are the same as interprofessional values and beliefs (Hammick et al., 2009, p. 20). However, health professionals must rise above socialization limited to a single profession-specific disciplinary framework in order to effectively collaborate interprofessionally (Stiles et al., 2014, p. 492).

Wherever the juncture in which it takes place, socialization involves personal change as one reforms or redefines a new professional self-identify (Saewert, 2017, p. 40). Given that interprofessional leadership is a necessary component of preparing the next generation of healthcare professionals for interprofessional practice, what do we understand about what it takes and what it is like to become an interprofessional leader in healthcare? What practices are involved?

Finding Shared Meaning in Leading Interprofessionally

FINDING SHARED MEANING

I think we must be very clear that interprofessionalism enhances and does not compromise or diminish the contributions of nurses to patient care or healthcare outcomes. As a nurse who is an interprofessional leader, I am very aware of and respect nursing's history. We have worked very hard and have waged many battles to get where we are today: the largest, most respected profession in healthcare. I believe that I am effective in the interprofessional space precisely because I understand this. I would say that my ability to visibly and consistently balance my advocacy and love for nursing with my advocacy and commitment to interprofessional care is finely tuned and discerning.

—*Gerri Lamb, PhD, RN, FAAN (2017)*

Purposefully combining knowledge, skills, and attitudes promotes competent interprofessionalism and is essential to leading interprofessionally. There is rising emergent interest in interprofessionalism, but the literature only fleetingly references leaders or leadership and little has been published on what effective leadership in interprofessional practice and education entails (Brewer, Flavell, Trede, & Smith, 2016, pp. 408, 412). And while many perspectives regarding leadership offer intriguing views of the concept, no definitive conceptualization exists (Weiss, Tilin, & Morgan, 2018, e-1538).

FINDING SHARED MEANING

You don't get very far in leading interprofessional teams if all professions do not trust that you value their expertise and advocate for patients and families first and foremost.

—*Gerri Lamb, PhD, RN, FAAN (2017)*

High-profile reports from within and outside the nursing profession have underscored the need for nursing leadership and nurse leaders to shape the future of nursing to improve the delivery of healthcare services and health-profession education (Hoffart et al., 2015, p. 375). Interprofessional education, practice, and collaboration allow nurses to present a solid definition of nursing's role, to expand their scope and knowledge base, and to establish a persisting presence in the future of healthcare (Clark & Hassmiller, 2013, p. 335). There is a vast and expanding need to radically improve healthcare delivery and substantially strengthen workforce capacity across the world, making leadership at all levels of nursing vital to meet current and future needs. Should there even be a question whether being interprofessional and leading interprofessionally must be a routine part of how we work together? If it is necessary, what competencies are needed?

Competencies for Leading Interprofessionally

COMPETENCIES FOR LEADING INTERPROFESSIONALLY

I think interprofessional leadership incorporates all the desired leadership characteristics and competencies. Providing meaningful leadership across professions has several unique components that I think are foundational and integral to success. Interprofessional leadership requires being able to communicate, coordinate, and collaborate across different professional cultures, languages, and ways of thinking—respecting them all—and to create an environment in which every individual and group believes or knows that their contribution is valued and essential. Leadership takes the Interprofessional Education Collaborative competencies to the group and organizational level.

—Gerri Lamb, PhD, RN, FAAN (2017)

> ## COMPETENCIES FOR LEADING INTERPROFESSIONALLY
>
> *Values play a critical role in creating the incentive to transcend professional boundaries and move into the spaces between professions. I have a very deep belief in the value of teamwork and collaboration; I believe they are essential for our ability to achieve the goals of healthcare and to address patient and family needs. This is the common ground, and I believe it is essential to navigating those in-between spaces.*
>
> —Gerri Lamb, PhD, RN, FAAN (2017)

> ## COMPETENCIES FOR LEADING INTERPROFESSIONALLY
>
> *What other competencies I think interprofessional leaders need: to know the field and have grounding in interprofessional theories and team science. I also think they need to be advocates for advancing team performance and best practices and aligning incentives that recognize team outcomes. I do think that understanding the professional–interprofessional interface is key to understanding how and why interprofessional leadership is unique.*
>
> —Gerri Lamb, PhD, RN, FAAN (2017)

What individual behaviors are evident and observable when one is leading interprofessionally (quantitative terms)? What subjective traits are associated with leading interprofessionally (qualitative terms)? Understanding and leveraging the conditions that enable us to work within the innovation-evidence-leadership framework will be integral to moving healthcare from its siloed and mechanistic structures to more dynamic, integrated, relational, and value-driven structures that can meet the needs of patients and providers today and in the future (Weberg & Davidson, 2017). Forming productive and efficient teams requires a knowledge base, interprofessional leadership, the use of best practices, and individuals who are well prepared to be collaborative and effective members of the team (Meleis, 2018).

The complex nature of our ever-changing healthcare environment necessitates interprofessional leadership skills as only one set of competencies that nurses and members of other health professions require (Stiles et al., 2014,). A study to investigate attributes of nursing leaders during a time of great organizational upheaval repeatedly mentioned six traits: being an optimistic visionary, having a moral center, being able to manage crisis with knowledge expertise, having a personal connection with nurses and participating in teamwork and communication, facilitating professional growth, and empowering others (Anonson, as cited in Anonson et al., 2009, pp. 19–20). It is hard to argue against the enduring timeliness and relevancy of these traits.

Nurses must embrace interprofessionalism for it to become a core competency of nursing practice, actively exchanging ideas about interprofessionalism and addressing any unwillingness to do so (Sommerfeldt, 2013, p. 522). Sommerfeldt further suggests that reluctance to these conversations places nurses at risk of losing decision-making influence in interprofessional healthcare reform, and in areas where nurse leaders model engagement by articulating the nursing perspective on the local and global stage. Leaders of innovation and change must habituate to new ways of being and doing (Weberg & Davidson, 2017). Leadership in the interprofessional space requires both the designated leader and others to be willing to share the responsibility of leadership and to be cognizant of group dynamics to work with widely diverse skills, values, and interests (Lee, as cited in Weiss et al., 2018, e-279). Designated leaders must also simultaneously assume responsibility for drawing out the leadership ability of other members by modeling these behaviors (Weiss et al., 2018, e-273). An emergent conceptualization of the competencies essential for nurses to lead interprofessionally includes the elements in figure 6-1.

Invests as a collaborative partner in achieving outcomes of value for patients, families, and the community

Draws out the leadership ability (values, intention, and vision) of all team members by modeling

Accepts the responsibility for actively contributing to relationship-centered, safe, effective, and quality health services

Champions negotiating through diverse disciplinary perspectives to achieve optimal patient outcomes

Communicates one's own disciplinary knowledge and roles to others in interprofessional interactions

Conveys a strong team orientation and the knowledge, skills, and attitudes that enable teams to be productive yet efficient and innovative

Influences and shapes team-based healthcare delivery with a respect and trustworthiness that considers context, setting, and disciplinary expertise

Leading Interprofessionally

Strives to arrive at common ground through deliberate actions and a high level of self, team and organizational awareness

Brings dual passions to the table—passion for one's own profession and passion for the intent of the team's work

Surpasses one's own disciplinary outlook to appreciate diverse perspectives and develop new mindsets

Examines one's approach to work and worldview by joining with others from different backgrounds and expertise

Focuses on the dynamic relationships between leadership values, culture, capabilities, and the organizational context

Lays a foundation for collaboration aimed at keeping patients safe, optimizing patient outcomes, enhancing quality, and containing or reducing costs

Engages with others with the eagerness and openness required to fully appreciate what others do and how others think

FIGURE 6–1.   Leading interprofessionally: essential competencies (© 2017 Karen J. Saewert, all rights reserved. Used with permission.)

Leading Interprofessionally: Strategies

> ### STRATEGIES FOR LEADING INTERPROFESSIONALLY
>
> *I work very hard to stay up on and understand system issues, opportunities, and potential barriers. It's impossible to work in the interprofessional space without an appreciation for and ability to demonstrate understanding of context and the factors that influence our ability to provide outstanding healthcare and enable all members of the team, including nurses, to practice to their highest level.*
>
> —*Gerri Lamb, PhD, RN, FAAN (2017)*

> ### STRATEGIES FOR LEADING INTERPROFESSIONALLY
>
> *You must be able to realistically evaluate when your profession's expertise is essential and when alternatives may be needed or possible.*
>
> —*Gerri Lamb, PhD, RN, FAAN (2017)*

What does leading interprofessionally involve? What strategies should you consider? There are abundant strategies proposed in the literature. That said, consider the importance of carefully aligning planned interventions with desired outcomes. While we may arrive at preferred outcomes through unforeseen and serendipitous means, it is the intentionality of our efforts to lead interprofessionally that is key. To offer greater visibility and justice to the work of the many, table 6-1 outlines suggested strategies that cover a wide range of approaches and considerations for leading interprofessionally. The table includes a source-retrieval crosswalk to aid in a personal examination of the literature.

TABLE 6-1.   Table 6-1. Suggested strategies for leading interprofessionally: source-retrieval crosswalk

Suggested Strategy	Source
Draw out the leadership ability of all team members by modeling. An interprofessional healthcare team can reach its full potential when each member assumes a leadership stance, recognizes the power of their unique professional expertise and personal qualities, and accepts the responsibility of actively contributing to relationship-centered, safe, effective, and quality health services.	Weiss, Tilin, & Morgan, 2018, e-273
Share the responsibility of team leadership. Be cognizant of group dynamics to work with widely diverse skills, values, and interests.	Lee, as cited in Weiss et al., 2018, e-279
Influence the development of new interprofessional education programs while enhancing the profile of nursing and strengthening current and future leadership capacity.	Hoffart, Brown, & Farrell, 2015, p. 375
Role mode a vision of change and challenge resistance, respectfully communicate and collaborate, and actively contribute to efforts to include interprofessional initiatives in the learning experiences of students and practitioners of all health professions.	Hoffart et al., 2015, p. 387
Be self-aware, self-regulating, and attuned to the diverse perspectives, needs, and abilities of one's following and to the requirements of the situation. Develop social and emotional intelligence, hone the ability to develop and maintain reciprocal relationships, exhibit willingness to empower others, and employ a balance of task-related and relationship-building behaviors.	Weiss et al., 2018, e-1891
Display an allegiance to group goals that supersedes personal goals. Develop a strong orientation toward others.	Weiss et al., 2018, e-2942–e-2943
Engage with others in mutual respect and commitment to team goals. Make optimum functioning the norm and make reflection an impetus for and result of learning.	Weiss et al., 2018, e-2884
Adjust to accommodate the views of others and negotiate disciplinary perspectives making all perspectives legitimate and meaningful to the progress of the patient. Institutional excellence and effective leadership of interprofessional teams depends on the integration of various points of view.	Weiss et al., 2018, e-3000
Practice interprofessional curiosity, active listening, and principled negotiation techniques.	Weiss et al., 2018, e-3000
Recognize that becoming an interprofessional leader is a process that may vary from that of becoming a leader within a profession and that it takes time and calls for self-reflection, deliberate actions, and a new mindset.	Stiles, Horton-Deutsch, & Andrews, 2014, pp. 488–489
Seek opportunities to join with others from different backgrounds and expertise to engage in self-examination of one's work and worldview.	Stiles et al., 2014, p. 489

Suggested Strategy	Source
Be mindful of the perspective one brings personally and professionally. Develop a keen sense of self and how one engages with others.	Stiles et al., 2014, p. 489
Engage others openly and with an appreciation for how they think.	Stiles et al., 2014, p. 489.
Bring one's passions to the table—passion for one's own profession and passion for the intent of the team's work. Effective interprofessional leaders work toward goals beyond the purview of any one profession.	Stiles et al., 2014, p. 489.
Design novel approaches to teaching and learning to move interprofessional education forward.	Hoffart et al., 2015, pp. 376–377
Exercise readiness to be flexible and adapt. Anticipate that leadership may change in settings where people work together interprofessionally as the service user's needs change.	Hammick, Freeth, Cooperman, & Goodsman, 2009, p. 54
Be action oriented and push forward remembering that change can be good.	Hoying, 2017, p. 175
Tap into abilities other than pure operational leadership behaviors to view and translate complex systems to better understand and enable nonlinear work flows.	Soriano & Weberg, 2017, p. 146
Unlearn in order to learn. Part of the learning process is unlearning, which involves letting go of old knowledge or old ways of doing business. The inability to unlearn can be detrimental to moving forward.	Hoying, 2017, p. 176
Listen with the intent to understand. This involves being curious and asking questions to gain additional perspectives while also creating connections and building relationships.	Stiles et al., 2013, p. 490
Foster a culture of openness to new ideas, a willingness to take risks, and other forms of breakthrough thinking and doing.	Hoying, 2017, p. 175
Link together shared leadership attitudes and practices in healthcare to emphasize the importance of promoting a strong team identity in interprofessional teams.	Forsyth & Mason, 2017, p. 297
Evolve one's communication skills to meet the intrinsically complex needs of interprofessional work. Learn to attend to others in particular ways.	Stiles et al., 2013, p. 489
Practice, practice, practice. Approach collaboration as a skill that does not necessarily come naturally but is learned and can be mastered with practice.	Stiles et al., 2013, p. 489
Promote strong team identification to encourage favorable attitudes to shared leadership.	Forsyth & Mason, 2017, p. 297
Get comfortable in navigating through uncertainty and complexity. Complex systems require problem solving and cooperative and collaborative interprofessional work in unclear or uncertain situations.	Kinnaman & Bleich, as cited in Stiles et al., 2014, p. 491

Thought Exercise

Examine the *Core Competencies for Interprofessional Practice: 2016 Update* (available at the link provided below). Once familiarized, list additional leadership competencies—aligned with one or more Interprofessional Education Collaborative core competencies—that you consider essential additions to this chapter's discussion. Consider inviting colleagues to the table of this conversation.

	Values/ Ethics for Interprofessional Practice	Roles/ Responsibilities	Interprofessional Communication	Teams and Teamwork
Core Competencies for Interprofessional Practice	Work with individuals of other professions to maintain a climate of mutual respect and shared values.	Use the knowledge of one's own role and that of other professions to appropriately assess and address the healthcare needs of patients and to promote and advance the health of populations.	Communicate with patients, families, communities, and professions in health and other fields in a responsive and responsible manner that supports a team approach to the promotion and maintenance of health and the prevention and treatment of disease.	Apply relationship-building values and principles of team dynamics to perform effectively in different team roles to plan, deliver, and evaluate patient- and population-centered care and population health programs and policies that are safe, timely, efficient, effective, and equitable.
Leadership Competencies				

Interprofessional Education Collaborative. (2016). *Core competencies for interprofessional practice: 2016 update*. Washington, DC: Author. Retrieved July 15, 2017, from http://www.aacn.nche.edu/education-resources/IPEC-2016-Updated-Core-Competencies-Report.pdf

Summary

CORE MESSAGE

For nurses, becoming leaders in interprofessional practice, education, and research is central to advancing the profession of nursing and to achieving the shared goals of all professions in healthcare, namely to improve health and healthcare outcomes.

—Gerri Lamb, PhD, RN, FAAN (2017)

So why should you care? What difference does this make to you? It has often been said that we all have a role to lead from wherever we stand. We all have influence, whether it be for the good or not so good. To be in this leadership role and say that you are going to keep the status quo is an abdication of the responsibility (Nelson, Tasson, & Hodges, 2014, p. 55) to dig deep with the courage and vulnerability needed to bring about system changes. Inarguably, we face complex issues in healthcare that are far reaching. The interprofessional leadership knowledge, skills, and values discussed in this chapter—and likely more—are essential to addressing these issues and warrant a high level of tenacity. Now is yet another time to bolster our determination as nurses and leaders in nursing to visibly lead interprofessionally in the increasingly interprofessional healthcare domain. The time and needs associated with leading interprofessionally wait for no one.

Communicating nursing knowledge and roles to others in interprofessional interactions is a nursing competency as well as an interprofessional one that requires the intentional attentiveness of nurses, nurse leaders, and nurse educators (Sommerfeldt, 2013, p. 519). A lack of theoretical frameworks suggests that leadership in interprofessional education and collaborative practice is undertheorized and undertested. This limits our understanding of leadership within the interprofessional context and makes it difficult to evaluate or share effective leadership practices (Brewer et al., 2016, p. 413).

Many theories, cases, and models have influenced current leadership strategies that can be applied to healthcare settings and can guide effective leadership focused on the dynamic relationships between leadership values, culture, capabilities, and the organizational context of a leader's developmental journey (Al-Sawai, 2013, p. 287). There is also great synergy between education in interprofessional and healthcare innovation; the knowledge, skills, and attitudes that enable innovative teams are also the foundation of high-functioning collaborative teams (Davidson, 2017, p. 449).

Cultivating an identity as a nurse and nurse leader that includes interprofessionalism requires intentionally learning, developing skills, and nurturing beliefs and attitudes that will allow you as a nurse to invest yourself as a collaborative partner in optimizing valuable outcomes for patients, families, communities, and populations. Fully partnering with other members of healthcare professions in redesigning healthcare in the United States and in global settings requires visionary interprofessional leadership (Nicholas & Breakey, 2015, p. 19).

Chapter Key Points

- For any of this to happen, conversations need to take place and actions taken.

- The hard work of thinking and doing differently has to be envisioned, tested, evaluated, re-envisioned, re-tested, and re-evaluated until we get it right.

- Greater transparency about how interprofessional leadership is conceptualized and theorized will advance rigorous development and testing of new and effective leadership models for the varied contexts in which interprofessional practice and education occur.

- It is never too late to become a better version of ourselves as nurses and exercise a deserved place in partnerships and in leading interprofessionally.

References

Al-Sawai, A. (2013). Leadership of healthcare professionals: Where do we stand? *Oman Medical Journal, 28*(4), 285–87. DOI: 10.5001/omj.2013.79

Anonson, J. M. S., Ferguson, L., MacDonald, M. B., Murray, B. L., Fowler-Kerry, S., & Bally, M. G. (2009). The anatomy of interprofessional leadership: An investigation of leadership behaviors in team-based health care. *Journal of Leadership Studies, 3*(3), 17–25. DOI: 10.1002/jls.20120

Arndt, J., King, S., Suter, E., Mazonde, J., Taylor, E., & Arthur, N. (2009). Socialization in health education: Encouraging an integrated interprofessional socialization process. *Journal of Allied Health, 38*(1), 18–23.

Brewer, M. L., Flavell, H. L., Trede, R., & Smith, M. (2016). A scoping review to understand "leadership" in interprofessional education and practice. *Journal of Interprofessional Care, 30*(4), 408–15. DOI: 10.3109/13561820.2016.1150260

Clark, P. N. & Hassmiller, S. (2013). Nursing leadership: Interprofessional education and practice. *Nursing Science Quarterly, 26*(4), 333–36. DOI: 10.1177/0894318413500313

Davidson, S. (2016). Leading innovation: The beginner's mind and mindful beginnings. *Nurse Leader, 14*(2), 96–97. DOI: 10.1016/j.mnl.2015.12.009

Davidson, S. (2017). Evidence-based education for healthcare innovation. In S. Davidson, D. Weberg, T. Porter-O'Grady, & K. Malloch (Eds.), *Leadership for evidence-based innovation in nursing and health professions* (pp. 441–73). Burlington, MA: Jones & Bartlett Learning.

Forsyth, C. & Mason, B. (2017). Shared leadership and group identification in healthcare: The leadership beliefs of clinicians working in interprofessional teams. *Journal of Interprofessional Care, 31*(3), 291–99. DOI: 10.1080/13561820.2017.1280005

Hammick, M., Freeth, D., Copperman, J., & Goodsman, D. (2009). *Being interprofessional*. Malden, MA: Polity Press.

Hoffart, N., Brown, E. J., & Farrell, S. E. (2015). Nursing leadership in interprofessional education. In S. Breakey, I. B. Corless, N. L. Meedzan, & P. K. Nicholas (Eds.), *Global health nursing in the 21st century* (pp. 375–89). New York, NY: Springer.

Hoying, C. (2017). Creating a business case for innovation. In S. Davidson, D. Weberg, T. Porter-O'Grady, & K. Malloch (Eds.), *Leadership for evidence-based innovation in nursing and health professions* (pp. 173–215). Burlington, MA: Jones & Bartlett Learning.

Kinnaman, M. L. & Bleich, M. R. (2004). Collaboration: Aligning resources to create and sustain partnerships. *Journal of Professional Nursing, 20*(5), 310–22. DOI: 10.1016/j. profnur.2004.07.009

Meleis, A. (2018). Preface. In *The interprofessional health care team: Leadership and development* (2nd ed., e-139–e-165). Burlington, MA: Jones & Bartlett Learning.

Moss, E., Seifert, P. C., & O'Sullivan, A. (2016). Registered nurses as interprofessional collaborative partners: Creating value-based outcomes. *Online Journal of Issues in Nursing, 21*(3). DOI: 10.3912/OJIN. Vol21No03Man04

Nelson, S., Tassone, M., & Hodges, B. D. (2014). *Creating the health care team of the future: The Toronto model for interprofessional education and practice*. Ithaca, NY: Cornell University Press.

Nicholas, P. K. & Breakey, S. (2015). Global health and global nursing. In S. Breakey, I. B. Corless, N. L. Meedzan, & P. K. Nicholas (Eds.), *Global health nursing in the 21st century* (pp. 3–24). New York, NY: Springer.

Pollard, K. C., Ross, K., & Means, R. (2005). Nurse leadership, interprofessionalism and the modernization agenda. *British Journal of Nursing, 14*(6), 339–44.

Rutherford-Hemming, T. & Lioce, L. (2018). State of interprofessional education in nursing: A systematic review. *Nurse Educator, 43*(1), 9–13.

Saewert, K. J. (2017). Beyond professional socialization. In E. E. Friberg & J. L. Creasia (Eds.), *Conceptual foundations: The bridge to professional nursing practice* (6th ed., pp. 38–43). St. Louis, MO: Mosby.

Soriano, R., & Weberg, D. (2017). Incorporating new evidence from big data, emerging technology, and disruptive practices into your innovation ecosystem. In S. Davidson, D. Weberg, T. Porter-O'Grady & K. Malloch (Eds.),*Leadership for evidence-based innovation in nursing and health professions* (pp. 145–71). Burlington, MA: Jones & Bartlett Learning.

Sommerfeldt, S. C. (2013). Articulating nursing in an interprofessional world. *Nurse Education in Practice*, *13*(6), 519–23. DOI: 10.1016/j. nepr.2013.02.014

Stiles, K. A., Horton-Deutsch, S. L., & Andrews, C. A. (2014). The nurse's lived experience of becoming an interprofessional leader. *The Journal of Continuing Education in Nursing*, *45*(11), 487–93. DOI: 10.3928/00220124-20141023-03

Weberg, D. & Davidson, S. (2017). Moving to the future of evidence, innovation, and leadership in health care. In S. Davidson, D. Weberg, T. Porter-O'Grady, & K. Malloch (Eds.), *Leadership for evidence-based innovation in nursing and health professions* (pp. 173–215). Burlington, MA: Jones & Bartlett Learning.

Weiss, D., Tilin, F., & Morgan, M. (2018). *The Interprofessional health care team: Leadership and development* (2nd ed.). Burlington, MA: Jones & Bartlett Learning.

Additional Resources

American Association of Colleges of Nursing. (2006). *The essentials of doctoral education for advanced nursing practice*. Washington, DC: Author. Retrieved from http://www.aacnnursing. org/Education-Resources/ AACN-Essentials

American Association of Colleges of Nursing. (2008). *The essentials of baccalaureate education for professional nursing practice*. Washington, DC: Author. Retrieved from http://www.aacnnursing. org/Education-Resources/ AACN-Essentials

American Association of Colleges of Nursing. (2011). *The essentials of master's education in nursing*. Washington, DC: Author. Retrieved from http://www.aacnnursing. org/Education-Resources/ AACN-Essentials

American Association of Colleges of Nursing. (2013). *Standards for accreditation of baccalaureate and graduate nursing programs*. Washington, DC: Author. Retrieved from http://www.aacnnursing. org/CCNE-Accreditation/ Resource-Documents/ CCNE-Standards-Professional -Nursing-Guidelines

Commission for Nursing Education Accreditation. (2016). *Accreditation standards for nursing education programs*. Washington, DC: National League for Nursing. Retrieved from http://www. nln.org/docs/default-source/ accreditation-services/ cnea-standards-final-february- 201613f2bf5c78366c7 09642ff00005f0421.pdf

Interprofessional Education
Collaborative. (2016). *Core
competencies for interprofessional
practice: 2016 update.* Washington,
DC: Author. Retrieved July 15,
2017, from http://www.aacn.
nche.edu/education-resources/
IPEC-2016-Updated-Core
-Competencies-Report.pdf

Mitchell, P., Wynia, M., Golden, R.,
McNellis, B., Okun, S., Webb, C.
E., . . . & Von Kohorn, I. (2012).
*Core principles & values of effective
team-based health care* [discussion
paper]. Retrieved from National
Academy of Medicine: https://nam.
edu/perspectives-2012-core
-principles-values-of-effective
-team-based-health-care/

Chapter 7

Leading in Informatics: Through the System Development Life Cycle

Jane Carrington, PhD, RN, FAAN

The Health Information Technology for Economic and Clinical Health (HITECH) Act of 2009 was the stimulus for some organizations to implement electronic health records (EHRs). Organizations that had already implemented EHRs used the criteria of the act and its concept of meaningful use to evaluate and extend their use of EHRs. Along with the advancement of health technology, the HITECH Act and the concept of meaningful use inadvertently challenged nursing leaders in healthcare organizations to examine their current roles and determine what changes would be required in light of EHR implementation and our new data-guided healthcare system. The role of chief nursing officer (CNO) had been established, and the role chief nursing informatics officer (CNIO) then emerged.

Change is a constant in organizations and it reveals the need to evaluate the system and the leaders within. Nursing leadership is not exempt from this exercise. A few myths have emerged since the HITECH Act: First, with a CNIO in place, the CNO does not have to know or deal with technology. Second, with EHRs successfully implemented, an organization no longer needs the CNIO. This chapter seeks to dispel these myths and offers suggestions as to how the CNO and CNIO along with unit-level nursing leaders can effectively work together using technology and the data it captures to guide nursing care toward better patient outcomes.

The systems development life cycle (SDLC) is used to achieve the goals of this chapter. The SDLC assists healthcare organizations in sustaining the health of their technology. The phases of the cycle are plan, analyze, design, implement, and maintain. Between each phase is the very important phase of evaluation. In the early years of technology implementation in healthcare organization, the philosophy was generally that the information systems department would select a vendor, compile a proposal, obtain agreement from the organization's administration, and go forward. Since then the technology has grown more sophisticated, from partial clinical systems (order-entry software separated from the clinical health-record system, for example) to complex, system-wide software solutions. These systems help guide, record, and evaluate patient care, while the data within the systems aid in broader analysis of a healthcare organization. Complex technologies within complex healthcare organizations can no longer be relegated to one department for decision-making through the SDLC, but rather the CNIO, CNO, and nursing management leaders together are essential for the success of the planning, analysis, decision, implementation, and maintenance of healthcare technologies.

Nursing Leadership in Healthcare Organizations

Nursing leadership within healthcare organizations has become better understood in the last decade due to the work of nursing systems and organization scientists. Because of the changes in healthcare, issues in reimbursement, and overall state of our nation's health, nursing leadership within healthcare organizations is critical to maintaining organizational stability.

The role of CNO evolved from the title of director of nursing and symbolically moved nurse leaders to executives in healthcare organizations. The CNO represents the nurses of an organization for the governing body or board of directors during key meetings within the organization. Here the CNO keeps the team apprised of the nursing work done in the organization. The CNO develops and communicates the vision and direction of nursing within the organization, keeping with national trends and consistent with best evidence. The CNO sustains the philosophy of the nursing governance, which gives a voice to the bedside nurses and those in other departments and roles. In collaboration with nurse managers, the CNO establishes goals and patient outcome targets. These role components and more are directly linked to the organizational goal of providing consistent quality care to patients.

The role of CNIO has evolved from the very early reckoning of technology in healthcare. These nurses were originally within the information systems department and served as analysts, connecting nurses, physicians, and administrators to the hardware and software of organization. With the HITECH Act of 2009, these nurses then became leaders in nursing informatics and from here the role of the CNIO emerged. The CNIO is responsible for integrating nursing science with computer science, information management, and analytical science to manage data, thus developing information and wisdom in nursing practice. The CNIO connects the technology and nurse workflows and also brings a vision to the organization involving technology, data, and nursing.

Nurse managers are responsible for the shift-to-shift and day-to-day operations on a nursing unit. These leaders ensure that nurses can perform their roles and that immediate patient issues are addressed. These leaders often emerge from the nursing staff, first serving as shift leaders and then becoming nurse managers. They link the nursing staff to the senior leadership and CNO. They also provide insights about workflow and technology to the CNIO.

These nurse leaders work together to identify system problems and solutions. Each brings specific contributions to the SDLC, and in the maintenance phase of the cycle these nurse leaders collaborate in decision-making to ensure the stability of the technology and organization.

Nursing Leadership and the Systems Development Life Cycle

The SDLC is a framework that guides the process of approaching a problem, seeking a solution, implementing that solution, and determining its success for an organization. In this chapter the SDLC demonstrates the collaboration between nurse leaders in a healthcare organization. As mentioned above, the SDLC consists of five phases: plan, analyze, design, implement, and maintain. Evaluation is often omitted from the model; however, this is an essential phase between each of the five others. The following describes each phase with detail and examples of the roles for nursing leadership—CNO, CNIO, and nurse manager.

Plan

The first phase is to plan. The goal of this phase is to determine the goals of the organization along with the problems the organization seeks to resolve, the possible solutions, and alternatives. A healthcare organization's administrative leaders review priorities and federal mandates for technologies and also threats to reimbursement. Important factors guiding this phase are budget constraints for the project, requirements within the plan to achieve the goals, the benefit of the solution to the organization, and the timeline with specific detail for each phase of the life cycle. In this stage the team develops and reviews a proposal including the specific goals for the organization and the timeframe, budget, and resources necessary to achieve the goals.

The CNO approaches this phase with a keen understanding of the patient care issues and any problems with desired outcome measures. The CNO also has an aggregated perspective of the staff nurses and nurse managers toward solving the problem and achieving the organizational goals. The CNIO approaches this phase with knowledge of the organization's technologies (hardware and software) and its data flow. The CNIO also has an idea of what new technologies or upgrades would help solve the problem as well as the data elements to extract from the database and methods of analysis for outcome measures.

Analyze

Next, organizational leaders complete a full analysis of the system including workflow, hardware, and software. The CNO leads the analysis of workflow including staff requirements, current admission and length-of-stay data, and so forth. The CNIO leads the analysis of work and technology or the software used to complete tasks and work. The CNIO knows the status of all software (contract dates and software upgrades, for example) and hardware (computers and servers, for example) that nurses use to complete tasks and work. The nurse managers contribute to the analysis with patient-level information about the problem and potential solutions.

The analysis should include a detailed understanding of current workflow for all tasks, from admission to discharge, in all nursing units. This includes processes from the time of order entry to achieving the results. Identify issues and items that work well. This process should reveal all aspects of the problem and may expose other issues that require a solution.

This is also a good time to update spreadsheets that contain the list of equipment including computers, cables, physical servers, and cloud servers. Itemize computers and list their memory and processing power. Assess physical servers for age, memory load, power, and documented downtime and service costs. Follow each cable in the network and verify upload and download speeds for digital imaging and other messages. Analyze each piece of software for the date it went live and the date that the vendor will no longer support it, and review current contracts including time frames, costs to be paid, and usability such as frequency of support calls. This updated information will assist in guiding the team toward the solution.

Design

During the design phase, the team develops and tests the solution. Building on the planning and analysis stages, here the CNO and nurse managers discuss the desired features of systems to address the problem, including specifics like screen layout, guiding rules of code for usability, potential codes, and system structure, for example. The CNIO understands the performance of the hardware and software for the intended solution, collects the desired functionality from the CNO and nurse leaders, and works with the programmers, vendor, and support staff to develop the technology solution to the problem.

Development during this phase of design is important and requires models and point-by-point discussions with all team members. During development, programmers develop code and designers engineer usable technology to meet the needs of the organization and solve the problem. This is when the input from nursing leaders (CNO, CNIO, and nurse manager) becomes part of the solution and helps meet the goals of the organization.

The CNIO may oversee the design phase and ensure that it is completed from two key directions: from the foreground and user to the technology and from technology to the user and to the background. From the foreground to user encompasses the organization as a system to the user and includes such items as policies and procedures, identified tasks and work, established plans for if-then cases, links from one department to the next for each task and work, interconnections between each user on a unit or department, and the connection to the patient. From the user to the background consists of all elements that exist behind the scenes and are essential for all hardware and software to function without issues to the user. The point at which these two directions of design meet is the user–technology interface and is well known as the key for human factors, or how people interact with technology. Design guided around these principles is associated with increased usability of the technology and improved patient outcomes.

Again, the CNIO may oversee the process of testing the solution. Software is generally tested in a test environment or simulated from the live environment. Constructing the layout of the design is followed by developing the test build. Here the components from design are built for testing. Developers test each facet of the design, looking for problems to be addressed and determining what actions break the system (causing malfunction or frozen screens, a missing step in workflow, and so forth). The philosophy is "better to break here than with an actual patient." This phase exposes design flaws in the technology and the organization and provides time to repair or modify the design.

Testing requires detail in planning, execution, and documentation; nothing should be taken for granted. Here, the plan for testing is laid out and the entire process is communicated to all involved. Each item is tested as planned and the process and outcomes are documented along with plans to address flaws. Design flaws can rarely be isolated to one component. Most flaws link to other elements of the system somewhat like the domino theory, one after the other having an impact from the one before.

Throughout the processes of designing and testing, the CNIO, CNO, and nurse leaders meet routinely to ensure that all features of design recommended by the CNO and nurse managers have been considered and all scenarios have been tested and outcomes documented. The CNIO, CNO, and nurse managers must agree on the design prior to moving to the next phase.

Following the testing of all systems, redesign of necessary facets, testing of the redesign, and finally reaching agreement that systems function as designed and support workflow, the organization then moves to implementation.

Implementation

The implementation phase includes teaching the end users to use the system and the new workflow, communicating key dates, and developing the process for feedback. The CNIO, CNO, and nurse managers work together to determine the schedule for training end users to use the new technology and the new workflow.

Teaching the end users to use the system has consistently been the weakest link in implementation. Include in the official training process some test cases that have the end users trial each part of the technology. Attempt to include all possible tasks and work that will be completed using this new technology, and allow extra time for end users who need it. This is a critical stage toward adoption of the technology.

Along with learning the new technology, end users also need to understand the new workflow. Here end users learn how they previously completed the task and work and then learn the new workflow. This phase of teaching can go along with the simulated training using the new technology and other mechanisms.

A small group of end users will emerge as early adopters of the technology and will in short order grasp how to use the new system and gain confidence in their ability to support other end users. A larger group of end users will emerge as willing to adopt the technology but will require additional time to learn the system and fully adopt the technology into their workflow. The last group of end users is about the size of the first and will resist education and adoption. CNOs and nurse managers should anticipate these end users and plan accordingly. For example, have the early adopters assist in end user support on the nursing units. Consider pairing the early adopters with the laggards or resisters to lower the barriers and educate them to use the system.

Communicating the key dates—agreed upon by the CNIO, CNO, and nurse managers—and the implementation plan to the end users and organization is critical. Key dates include training, dates the technology goes live for unit or department, and dates of switching from one system to the next (from one EHR vendor to another, for example). These dates can be adjusted with effective communication; however, changes should be based on real issues in order to not lose the confidence of the end users.

End user feedback from learning the system is critical. Listening to the end users bolsters their buy-in, and they provide a perspective from the front lines of using the technology that testing and simulation may not have duplicated. A situation may emerge that was not considered in testing, and system flaws may not be detected without feedback from the end users.

Implementation also involves generating reports and data to evaluate the organization and processes as requested by the CNO and nurse manager and recommended by the CNIO. Each administrator can view the data and determine how well the processes function. Administrators can also extract data to assist in evaluating outcomes and should be educated to the full use of the system, data flow within the system, and reporting functions.

The CNIO should highly recommend that the CNO and nurse managers attend the training for the new system and workflow. Each should become knowledgeable of the system.

Maintenance

The system moves to maintenance a few weeks or a month after implementation. This phase is identified by the reduction in support calls from the end users, reduction in calls for support from the vendor, and cessation of unanticipated system issues. Here the new workflow becomes the new normal and is set for adoption by the organization. The goal of this stage is to sustain elements of the system and work with the vendor to keep the system functioning as designed. Here is where the organization communicates with the vendor for anticipation of upgrades and sunset dates, or when the vendor will no longer provide support for the software. It also deals with unexpected issues with technology, downtime, and so forth.

It is at this stage that the team could falsely think the work is done. Implementation of technologies and changes in workflow can raise new questions about outcomes, organizational measures, and direction for new technologies. Here the relationship between the CNIO and CNO is critical to continuously evaluating organizational goals, workflow, systems, and technology.

It is also during this phase that vendors provide system updates that could require the team to reevaluate and start at the beginning of the SDLC. Unfortunately even with the best and detailed planning, hardware fails, software crashes, and server solutions can be problematic. Many would refer to this phase as crucial to sustaining an organization's enterprise. The CNIO is critical to understanding the issues, communicating them to the CNO and nurse leaders, and developing a plan to avoid threats to patient safety.

There are two important points about this phase of the SDLC: First, this is the phase when all other technologies and prior solutions work together toward organization goals. The organization is continuing with the entire enterprise while sustaining itself with the most recent solution. Both static and chaotic organizations will experience new problems and establish new goals. Second, an organization can experience multiple SDLCs at once when there are multiple problems. One solution may be in maintenance and another in planning or analysis, for example, at the same time. Naturally, there are solutions in SDLC that are deemed minor when compared to others. An organization determines the schedule based on the critical nature of the problem, resources, and cost.

Evaluation

Evaluation is the last part of each of the phases of the life cycle. During this process, each element of the phase is reviewed and ideally determined to be satisfactory and ready to progress. If a phase is reviewed and deemed unsatisfactory or incomplete, then it continues or is repeated. Communication between the CNIO, CNO, and nurse managers should establish measures to determine success at one phase to move to the next.

Chief Nursing Information Officer, Chief Nursing Officer, and Nurse Manager

Throughout the SDLC, the success of each phase and evaluation relies on the relationship between the CNIO, CNO, and organizational nurse managers. This group of nurses is well positioned to work together because each understands nursing, nursing care, nursing workflow, and how technology supports nurses. Each adds a unique perspective to the team. The CNIO is the expert of current technology in the organization, the technology available and in development, federal regulations influencing the use of technology, data analysis, and nursing informatics research toward increasing our understanding of how nurses use technology. The CNO has expertise in organizational health and national trends in nursing and also an understanding of the organizational goals both short and long term. Nurse managers are experts in the day-to-day operations of care delivery, are charged with sustaining organizational health, and are first in line to the nurses who are providing care. Together these nurse leaders can uniquely contribute to the SDLC for the organization.

The goal of this chapter is to dispel two myths about nurse leaders within healthcare organizations: First, with a CNIO in place, the CNO does not have to know or deal with the technology. Second, with EHRs successfully implemented, an organization no longer needs the CNIO.

It is not uncommon for nurse leaders to say, "I have a CNIO; I don't need to know the technology" or "I don't have time to know the technology." The role of the CNO, as mentioned above, includes understanding nurses and their workflow. At a micro level, CNOs need to understand EHRs and other technologies involved in patient care to effectively address technology–nurse mismatches including issues with the user–technology interface. No, the CNO is not directly entering data in an EHR, for example, but the CNO must understand how their nurses are using technology to anticipate and address issues.

The second myth manifests in conversation with phrases like "we have our EHR implemented, so we don't need the CNIO and nurse informaticists." The role of the CNIO and the informatics team is enormous with technology and care. These nurses strive to effectively work with nurses to understand features and functions of technology to enhance workflow. These nurses also have significant contributions to the SDLC. Having nurses with expertise in informatics is a strength for organizations, with the possibility of multiple SDLCs ongoing and overlapping and with the ongoing work during maintenance and beyond. Led by the CNIO, this team works to convert the collected data from all technologies within the organization into information and wisdom to guide practice.

In addition, the CNIO is a representative at national meetings and conferences to advocate for the organization and learn how others are coping with problems and solutions. This information strengthens an organization's ongoing SDLC efforts.

Effective Collaboration

If the CNO is encouraged to understand the technology and workflow and the CNIO is supporting technology to enhance nurse workflow, how do these nurse leaders work together without stepping on each other's toes? The roles of the CNO and CNIO are not mutually exclusive. Each shares in domains of technology and patient care; however, their perspectives and approaches differ.

The CNO's perspective is largely focused on nursing and delivery of care, and therefore the CNO supports nurses and those involved in patient care. The CNO can demonstrate support by attending a technology-education session prior to implementation to learn the system and then attending other sessions to be visible to the nursing staff, working with nurse managers to staff beyond typical constraints during the implementation, and being visible on nursing units, seeking nurses' perspectives and providing encouragement during the SDLC.

Along with the CNO, the CNIO should be equally visible on nursing units to learn the perspectives of nurses before and during the SDLC for each problem. CNIOs can also attend training sessions, demonstrating support for the trainees. CNIOs should also be visible on nursing units throughout the SDLC and especially when the new technology goes live, providing support. The CNO and CNIO should meet regularly to land and remain on the same page for the organization.

There is overlap here with the CNO and CNIO, demonstrating again the mutual work of these two nurse leaders. Nurse managers can be effective by working with both administrative nurse leaders to assist the nursing staff during the phases of the SDLC. Transparency leads to greater trust and confidence from problem to maintenance.

Summary

This chapter seeks to dispel two myths in nursing leadership. The first myth is that the CNO does not have to know or deal with technology. However, healthcare is now firmly in the era of data evaluation of care and is entering that of data-driven care. The CNO is now guided by data and data-driven measures to establish goals for the organization and to meet outcome goals. Data comes from an organization's technology, and the value of data is dependent upon how the end users (nurses, for example) enter the data. Therefore, the CNO should be keenly aware of the technologies within the organization, the flow of data, and the methods for evaluating those data to guide decision-making.

The second myth is that with the successful implementation of the EHR or other technology, an organization no longer needs the CNIO. But the CNIO guides an organization in turning data flow into information and knowledge into wisdom for patient outcomes. The CNIO guides a team of nurse informaticists to manage the data flow. This team also works with nurse managers and the CNO to identify problems and sustain solutions through each SDLC. The CNIO is also uniquely positioned to communicate with vendors to negotiate and learn upcoming changes to current systems.

Chapter Key Points

- There are two myths permeating in healthcare organizations: first, the role of the CNO does not include efficiency with technology, and second, with technology in place, the CNIO is no longer essential to an organization.

- Each problem-stimulated SDLC requires both CNO and CNIO to be very involved, and complex and dynamic healthcare organizations often endure multiple SDLCs at one time. The maintenance phase is the time of ongoing organizational stability with the designed technological solution.

- Technology provides data and data guide the organization.

- Technology monitors patient status, stores patient data, interprets data, and reports data so that nurse leaders and administrators can effectively evaluate practice with data by measuring patient outcomes.

- Technology has become ubiquitous in healthcare and society. Therefore, technology is involved in all phases of patient care.

Chapter 8

Purposeful Diversity in Leadership: A Call to Action for All Nurses

Gaurdia Banister, PhD, RN, NEA-BC, FAAN
Melissa Joseph, MSN, RN, NE-BC

If not now, when? If not us, who?

—George Romney ("Nation," 1963)

Organizations and their leaders must be sensitive and aware of their feelings and reactions toward those they perceive to be different. This sensitivity is critical to advancing a workplace that promotes inclusivity and to reducing barriers and obstacles that impede diversity. The website for Queensborough Community College gives the following definition of diversity:

The concept of diversity encompasses acceptance and respect. It means understanding that everyone is unique and recognizing our individual differences. These can be along the dimensions of race, ethnicity, gender, sexual orientation, socio-economic status, age, physical abilities, religious beliefs, political beliefs, or other ideologies. It is the exploration of these differences in a safe, positive, and nurturing environment. It is about understanding each other and moving beyond simple tolerance to embracing and celebrating the rich dimensions of diversity contained within each individual. (Queensborough Community College, n.d.)

The purpose of this chapter is (1) to provide an overview and background of diversity and health disparities; (2) to examine leadership practice at the bedside, middle-management, and executive levels; (3) to showcase leaders through exemplars who have leveraged their sphere of influence both personally and professionally to drive successful clinical and organizational outcomes, to create change, and to establish a legacy for the future; and (4) to provide a plan of action to advance diversity at all leadership levels.

Background

The composition of the United States population is changing. According to the US Census Bureau, by 2044 more than 50% of Americans will likely belong to a minority group, and by 2060 nearly one in five of the nation's total population is expected to be foreign born (Colby & Ortman, 2015). As the country has become more diverse, so has the patient population in various healthcare settings where nurses practice every day. A natural progression of this change is that the workforce diversity in healthcare would also evolve. And although the workforce is becoming more diverse, more progress is needed as minority nurses are still underrepresented nationwide. Nurses from minority backgrounds represent less than 20% of the registered nurse workforce (Phillips & Malone, 2014).

Achieving racial, ethnic, cultural, and gender diversity is a major priority in healthcare, as it relates to efforts to mirror the workforce to the patient population it serves. According to *The Registered Nurse Population: Findings from the 2008 National Sample Survey of Registered Nurses* report, white women remain overrepresented by comparison to the country's population despite the nursing workforce becoming more diverse. The next largest group of nurses are Asian, Native Hawaiian, and Pacific Islanders followed by non-Hispanic Blacks and then Hispanics and Latinos (U.S. Department of Health and Human Services, 2010). Furthermore, the number of men in nursing, while significantly increasing, lags the general population. Of the 2010 census population, men make up 49.2% of the population (Howden & Meyer, 2011) yet the male workforce among registered nurses is 12% (Hess, 2017). We need a call to action to further diversify the nursing workforce in order to truly reflect the patient population.

The next time you walk into a staff meeting, classroom, patient care unit, or leadership meeting, look around. What do you see? Take inventory of it. As mentioned earlier, there is a mismatch between those who deliver care and those who receive it. This mismatch pushes efforts to improve care and reduce health disparities toward an uncertain outcome. Achieving health equity, eliminating disparities, and improving the health of all people is a priority for the country. The Center for Disease Control and Prevention (CDC) states in its publication *Promoting Health Equity* (Brennan Ramirez, Baker, & Metzler, 2008) that health equity is achieved when every person has the opportunity to "attain his or her full health potential" and no one is "disadvantaged from achieving this potential because of social position or other socially determined circumstances" (p. 6). Health disparities, or inequities, are types of unfair health differences closely linked with social, economic, or environmental disadvantages that adversely affect groups of people (Brennan et al., 2008, p. 5). For example, African American patients who present for healthcare often experience higher rates of complications and mortality than white patients; this disparity is even higher when the hospital they are treated at lacks a diverse workforce (Okafor, Stobaugh, van Ryn, & Talwalkar, 2016). Countless organizations concur with this belief, and health equity is fundamental to the provision of exemplary nursing care.

According to Gallup, in 2016 Americans had ranked nurses as the most trusted profession for 15 years in a row (Norman, 2016). Trust is a value that is sacred in the healthcare profession and can help us forge trusting relationships with our patients. Diversity plays a role in trust. It strengthens access to healthcare for underserved patients, increases racial and ethnic minority patient choice and satisfaction, and ultimately improves the competence of the healthcare workforce to efficiently attend to the needs of all Americans (Health Professionals for Diversity Coalition, n.d.).

It is not only important to increase diversity within the nursing workforce, but it is also imperative to recognize the underrepresentation
of American nurse executives from ethnic or racial minority groups in
nursing-leadership roles. The trends in the United States indicate there
are opportunities to address the lack of diversity in nursing-leadership
roles. According to Fisher (2015), the US trends in hospital and healthcare
leadership reveal that nearly 50% of not-for-profit hospital governing
boards lacked racial and ethnic minorities in 2013 and only 28% of hires
in hospital and health-system C-suites were women in 2014. Advancing
diversity in nursing leadership is essential and can be beneficial to
improving the health of our communities.

Chapters 2 and 6 mention the landmark report that was released by the
Institute of Medicine (IOM) and sponsored by the Robert Wood Johnson
Foundation titled *The Future of Nursing: Leading Change, Advancing
Health*. Recognizing the increasing diversity of the patients needing care
as one factor, the report offered a vision for the future of healthcare and
proposed four key messages for nurses and the nursing field. Nurses
practicing at the full extent of their education and training, achieving
higher levels of education, participating as full partners with other healthcare professionals in redesigning healthcare, and improving systems for
better data collection with the goal of effective workforce planning were
detailed in the report (IOM, 2011). Additionally, the report indicates that
a challenge for nursing is the lack of diversity compared to the general
population and that a more diverse workforce will provide more culturally competent care and better meet the healthcare needs of the increasingly diverse healthcare community (IOM, 2011). Furthermore, the report
goes on to support increasing the diversity of baccalaureate and doctoral
education, which are vital as one progresses into leadership roles.

Delivering quality healthcare is challenging. With advancements in
technology, pressures to reduce costs, hundreds of quality measures,
the demands for innovation, and as outlined in this chapter the increasingly diverse patient population, effective leadership is key. "Complex
environments require that leaders not only know more but that they be
able to change how they think and become more conscious about how
they feel" (Gerardi, 2017, p. 8). As it relates to diversity, "if we all look the
same, we limit our ability to learn about how we can improve the practice
of nursing" (IOM, 2011, p. 1). In an article that asks the question, Does
US healthcare need more diverse leadership? (Henkel, 2016), the author

suggests that diversity strengthens an organization by increasing the richness of ideas that can be used to address and solve challenging problems. His perspective is reinforced by Scott Page, a professor of complex systems, political science, and economics at the University of Michigan who examined the empirical evidence related to diversity and found that "diverse perspectives and tools enable collections of people to find more and better solutions and contribute to overall productivity" (2008, p.13).

Bedside Practice

Diversifying the nursing workforce is a high priority. Nurse leaders are encouraged to learn and understand how to manage a racially and culturally diverse staff. Along with the efforts to diversify the nursing workforce, we should explore the work–life experiences of nurses of diverse backgrounds who work in complex healthcare environments. The day-to-day lived experiences of nurses from different backgrounds involve fitting in, belonging, being accepted, proving oneself, and personal career development (Vikic, Jesty, Matthews, & Etowa, 2011). Other challenges include educating coworkers, directly confronting issues including patient-related experiences such as one's care being refused by a patient, and even being called inappropriate names.

Creating cultural awareness in practice environments is important. It entails creating a space where people feel comfortable speaking up and voicing concerns. Bedside staff nurses can help by creating an environment of acceptance, engagement, and trust. The value of trust remains a common thread through patients, communities, and populations. Bedside staff nurses are confronted with how to best manage situations when faced with prejudicial matters from patients. Lim and Borski (2015, para. 5) offer some options to cope such as "avoid a possible confrontation or ignore the patient's aggression, either verbal or physical or have the patient re-assigned or the nurse request a different assignment," however, nurses should take into consideration how these options influence patient health outcomes and staff job satisfaction.

Nurses working at the bedside provide care for patients from all walks of life. There is an expectation for nurses to deliver culturally competent care. The American Academy of Nursing and the Transcultural Nursing Society (2010) established standards of practice for culturally competent nursing care. The standards are based on the idea that every individual

NURSE LEADER EXEMPLAR

Bedside Registered Nurse

Farah Abellard, MSN, RN, is a clinical nurse of Tower 10BA, an acute care medical unit at Brigham and Women's Hospital. Farah has been in her role as a clinical nurse for six years.

In her early years, Farah knew she wanted to be a nurse. Born in Haiti, raised in the Caribbean nation part of her life, and now living in the United States, she is aware of what life would have been like if she had stayed in Haiti. Farah values diversity. She is proud of her Haitian American heritage. She acknowledges that she doesn't have it easy and that she is in a constant pattern of continuous improvement. Farah also shared that she does not believe that her nursing program adequately emphasized the importance of diversity or that it prepared her to succeed in a racially homogeneous environment as a person of color.

Farah applies the Brigham and Women's Hospital's professional practice model in her practice at the bedside. She believes that advancing diversity should be important to all nurses because we live in a heterogeneous world. Patients are different, and our coworkers come from diverse backgrounds. Farah is intentional about expanding her lens on diversity by traveling, seeing and interacting with different cultures, trying to speak different languages, and listening to her patients and her coworkers. She also engages with her nursing director to understand different perspectives through a nonjudgmental practice.

Receiving mentorship and support from another nurse of a diverse background helped ease her transition from student nurse to nurse clinician. The experience also increased her awareness of diversity. Farah had a preceptor who sat down with her and shared some hard reality–based insights such as, "When you get to the floor, everybody could be going out drinking afterwards, [and] you may or may not get invited to attend. Patients could refuse you because of what you look like." Farah admitted to experiencing this early on. It was particularly trying at the time because as a young person who immigrated from Haiti, "I didn't see color." She also reflected on how her parents didn't raise her "to see color." Farah believes it is important for her to teach others about diversity and inclusivity.

Farah recently conducted some research and presented on the perceptions of diversity and inclusion among the nursing staff at the hospital. The focus of her research was on raising awareness about diversity and inclusivity at the Brigham and Women's hospital. However, she quickly realized that people often didn't want to be confronted with such a topic because it made them feel uncomfortable.

Farah shared an encounter in which a patient verbally expressed refusal to have African Americans or people of color, those from different backgrounds, caring for him. People did not know what to say or how to respond. Farah stands by her belief that patients open up more when people that look like them are taking care of them as they tend to share more.

In reflecting on her hospital's commitment to diversity and inclusion, along with other efforts, she explained the hospital has hired a chief diversity officer to assess, teach, and develop a plan related to diversity and inclusion. Programs such as the Roxbury Community College and Brigham and Women's Hospital collaborative show that there is some commitment to diversity. Farah shared that she is a mentor to college students attending the program. She believes in voicing her opinion, speaking up, and advocating for patients, others, and herself.

In closing, Farah shared some advice: If you are passionate about advancing diversity, know that it is not easy. The mission can be uncomfortable and the resulting interaction awkward. Yet Farah encourages those interested in advancing the cause of diversity to keep going. She believes it is imperative for people to understand how important the work is. When people don't think diversity is important to them, it doesn't mean they are racist. As Farah mentioned, "It's just something they do not think about." She highlighted programs in place to help support diversity such as the Clinical Leadership Collaborative for Diversity in Nursing between Roxbury Community College and Brigham and Women's Hospital.

—F. Abellard, personal communication, August 30, 2017

should receive fair and equal care and participate in healthcare options. Cultural competence improves the quality of healthcare for patients, communities, and populations (Saha, Beach, & Cooper, 2008, p. 1275).

Intercultural care encounters during hospitalizations are challenged by language barriers, lower health literacy, and psychosocial and socioeconomic factors. A descriptive study was conducted to discover nurses' experiences when they care for patients from cultures different than their own and their perception of what helps them deliver culturally competent care (Cang-Wong, Murphy, & Adelman, 2009). The findings indicate that nurses draw on past experiences inclusive of those with family and friends, education and training, travel experience, and information learned from the internet. It is imperative to educate nurses and raise their level of awareness. Bedside nurses have a responsibility to contribute to creating an environment of cultural awareness. It is essential that everyone on the team feels accepted and like they belong. Sometimes, bedside nurses remain silent when others make derogatory comments. Fitzgerald, Myers, and Clark (2017, para. 13) report "silence indirectly perpetuates and contributes to the injustice, leading one to be a guilty bystander." The authors conclude "civil and healthy workplaces are created by the ordinary, everyday actions of individual nurses" (Fitzgerald, Myers, & Clark, 2017, para. 4). Bedside staff nurses should be equipped with the skills to be effective advocates within the healthcare environment for colleagues, patients, and families. Establishing an infrastructure to promote diversity and to address cultural and racial concerns in the workplace is paramount. Structures such as mentorships, buddy systems, and open forums are just some examples to help with establishing an infrastructure but to also assist with helping a peer.

Middle Management

Nurse managers and nurse directors are the frontline nurse leaders in various healthcare settings. The titles of nurse manager and nurse director are common and sometimes used interchangeably. They are classified as middle management in organizations. Their role is multidimensional, as these individuals interact with patients, families, nursing staff, and other professional colleagues; the role is also fast paced and it involves multitasking. They are responsible for nursing staff, nursing practice, and quality of care delivered to patients. They are expected to create and support an environment that elevates professional practice and enhances employee engagement (Cipriano, 2011). Additionally, the role is notably one of the most difficult in healthcare as these professionals commonly deal with staff concerns, interdisciplinary and nursing staff relationships, and patient care issues.

The context of healthcare environments has changed with increasing patient acuity, decreased length of stay for patients, and the increased demands of regulatory and policy changes (Sherman, Schwarzkopf, & Kiger, 2011). Along with these changes, the role of nurse manager has become more complex and the demands of the role continue to evolve. Nurse managers are responsible for managing up and down to sustain their relationships with their bosses and their employees. Concomitant with the process of managing employees is a commitment to create and support an organizational philosophy that promotes an environment supportive of both patient and staff diversity (University of Indianapolis, 2017). Diversifying the nursing workforce is a vital priority for the United States. With this priority in the forefront, nurse managers need to understand how to manage a racially and culturally diverse workforce.

Nurse managers are invited to think differently about diversity and inclusion. Given the direction of the country becoming more diverse and given the generational gaps, nurse managers are encouraged to know how to neutralize tension, problem solve through conflicts, and recruit and retain staff with attention to diversity (Muchmore, 2017). Hunt (2007) researched ways to offer practical strategies for supporting overseas-trained nurses and managing cultural diversity in the health workforce. Although this research is related to overseas-trained nurses, these strategies can apply to managing a racially and culturally diverse nursing workforce. Hunt (2007) conducted a research workshop asking participants to discuss and explore the challenges to managers when managing a culturally diverse staff. The discussion resulted in four main themes: "assumptions and expectations; education and training to include cultural sensitivity, equality and human rights; performance management; and transparent human resource management processes" (Hunt, 2007, p. 2252). The research study concluded that in order to effectively manage a culturally diverse workforce, one should have an "intrinsic motivation to develop the cultural competence" (Hunt, 2007, p. 2252) to engage employees of different backgrounds and ethnicities.

Bedside nurses of diverse backgrounds experience many challenges with integrating into a predominantly white profession. Some of their struggles include fitting in with other colleagues in their respective units, facing patients who refuse to receive care from them, or enduring racial epithets or unequal distribution of teamwork or patient-assignment workload. Nurse managers should be aware of some of the day-to-day struggles that diverse nurses face and how to best support them and create a supportive work environment. Other dynamics that diverse frontline staff may experience include conflicts related to promotions, achievements, and accomplishments. Nurses should have opportunities to engage in leadership activities and should believe that they are capable and encouraged with nurse-management support.

NURSE LEADER EXEMPLAR

Nurse Director

Kathleen M. Myers, MSN, RN, CNE-BC, ONC, ANP-BC, ACNP-BC, is a nursing director of White 6, an acute care orthopedic and urology unit, and the director of the inpatient orthopedic nurse practitioner program at Massachusetts General Hospital. Kathie has been a nursing director for the past 39 years. For as long as she can remember, she has been committed to advancing diversity.

Kathie describes herself as a white girl with blond hair. She grew up in Somerville, Massachusetts, a town very close to Boston. In describing her family, she talked about her mother, who valued diversity by volunteering her time in diverse communities and exposing her children to this. She went to a private, all-girls Catholic school and says she was a little naive. She does not remember seeing anyone who was black when she attended nursing school, and the population was 99% female. Confounding this, according to Kathie, was that Boston was perceived as a racist city, and she would say to people that wasn't true, or she certainly did not want it to be true.

Kathie expressed pride in possessing both clinical competence and leadership acumen. She described her leadership style as transformational and consultative. She described the culture of trust she's built on her unit: she trusts her staff and they trust her. She has consistently superior clinical outcomes, but when things are not going well, she is the first to say what needs to be improved, whether it be cleaning a bed, getting a patient out of bed, or more.

She discussed multiple initiatives to advance diversity she's been involved in throughout her leadership career. In describing part of her impetus, Kathie said, " I've always looked around, and for our population that we serve or anywhere, we don't have the same type of people caring for people that we care for . . . I don't mean all black people go to a black hospital, it's for the catchment area, for the culture, for broadening the horizons of the profession at every level." She went on to say that she "wanted to really make a difference for people and not have them feel that it was due to the color of their skin."

What is important to note in talking with Kathie is her tenacity and her hands-on approach to this important work. She described in detail mentoring multicultural nursing students throughout her career. She talked about helping them find financial resources, identifying employment opportunities to help them learn clinical skills, holding study sessions for NCLEX preparation, and directing students to resources that would help improve their language skills since English was a second language for many of them.

She also emphasized that she learned as much from these nurses as they learned from her.

In describing one nurse that she mentored, Kathie stated, " Come hell or high water, I'll get her through the bachelor's program . . . but when you see people who are struggling and want to be successful, [that's] where can we be the most helpful. And it's not always money. Sometimes it's just time." She has purposely sought out diverse applicants and purposively hired. She has also directed diverse nurses to professional organizations and encouraged them to serve as role models for others.

Kathie has always pushed the boundaries. She talked about showing up at different forums and, as an example, talked about attending a Latino nurses' conference where she was the minority. She was asked why she was there, but according to Kathie, " I really did feel that we could make a difference, and [I] made friends and had people then that we could recruit to help with some of our [diversity] initiatives." She also spoke about barriers that she faced at times including lack of leadership support, a dearth of diverse candidates for hire, and peers who did not share her vision and values, but she didn't let this stop her.

As the complexity of care evolves, Kathie more recently has been assisting diverse nurses with pursuing advanced degrees in nursing. According to Kathie, "We still see very, very few diverse nurses in nursing director positions [or] associate chief positions."

In closing, Kathie had this advice for other nurses: " You have to keep working on [diversity] all the time . . . . I'm helping to bring people along who are going to take care of patients the way I think that people should be taken care of and how people should be treated. We need to have people who look like our patients . . . so that we can truly make this profession the best we can."

—K. Myers, personal communication, August 7, 2017

Executive Leadership

A commitment to advancing diversity and inclusion in executive nurse leadership is essential. It is the executive leader that helps drive the culture of an organization. Culture can be defined "as an integrated pattern of learned beliefs and behaviors that can be shared among groups and include thoughts, styles of communicating, ways of interacting, views on roles and relationships, values, practices and customs"(Smedley, Stith, & Nelson, 2002, p. 201). In nursing, achieving Magnet Recognition from the American Nurses Credentialing Center (ANCC) exemplifies a culture of excellence and high-quality patient care. Cultures in Magnet hospitals show more satisfied staff, lower turnover and vacancy rates, better patient outcomes, improved patient satisfaction, and more autonomy for nurses over their practice (Drenkard, 2010).

In *Guiding Principles for Diversity in Health Care Organizations* from the American Organization of Nurse Executives (2011), diversity and inclusion are fundamental to creating a healthy practice environment. These principles contend that misinterpretations about diversity could lead to an environment that lacks innovation or risk taking. They further state that leaders must facilitate work environments where there is open communication and an appreciation of differences as a source of strength and pride. Leveraging diversity can increase creative approaches to challenges. Diverse leaders often have experiences and insights that have given them behaviors and skills to bridge a cultural gap through cross-cultural communication and role modeling in teaching, research, and clinical practice.

It is important not only for nurse leaders to understand the needs and concerns of the diverse communities that they serve but also for their workforce to reflect and align with the demographics of the community. Potential benefits of attracting and retaining diverse leaders include improving cultural competency and cultural sensitivity in healthcare settings and improving health disparities (Health Research & Educational Trust, 2013). Furthermore, evidence indicates that racially, ethnically, and socioeconomically diverse healthcare providers are more likely to practice, care for patients, and advocate for patients in communities with similar populations, improving patients' access to care and the quality of care they receive ("Promoting Diversity," 2016).

"If you don't have a seat at the table, you're likely on the menu." Have you ever heard this quote before? In 2015 the percentage of minorities on boards was below 20% and the percentage of minorities in executive leadership positions was near 10% (Institute for Diversity in Health Management & Health Research and Educational Trust, 2015, p. 8). According to Phillips and Malone (2014), "minority nurses in influential leadership roles are more likely to be better positioned to directly influence resource allocation and the recruitment and retention of a diverse workforce, and shape organizational and national policies aimed at eliminating health disparities" (p. 48). Influential positions include academic deans and faculty, positions at all levels of government, health-policy roles, business owners, researchers, and leadership roles in professional, nursing, and healthcare organizations. It is not enough to be aware of diversity; we must also be intentional and purposeful. Some healthcare organizations have been deliberate in establishing goals for diversity and inclusion. Some goals include purposefully identifying diverse and talented individuals for promotion, making diversity and inclusion part of the performance expectations, and requiring diversity-and-inclusion training for cultural competency. Other goals include some that may not be so overt such as self-awareness and awareness of the psychosocial and emotional factors that form one's own psychosocial and cultural identity. Efforts such as these help organizations be proactive and deliberate in choices related to recruitment and retention around diversity.

NURSE LEADER EXEMPLAR

Executive Leader

Elias Provencio-Vasquez, PhD, RN, FAAN, FAANP, is an executive leader who is currently the dean of the School of Nursing at The University of Texas at El Paso. He is the first Latino male to earn a doctorate in nursing and to serve as a dean of a nursing school in the United States. He is a pioneer in creating innovative nursing approaches for mothers with substance-use disorders and for their children. Provencio-Vasquez recognizes that he is a role model for aspiring nurses who are men and who are racial or ethnic minorities.

Eli believes that diversity and inclusion are important as an executive leader because it provides not only a sense of belonging but also a sense of value. Eli is a Hispanic American who started his nursing career in the early 1980s. While there is much discussion about diversity and inclusion today, he remembers when it wasn't even discussed. He started his career at a community college, where many underrepresented minorities get their start. There, he stated, "I could prove myself and get the confidence that I belonged. . . . I think my educational path really has a lot to do with who I am as a leader and who I am today as a nurse."

Eli said that diversity was key to his career success. It was women who served as mentors throughout his career. They encouraged him to further his education and gave him opportunities to grow and develop as a leader. These women also stood by him when he made mistakes, which he learned

(*continued*)

from and tried not to make the same mistakes again. He plays it forward by mentoring others, identifying up-and-coming students who are "bright and have grit" and embody servant leadership. He's gotten feedback from diverse students that it was important for them to see role models who looked like them because they knew then that they would be accepted and it gave them hope for the future. This is also true to managerial and executive nurse-leadership roles, according to Eli. "We are seeing more CNOs and deans that are from minority populations. I think this opens up a lot of doors for other people to say, 'I can make it.'"

He went on to state that diversity is important because we, as nurses, take care of diverse patient populations. From a patient's perspective, sometimes it is more comfortable or comforting to have someone that looks like them providing care. He believes that diversity adds value to doing thing differently and having differing perspectives. He stated: "I think that patient care is different when you have diverse staff workforce, not only within a unit but certainly within a hospital. Whether diversity is gender or ethnicity or race, it really adds to the richness of the environment and the patient care that you give."

There have been challenging times for Dr. Provencio-Vasquez as a Hispanic nurse. He described a time when a faculty member in one of his previous positions publicly stated that he was only hired because he was Hispanic and male. From that experience, he decided to work harder to prove his worth to be there. He went on to say, "Most of my career I was included because I didn't walk away being bitter or angry about not being included."

Where he is currently dean in El Paso, Texas, Eli reflected that diversity is "sort of backward." He has worked hard to ensure that the faculty and students reflect the majority demographics of the Mexican American population in El Paso. He goes on to say that he is particularly proud that he has recruited many male faculty—probably one of the largest number in the country. He is committed to ensuring that everyone feels included, is represented, and has a voice. He has fewer African American and Caucasian faculty, but he is purposeful in ensuring that they are a part of all major decisions.

A commitment to community services and social justice is a priority for Eli, whether as a leader at the bedside or in a managerial or executive leadership role. Early in his career, he made over 500 home visits to African American patients as a pediatric and neonatal nurse practitioner. He's worked in the Hispanic communities in Miami and El Paso. He's engaged community organizations to understand their needs and offer resources.

Dr. Provencio-Vasquez believes that you must be passionate about advancing diversity and that it must be purposeful: "You must demonstrate that it is important to you and that you value it."

—E. Provencio-Vasquez, personal communication, August 23, 2017

Reflective Questions for the Reader

Examining diversity can be challenging and emotionally charged. Self-reflection is a starting point to begin to understand one's own beliefs and values. Swanson (2004) suggests that some starting options include having more conversations, exploring areas of similarities rather than differences, being fully present by listening and seeking full understanding, and taking risks by being vulnerable. Furthermore, acknowledging one's own prejudices and biases is key. True leadership at all levels of practice requires that we act on what matters most: providing exemplary care for our patients, creating a practice environment that is inclusive, and creating a culture where all can excel.

Here Are Some Other Questions to Consider

1. Do you value diversity, and what are your personal beliefs?

2. Who is in your sphere of influence or circle of friends? Do they all look and sound like you?

3. Who are you mentoring?

4. Are you curious about those who look and sound different from you?

5. Are you open to multiple ideas, suggestions, and viewpoints?

6. When was the last time you said, "I don't understand; I want to learn more"?

7. How knowledgeable are you about health disparities and social determinants of health?

8. How does your background influence your comfort level with others from different backgrounds?

Addressing these questions openly and honestly is the first step in becoming more aware of your perceptions.

Summary

Claiming to understand diversity and being committed with words is not enough. It is time to move from collective good intentions to collective actions. Diversity and inclusivity are foundational to our clinical and leadership practice. Scherman (2017) states that "the most effective healthcare professionals are those who maintain a steady commitment to continually learn and progress in their field" (para. 21). While we have made demonstrative steps toward diversifying the nursing workforce, we can do more.

In this chapter, we reviewed the background and demographics of diversity and inclusion while sharing information about their impact on health disparities and how they relate to the healthcare workforce. We discussed many strategic opportunities within the healthcare climate and we discussed how the influence and the direct actions of organizations and agencies have diversified the nursing workforce. This chapter provided you with an opportunity to read about exemplars through the lens of a bedside staff nurse, a nurse manager, and an executive nurse leader who shared insights into the lived experiences of their roles. We have shared a plethora of information with you and now the question is, What is your next step? It behooves us all as nurses to respond to the opportunity. Table 8-1 provides a list of things that you can do to contribute to diversifying the workforce, helping make diversity a welcomed asset to nursing. Please keep in mind that these categorizations are not mutually exclusive.

TABLE 8-1.　What can you do?

Bedside Staff Nurse	Middle Management	Executive Leadership
Create an environment where staff feel valued, appreciated, and respected.	Create an environment where staff feel valued, appreciated, and respected. Make diversity a strategic goal.	Create an environment where staff feel valued, appreciated, and respected.
Diversify social circle to include more minority persons.	Diversify social network to include more minority persons; deepen your experiences across race.	Diversify social network to include more minority persons; deepen your experiences across race.
Conduct a self-check for in-group favoritism (a bias that favors your group).	Mentor minorities and provide opportunities for professional development that include leadership training.	Mentor minorities and provide opportunities for professional development that include leadership training.

Bedside Staff Nurse	Middle Management	Executive Leadership
Deepen your experiences across race.	Conduct a self-check for in-group favoritism (a bias that favors your group).	Make diversity a strategic goal. Create a vision. Establish organizational sensitivity.
Speak up and voice concern to avoid being a guilty bystander.	Promote from within for recruitment and retention.	Promote from within for recruitment and retention.
Seek out young people graduating from high school and college to expose them to healthcare as a career.	Seek out young people graduating from high school and college to expose them to healthcare as a career.	Provide internships or fellowships for graduate students.
Find networking opportunities.	Select minority individuals to shadow you in your role.	Commit to finding diversity leaders.
Mentor someone that does not reflect the same background as you.	Serve on a board.	Invest in leadership development to retain high performers.
Ensure diverse voices are involved in making decisions.	Ensure diverse voices are involved in making decisions.	Ensure diverse voices are involved in making decisions.
Serve on a board.	Hire staff nurses from diverse backgrounds.	Utilize metrics.
		Offer diversity training.
		Impact policy-making and resource allocation at the local, state, and federal level.

We all should know that diversity makes for a rich tapestry, and we must understand that all the threads of the tapestry are equal in value no matter what their color.

—Attributed to Maya Angelou

Chapter Key Points

- The time is now for individuals and communities to seize the moment to create opportunities for transparent conversations and real actions to produce outcomes that will change the disparity dynamic.

- Disparity has existed for a long time, and when it comes to health disparities, the United States is only outranked by Chile and Portugal (Khazan, 2017).

- Nursing has an opportunity as the most trusted profession to not only lead the change but also be the change others need to see.

References

Angelou, M. (2017). *Maya Angelou quotes.* Retrieved from https://www.goodreads.com/quotes/67256-we-all-should-know-that-diversity-makes-for-a-rich

American Organization of Nurse Executives. (2011). *AONE guiding principles for diversity in health care organizations.* Washington, DC: Author.

Brennan Ramirez, L. K., Baker, E. A., & Metzler, M. (2008). *Promoting health equity: A resource to help communities address social determinants of health.* Atlanta, GA: U.S. Department of Health and Human Services, Centers for Disease Control and Prevention. Retrieved from https://www.cdc.gov/nccdphp/dch/programs/healthycommunitiesprogram/tools/pdf/sdoh-workbook.pdf

Cang-Wong, C., Murphy, S. O., & Adelman, T. (2009). Nursing responses to transcultural encounters: What nurses draw on when faced with a patient from another culture. *The Permanente Journal, 13*(3), 31–37.

Cipriano, P. F. (2011). Move up to the role of nurse manager. *American Nurse Today, 6*(3). Retrieved from https://www.americannursetoday.com/move-up-to-the-role-of-nurse-manager/

Colby, S. L. & Ortman, J. M. (2015). *Projections of the size and composition of the U.S. population: 2014 to 2060* (No. P25-1143). Report prepared for U.S. Census Bureau. Retrieved from https://www.census.gov/content/dam/Census/library/publications/2015/demo/p25-1143.pdf

Douglas, M. K., Rosenkoetter, M., Pacquiao, D. F., Callister, L. C., Hattar-Pollara, M., Lauderdale, J., ... Purnell, L. (2014). Guidelines for Implementing Culturally Competent Nursing Care. *Journal of Transcultural Nursing, 25*(2), 109–21. Retrieved from https://tcns.org/standards/

Drenkard, K. (2010). Going for the gold: The value of attaining magnet recognition. *American Nurse Today, 5*(3), 50–52.

Fisher, N. (2015). 3 Surprising hospital leadership trends. *Forbes.* Retrieved from https://www.forbes.com/sites/nicolefisher/2015/03/20/3-surprising-hospital-leadership-trends

Fitzgerald, E. M., Myers, J. G., & Clark, P. (2017). Nurses need not be guilty bystanders: Caring for vulnerable immigrant populations. *Online Journal of Issues in Nursing, 22*(1). DOI: 10.3912/OJIN.Vol22No01PPT43

Gerardi, D. (2017). Using coaches and mentors to develop resilient nurse leaders in complex environments. *Voice of Nursing Leadership, 15*(4), 8–12.

Health Professionals for Diversity Coalition. (n.d.). *Fact sheet: The need for diversity in the healthcare workforce.* Retrieved from http://www.aapcho.org/wp/wp-content/uploads/2012/11/NeedForDiversityHealthCareWorkforce.pdf

Health Research & Educational Trust. (2013, June). *Becoming a culturally competent health care organization.* Chicago, IL: Illinois. Health Research & Educational Trust Accessed at http://www.hpoe.org/resources/ahahret-guides/1395

Henkel, G. (2016, June). Does U.S. healthcare need more diverse leadership? *The Hospitalist.* Retrieved from http://www.the-hospitalist.org/hospitalist/article/121639/does-us-healthcare-need-more-diverse-leadership

Hess, R. G. (2017, March 17). Making the case for more men in nursing [blog post]. Retrieved from https://www.nurse.com/blog/2017/03/17/making-the-case-for-more-men-in-nursing/

Howden, L. M. & Meyer, J. A. (2011, May). *Age and sex composition: 2010* (No. C2010BR-03). Report prepared for U.S. Census Bureau. Retrieved from https://www.census.gov/prod/cen2010/briefs/c2010br-03.pdf

Hunt, B. (2007). Managing equality and cultural diversity in the health workforce. *Journal of Clinical Nursing, 16*(12), 2252–2259. DOI: 1111/j.1365-2702.2007.02157.x

Institute for Diversity in Health Management & Health and Health Research and Educational Trust. (2015). *Diversity and disparities: A benchmarking study of U.S. hospitals in 2015.* Retrieved from http://www.diversityconnection.org/diversityconnection/leadership-conferences/2016%20Conference%20Docs%20and%20Images/Diverity_Disparities2016_final.pdf

Institute of Medicine. (2011). *The future of nursing: Leading change, advancing health.* Washington, DC: National Academies Press.

Khazan, O. (2017, June 5). America's health inequality problem. *The Atlantic.* Retrieved from https://www.theatlantic.com/amp/article/529158/

Lim, F. & Borski, D. (2015, September). Defusing bigotry at the bedside. *Nursing, 45*(10), 40–44. DOI: 10.1097/01.NURSE.0000469238.51105.20

Muchmore, S. (2017). Why hospitals should pursue diversity beyond the hiring process. *Healthcare Dive.* Retrieved from http://www.healthcaredive.com/news/why-hospitals-should-pursue-diversity-beyond-the-hiring-process/448665/

Nation: If not now, when? If not us, who? (1963, September 20). *Time, 82*(12). Retrieved from https://medium.com/@pammoran/in-1963-according-to-time-magazine-george-romney-spoke-to-the-michigan-legislature-and-used-the-591047638207

Norman, J. (2016, December 19). Americans rate healthcare providers high on honesty, ethics. *Gallup News*. Retrieved from http://news.gallup.com/poll/200057/americans-rate-healthcare-providers-high-honesty-ethics.aspx

Okafor, P. N., Stobaugh, D. J., van Ryn, M., & Talwalkar, J. A. (2016). African Americans have better outcomes for five common gastrointestinal diagnoses in hospitals with more racially diverse patients. *The American Journal of Gastroenterology, 111*(5), 649–57. 1DOI: 0.1038/ajg.2016.64.

Page, S. E. (2008). *The difference: How the Power of Diversity Creates Better Groups, Firms, Schools, and Societies.* Princeton University Press.

Phillips, J. M. & Malone, B. (2014). Increasing racial/ethnic diversity in nursing to reduce health disparities and achieve health equity. *Public Health Reports, 129*(suppl. 2), 45–50. DOI: 10.1177/00333549141291S209

Promoting diversity. (2016). In S. H. Altman, A. S. Butler, & L. Shern (Eds.), *Assessing progress on the institute of medicine report The Future of Nursing* (pp. 109–34). Washington, DC: National Academies Press.

Queensborough Community College. (n.d.). *The Queensborough Community College definition of diversity*. Retrieved from http://www.qcc.cuny.edu/diversity/definition.html

Robert Wood Johnson Foundation. (2010). *Federal survey finds nursing population is bigger, more diverse.* Retrieved from https://www.rwjf.org/en/library/articles-and-news/2010/01/groundbreaking-new-survey-finds-that-diverse-opinion-leaders-say.html

Saha, S., Beach, M. C., & Cooper, L. A. (2008). Patient centeredness, cultural competence and healthcare quality. *Journal of the National Medical Association, 100*(11), 1275–85.

Scherman, J. M. (2017). *Is a lack of cultural diversity in healthcare harming our patients?* Retrieved from Rasmussen College: http://www.rasmussen.edu/degrees/nursing/blog/lack-of-cultural-diversity-in-healthcare/

Sherman, R. O., Schwarzkopf, R., & Kiger, A. J. (2011). Charge nurse perspectives on frontline leadership in acute care environments, *ISRN Nursing, 2011*, 164052. DOI: 10.5402/2011/164052

Smedley, B. D., Stith, A. Y., & Nelson, A. R. (Eds.). (2002). *Unequal treatment: Confronting racial and ethnic disparities in health care.* Washington, DC: National Academies Press.

Swanson, J. W. (2004). Diversity: Creating an environment of inclusiveness. *Nursing Administration Quarterly, 28*(3), 207–11.

U.S. Department of Health and Human Services. (2010). *The registered nurse population: Findings from the 2008 National Sample Survey of Registered Nurses.* Retrieved from https://bhw.hrsa.gov/sites/default/files/bhw/nchwa/rnsurveyfinal.pdf

Vukic, A., Jesty, C., Matthews, V., & Etowa, J. (2012). Understanding race and racism in nursing: Insights from Aboriginal nurses. *ISRN Nursing, 2012*, 196437. DOI: 10.5402/2012/196437

Additional Resources

Brigham and Women's Hospital and Roxbury Community College Partnership: https://give.brighamandwomens.org/stories/nursing-partnerships-launch-careers/

Clinical Leadership Collaborative for Diversity in Nursing: https://www.umb.edu/academics/cnhs/partnerships/clinical_leadership_collaborative

Dotson Bridge and Mentoring Program http://internal.simmons.edu/students/snhs/nursing/program-and-leadership-opportunities

Magrath, P. (2012). Nursing Career Lattice Program, Children's Hospital Boston [blog post]. Retrieved from http://blog.diversitynursing.com/blog/bid/113401/The-Nursing-Career-Lattice-Program-and-Diversity-Cultural-Competence-at-Children-s-Hospital-Boston

Minority Nurse Leadership Institute: http://nursing.rutgers.edu/mnli/index.html

Myers, V. A. (2011). *Moving diversity forward: How to go from well-meaning to well-doing.* Chicago, IL: American Bar Association.

Witt/Kieffer. (2007). *Advancing diversity leadership in health care.* Oak Brook, IL: Author. Retrieved from http://www.diversityconnection.org/diversityconnection/membership/Resource%20Center%20Docs/Advancing%20Diversity%20Leadership%20In%20Health%20Care.pdf

Chapter 9

Leading the Growth of Innovations

Joan M. Vitello-Cicciu, PhD, RN, NEA-BC, FAHA, FAAN
Barbara Weatherford, PhD, RN
Kathleen Bower, DNSc, RN, FAAN, CMAC

Healthcare organizations are becoming more complex, undergoing major shifts, and as a result the need for transformation, creativity, and innovation is critical. These complexities include the shift from volume-based systems to value-based systems, the shortages of healthcare professionals, emergence of complex technologies, burgeoning of information technologies, existence of varied treatment modalities, and the constant demand by payers to manage quality and cost and to add value. Nursing is in the center of that complex, transformative environment and indeed faces its own unique challenges. These include creating new models for the delivery of care, incorporating informed, evidence-based practices into the care of patients and their loved ones, and keeping abreast of and learning about all the new technologies, medications, and emerging personalized modalities. Moreover, there may be an impending shortage of nurses regionally or in certain specialty areas as the baby boomers retire. This will create turnover and the need for nursing leaders to continually build cohesive, innovative teams (Auerbach, Staiger, Muench, & Buerhaus, 2013).

Some feel that there is an increased urgency for innovation in healthcare. For example, Newbold and Stover-Hopkins (2013) reinforce this need by stating, "We have no way to invest in the future if we do not invest in innovation" (p. 1). Garcia, Meek, and Wilson (2011) further emphasize that innovation is a way to provide for "a viable advantage in a highly competitive environment by allowing for the management of change and increasing leadership satisfaction" (p. 243). Porter-O'Grady (2007) further substantiates the need: "In today's healthcare environment, the characteristics and content of leadership are changing dramatically. Current leaders must be creative, innovative and highly adaptive to the critical and substantial changes affecting health care" (p. 44). And finally, Cianelli, Clipper, Freeman, Goldstein, and Wyatt (2016) highlight the need for innovation by stating, "While such high stakes require hospitals and healthcare centers to deliver clinical care within a tight structure of quality and risk management, the leaders of these organizations must begin to think innovatively to grow, expand, and solve problems amid delivery system reforms"(p. 4).

Moreover, there are some who believe that healthcare is headed for more "disruptive innovations" (Christensen, 1997; Christensen & Raynor, 2003), which are more radical and transformative changes that can signifi-cantly change an entire field. Examples of such disruptions are when cellular phones disrupted fixed landlines, the Swiffer disrupted the mop and bucket, and computers disrupted typewriters (Blackeney, Carleton, McCarthy, & Coakley, 2009; Christensen & Overdorf, 2000; Sitterding & Marshall, 2017). More recent disruptions include Uber disrupting taxis and Amazon disrupting on-site retail shopping. Disruptive changes in healthcare include medical and surgical homes, retail medical clinics, electronic medical records, and advances in genomics/genetics leading to precision and personalized medicine that will disrupt how certain illnesses are treated (Collins & Vamus, 2015; Jarousse, 2012). These disrup-tive innovations have clearly changed and will continue to change the way we conduct our lives and provide healthcare in the future.

Blackeney et al. (2009) argues that innovation itself is disruptive to an organization simply because those who are initiating the innovation process (i.e., divergent thinkers) think differently from their peers, ask new and diverse questions, challenge the status quo, make mistakes more frequently and learn much from these mistakes, provoke conflict, controversy, and resistance, and have the potential to significantly improve patient care. Divergent thinkers have the ability to make mental connections between unrelated matters (Mauzey & Harriman, 2003). They differ from convergent or linear thinkers, whose thinking leads to discovering discrete answers or specific solutions. Convergent thinking is more valued in healthcare; for example, prescribing the correct medication, utilizing the nursing process, and doing a physical exam require convergent thinking (Blackeney et al., 2009).

This chapter seeks to provide an overview of innovation by defining it and then describing leaders of innovation in the context of a research study conducted by the authors on the characteristics of nursing leaders of innovation and in the nursing literature. We then discuss those ways of planting the seeds for an innovative culture and examine the characteristics that must be cultivated to cause creativity and innovation to sprout as well as those that need to be pruned. We highlight through an exemplar case study how nursing leaders of innovation will fertilize the development of aspiring and current nursing leaders through evidence-based pedagogical approaches and how they can ensure continuous blossoming of innovations.

Definitions of Innovation

There are many definitions for innovation that can be found in the social sciences, business, engineering, healthcare, and organizational literature:

- "Innovation is a process and should not be treated as primarily an outcome but as an independent variable with multiple positive and negative outcomes during its process" (Seelos & Mair 2012, p. 49).

- "Innovation brings into existence something new that can be sustained and repeated, and which has some practical 'in the world' value or utility. It can be creating new tools, products or processes . . . to accomplish something that wasn't able to be accomplished previously" (Selman, 2002, p. 2).

- "Innovation can be viewed as a process for inventing something new or improving upon something that already exists with three highly interdependent components: individual or team creativity, the innovation itself and the environment" (Blackeney et al., 2009, pp. 1–2).

- "Innovation is the multi-stage process whereby organizations transform ideas into new/improved products, services or processes in order to advance, compete and differentiate themselves in their marketplace" (Baregheh, Rowley, & Sambrook, 2009, p. 1334).

- "Innovation is understood as the process of constantly improving knowledge, which leads to new ideas, further knowledge or other practices applicable in working life" (Nuotio, Kairisto-Mertanen, Penttila, & Putkonen, as cited in Kairisto-Mertanen, Penttilä, & Nuotio, 2011, p. 26).

- "Innovation is something new or perceived new by the population experiencing the innovation that has the potential to drive change and redefine healthcare's economic and /or social potential" (Weberg, 2009, p. 236).

- "Innovation is the application of creativity or problem solving that results in a widely adopted strategy, product or service that meets a need in a new and different way. It is deliberatively using knowledge to create novel approaches and services to solve problem and transform systems" (Lachman, Smith Glasgow, & Donnelly, 2006, pp. 205, 208).

What is striking with these definitions is that they do distinguish invention from innovation. Invention is when an idea for a new product or process occurs; innovation is when that idea or process is carried out into practice. There appears to be a long lag time between invention and innovation. According to Fagerburg (2005), this lag could be attributed to an insufficient need or to an inability to produce or market because a vital component is lacking or complementary factors are not yet available (p. 5). It is also evident from these aforementioned definitions that innovation incorporates learning and building knowledge to turn these ideas into new products or processes.

So how can we innovate in healthcare when those of us who have been in healthcare for a long time know that it is so risk averse, quality driven, heavily regulated, and lacking in downtime these days? According to Jarousse (2012), the place to start is at the top of the organization, where passionate leaders must set the vision for the organization and allocate the necessary resources to facilitate innovation from within. In particular, nursing leaders who lead at the point of care or in an academic setting must co-create environments where creativity and innovation can be cultivated, can flourish, and can be sustained. Malloch (2010) emphasizes the need to develop and have innovative leaders to intentionally guide, assess, integrate, and synthesize technology into the human work of patient care. We refer to these leaders as nursing leaders of innovation—especially those leaders who exhibit the competencies that were elucidated in our research study, which we highlight in this chapter.

Nursing Leaders of Innovation

When we denote nursing leaders of innovation, we are not referring to those who are innovators but to those leaders who coordinate and facilitate innovation in their sphere of influence. These could be nurse managers, nursing directors, associate chief nursing officers, chief nursing officers, vice presidents of patient care services, and deans and associate deans for innovation. These leaders do not need to be innovators themselves, but they do need to be committed to co-creating environments that allow innovations to flourish. *Innovative leadership/ leader* is another term described in the nursing literature. We use *nursing leaders of innovation* when referring to our research study and *innovative leadership/leader* when the term is used in the nursing literature.

An innovative leader is defined by Malloch and Porter-O'Grady (2009) as an individual who creates the context for innovation to occur by creating and implementing the necessary roles for innovation, ensuring that decision-making structures are in place, having the necessary physical space, forging partnerships and networks, and securing the equipment that supports innovative thinking and testing (p. 112). These leaders, according to Malloch (2010), must provide rewards for innovative work by constantly being aware of the inevitable and by valuing change. These innovative leaders are constantly scanning the external environment for changes, new technologies, new processes, and others' innovations to determine their impact on the internal environment (p. 6).

An innovative leader would then, according to Malloch (2010), use the trimodal work products of operations, innovations, and transition to "more effectively advance the work of the organization and create a context whereby critical thinking is valued, improvement is rewarded, and more importantly that individuals feel safe in recommending or initiating innovative ways of working and producing outcomes, which leads to a workplace environment that supports quality, creativity, new thinking, a willingness to challenge long standing rituals and assumptions and the means to transition between current to future focused state" (p. 3). Weberg (2017) further posits the following: "The innovation leadership gap originates from a difference between traditional notions of leadership that are grounded in command and control and linear assumptions, and the idea of complexity or innovative leadership which is based on assumptions of teams, network effects, and unpredictability . . . This can be translated to mean that leaders must facilitate teams that can work together to create novel changes" (p. 46).

Nursing leaders of innovation are critical as we need to create new approaches to population health, care delivery models, care across the continuum and across sites, and staff and patient engagement. The work of these healthcare leaders is now to be "fully aware of those circumstances and conditions that call each to discern the reality of their work, the challenges associated with doing it and the changes necessary to sustain it" (Porter-O'Grady & Malloch, 2017, p. 167).

These nursing leaders of innovation must have the requisite competencies to lead innovation in their respective organizations either in service or academic settings. This type of leadership requires shifting process and practice, creating new cultures, and adjusting clinical behaviors to set an increasingly technology-based framework for practice. Leaders of innovation must set the table by providing the context for care (environment, resources, and culture) and inviting in various stakeholders to create environments that embrace innovation (Weberg, Braaten, & Gelinas, 2013).

Leaders of Innovation in Nursing Study

Peter Drucker (1985) differentiates innovation as the work of knowing rather than doing. So what does a leader of innovation need to know? This was one of several questions that we pondered as nurse researchers when we embarked on our research study. We also wondered if key characteristics of leaders of innovation could be identified and differentiated from general leadership competencies. A subsequent question was whether innovative leadership competencies could be taught. We initiated our Delphi study to identify the key characteristics of nursing leaders of innovation in order to develop competencies and the requisite knowledge, skills, and attitudes (KSAs) that could guide the development of future educational programs. Our two research questions were as follows: (1) What are the key descriptors found in the literature used to describe behaviors or attributes of leaders of innovation in nursing?

(2) To what extent do experts agree on competencies for leaders of innovation in nursing?

We invited 40 nursing experts who were either innovators themselves or were innovative leaders to participate in the study, and 38 participated. Using literature from nursing, healthcare, and business, researchers identified 139 descriptors of innovative-leadership behaviors. We used a three-round Delphi survey for data collection. In the first round, study participants were asked to rate which of these 139 descriptors aptly described the leader-of-innovation behaviors using a scale of 1–5 (1 = strongly disagree; 5 = strongly agree). It became clear to us after completing an extensive review of the nursing literature that we must be able to differentiate general leadership competencies from innovation competencies. Therefore, in the second and third round, respondents were asked to differentiate between innovative and general leadership behaviors. Round two yielded 106 characteristics with an 85% consensus rate. The third round yielded 29 innovative leadership behaviors. The researchers clustered these behaviors into five overall themes: (1) *disruptive change*, (2) *innovation and creativity*, (3) *experimentation and design thinking*, (4) *risk taking*, and (5) *translating innovation into operations*.

We then took the 29 competencies that fell under the five themes and developed the requisite KSAs for each of them in the hopes of guiding curriculum and program development to educate nurse leaders as leaders of innovation in academic and practice settings. An example of one of the domains of risk taking and the related KSAs can be found in table 9–1. We are in the process of writing this completed research study for publication and have also written an article on innovation-leadership competencies (Weatherford, Bower, & Vitello-Cicciu, 2018).

TABLE 9–1. Risk taking (E) and the associated competencies

Risk Taking	Associated Competencies
E.1	Able to embrace failure as a learning opportunity.
E.2	Able to make risky decisions.
E.3	Asks the best questions.
E.4	Breaks open entrenched and intractable problems.
E.5	Supports positive deviance behaviors for innovation.

We believe that nursing leaders who possess these competencies should be considered leaders of innovation. We also use a metaphor associated with gardening, as these leaders need to be planting the seeds for an innovative culture, cultivating the characteristics that facilitate creativity and innovation, pruning weeds that destroy the growth of an innovative culture, fertilizing the development of the leaders of innovation and the innovation itself, and ensuring that there is continuous blossoming of innovation. We delve into these in the following sections.

Planting the Seeds for an Innovative Culture

One of the most important characteristics for the leader of innovation in both the practice and academic setting is to plant the seeds with his or her team to nurture a *compelling shared vision for innovation* and *shared value for a creative and innovative culture* (Melnyk & Davidson, 2009; Weatherford et al., 2018; White, Pillay, & Huang, 2016). This does not occur overnight, and it takes courage and perseverance on the part of the leader of innovation in preparing the context for innovation to occur. It may occur more rapidly if the leader can engage staff in discussion, champion the value that innovation can bring to patient care, and artic- ulate the role that nursing can play in creating a culture that supports innovation. Safety is also an important factor in sprouting creative ideas. If the staff do not feel safe in voicing their opinions and out-of-the-box thinking, then innovation will not be propagated (White et al., 2016).

As we found in our study and substantiated in the nursing literature, it is critical that the nursing leader of innovation is able to have an optimist view of the future and the unknown even during these transformative changes (Malloch & Porter-O'Grady, 2009; Weatherford et al., 2018). The necessary skill is to communicate positive thinking about the unknown and to foster future-focused thinking to cultivate new ideas.

We believe, as do Porter-O'Grady and Malloch (2017), that the most important nursing leaders of innovation are at the point of intersec- tion between the system and its point of service (the first-line leaders). This is the place where innovation is translated into operations and where design and action are realized. This intersection is where the dance of stability and risk and the challenge of change is most difficult. It is because risk-taking can be dangerous to patient care that adher- ence to regulatory mandates and the fear of failure are in opposition to innovation. However, it is here at this point of service (care) where the most opportunities abound (Porter-O'Grady & Malloch, 2017, p. 157). Lastly, the leader of innovation's willingness to plant the seeds for an innovative culture must also be valued and supported by senior nursing leaders in the organization such as the chief nursing officer or the dean of a school of nursing. They also must be given the necessary resources (i.e., time, techniques, materials, additional personnel, additional information, financial backing) when necessary.

The role of the chief nursing officer (CNO) is also to lead the innovation by creating the context of care—that is, the environment, resources, and culture that drives care (Weberg et al., 2013, p. 35). Five themes related to the development of innovative behaviors of the CNOs have been identified and consisted of:

1. Diverse views and talents are a key and require the CNO to understand the importance of diverse views in order to innovate and produce optimal outcomes.

2. The role of the leader is to set the table for innovation by ensuring that there are 10 heterogeneous faces around the table as articulated by Kelley (2005) and consisting of the anthropologist, experimenter, cross pollinator, hurdler, collaborator, director, experience architect, set designer, caregiver, and storyteller. These 10 faces or diverse views are needed to innovate.

3. Leaders become innovative agents for change and innovation by building confidence in constant change and explaining the purpose and context of change among those they lead.

4. Leaders should plan for possibilities instead of strategic planning, setting smart goals through scenario planning instead of devising strategic plans.

5. Leaders must manage polarities as innovation is about doing and being different. However, as with any change there usually exist opposing forces to the change, and the CNO must appreciate the possibilities and similarities among the opposing forces. (Weberg et al., 2013, pp. 34–35)

Cultivating the Characteristics That Facilitate the Sprouting of Creativity and Innovation

The literature contains many characteristics, competencies, skills, or strategies that the innovative leader must embody or embrace (Adams,

1994; Blackeney et al., 2009; Cianelli et al., 2016; Clark, 2013; Malloch, 2010; Malloch & Porter-O'Grady, 2009; Melnyk & Davidson, 2009; Pillay & Morris, 2016; Porter-O'Grady, 2009; Porter-O'Grady & Malloch, 2017; Weberg, 2017; Weberg & Davidson, 2017; Weberg et al., 2013; White et al., 2016). The following highlights the themes we discovered in our research as well as those delineated in the nursing literature.

An essential characteristic that we found in our study and in the literature is that the leader of innovation or the innovative leader must enrich his or her own *risk-taking* competencies. Risk taking involves being able to embrace failure as a learning opportunity, make risky decisions, ask the best questions, embrace positive deviance behaviors, and break open entrenched and intractable problems (Horth & Buckner, 2014; Porter-O'Grady & Malloch, 2017; Weatherford et al., 2018; White et al., 2016).

Some of the KSAs that foster competencies such as embracing failure require that the nursing leader of innovation be able to clarify how failure is defined, reframe failure as a learning opportunity, and create a nonpunitive environment when failure occurs. This takes courage on the part of the leader; the leader's reputation is at stake when failure occurs. To mitigate the risk, the leader must be able to analyze the level of risk in decisions, employ course-correction tactics in the midst of failures, verbalize an appreciation of the need to support risk taking, and acknowledge the tension that may exist in risky decisions. In order to develop the competency of asking the best questions, the innovative leader must foster curiosity in others, encourage others to feel safe in asking questions, and employ strategies to reach consensus on what is the right question to consider for innovation (Malloch & Porter O'Grady, 2009; Porter-O'Grady & Malloch, 2017; Weatherford et al., 2018; Weberg, 2017).

Positive deviance includes the behavioral characteristics of a team or an individual who disrupts the status quo by using uncommon but honorable strategies and who successfully determines and sustains better solutions to problems than their peers (Jaramillo et al., 2008; Melnyk & Davidson, 2009). According to Jaramillo et al. (2008), "Positive deviance is a method for transforming the culture to incubate creativity and grow innovators from within the organization" (p. 34). Often these positive deviants can achieve what their peers consider unachievable, and their new ideas need to be welcomed and cultivated (Melnyk & Davidson, 2009).

Our study validated that the leader of innovation must be able to discern and reinforce that positive deviance behavior is facilitated by practicing behavioral change rather than just knowing about it. And the leader must also be able to motivate others to adopt the positive deviance behavior, evaluate the scalability of the behavior to large numbers of individuals, and simultaneously appreciate that an uncommon positive deviant behavior can be adopted because it is already practiced by a few within a certain context. An example of a positive deviance behavior that an innovative leader should have recognized was when Ignaz Philip Semmelweis, a Hungarian physician in the mid-1800s, applied a rigorous hand-washing and scrubbing procedure in the doctor's ward with a powerful antiseptic that resulted in a dramatic decline in puerperal fever from 17% to 1%. It took four decades for his ideas and behaviors to be adopted (Jaramillo et al., 2008).

Another characteristic of a nursing leader of innovation is the ability to bring about change, and in fact we found in our study that *disruptive change* stimulates innovation. The leader must possess a positive and open attitude for change, must know that innovation disrupts the norm and brings about a change, and must be able to outline complex change theory for the staff. The leader must also verbalize that change doesn't happen in silos, acknowledge that disrupting existing processes is part of innovation development, and recognize that small steps of change may influence the sustainability of organizational change (McDonough, 2009; Weatherford et al., 2018; Weberg & Davidson, 2017).

Design thinking and experimentation are also important characteristics that cultivate creativity and innovation. Design thinking is akin to divergent thinking in that it requires individuals to use divergent thinking to stimulate ideas for innovation. This type of thinking is driven by deep engagement with customers, clients, and communities or in the case of healthcare with patients, significant others, and specialized targeted populations with chronic diseases (Seelos & Mair, 2012). The resulting human-centered designs are therefore built out from the needs of the users and are more effective and more widely embraced than those developed in other ways (Datar, 2017).

Design thinking is a prototype-driven process for innovation that can be used to develop new products, services, and business designs (Pillay & Morris, 2016). It is the process of questioning, observing, and experimenting to facilitate the capture of valuable information and to develop new ideas. It is important that nursing staff explore pain points when questioning and observing. These are the moments when a patient or a customer experiences frustration, difficulty, or uncertainty when using a product, service, or the like. Pain points indicate that a patient or customer has some unmet need. Pain points can be either explicit and elicited during questioning or latent, in which case they could be discovered through observation (Datar, 2017). Design thinking requires experimentation in order to comprehend how things work, testing to explore valuable insights that may emerge in the experimentation process (Brown, 2008).

The leader of innovation must verbalize that experimentation with new ideas or initiatives (idea testing) promotes creativity and innovation, and they must also understand that idea testing is enhanced through sharing of interprofessional resources and technology (Weatherford et al., 2018). Leaders must act like coaches during experimental phases and acknowledge the worth of maintaining a safe environment during experimentation, as some individuals may become uncomfortable with any experimentation. With experimentation there must also be a tolerance for failure, according to Cianelli et al. (2016), as such tolerance accepts that "the path to success is paved with many failures . . . and that leaders must condition themselves and their team members to accept failure as the pathway to innovation" (pp. 8–9). During any idea testing it is incumbent on the leader to maintain a strong oversight of safety and quality to ensure that all ideas are well tested before adoption into clinical practice.

Our study also revealed another important characteristic: the innovative leader must possess the ability to *translate innovation into operations*. A leader demonstrates this competency by being able to articulate the process of integrating a specific innovation into operations, by analyzing its impact, by using metrics to measure the outcomes, and by supporting the importance of technology that assists in translating an innovation into operations when applicable. Another competency is ensuring that financial resources are available for innovation work by first acknowledging the need for financial resources, procuring them, and then allocating them. Lastly, the innovative leader must implement roles to address the new world order during innovation. One must assess what new roles are needed, evaluate the effectiveness of those new roles, and consider the impact of the new roles on all stakeholders (Weatherford et al., 2018).

Cianelli et al. (2016) also identified agility and flexibility as two other important characteristics:

> *These characteristics refer to the ability to adapt quickly to rapidly developing trends, treatments, regulations, and changing market conditions. Agility is defined as the capability to adjust swiftly in response to global market changes. Flexibility describes the ability to provide different outcomes with the same resources by expanding, contracting and shifting them to meet emerging needs.* (p. 9)

They suggest that leaders hire employees who are able to quickly adapt to change and who can anticipate changes by scanning the literature and other work environments for new trends. We witnessed the need for agility and flexibility when we in healthcare were threatened with new emerging diseases like Ebola.

This section discussed what cultivates the characteristics that enable creativity and innovation to spout. However, there are also characteristics that can easily derail or destroy innovation. Thus it is imperative for the innovative leader to prune the weeds that can destroy an innovative culture.

Pruning the Weeds That Destroy an Innovative Culture

Obviously if any of the aforementioned characteristics that need to be embodied by the innovative leader is lacking, then creativity and innovation may not develop in that specific setting. In addition, Malloch (2009, p. 8) specifically warns about the need to minimize trash talk that consists of discussing remote possibilities (one-in-a-million, rare possibilities) or negative fantasies that could derail creative thinking.

As researchers, we believe that a leader of innovation must not possess command-and-control leadership practices as such practices will constrict any new ideas and not allow innovation to sprout, as individuals will not feel free to voice their ideas. Instead we encourage leaders to be authentic, to possess emotional intelligence, and to be transformative in their leadership style to develop supportive innovative cultures. Such leaders are often found in Magnet organizations.

Other common weeds that destroy innovation consist of a staff's fear of failure, poor team communication, inadequate education or preparation of the staff, lack of pretesting, lack of engagement of key stakeholders, rigid implementation rules, lack of a cohesive team, new ideas that have not been integrated into the system of care, criticism from other peers should an innovation fail, inability to communicate the value of innovation among team members, and lack of resources and time (Cianelli et al., 2016; Clement-O'Brien, Polit, & Fitzpatrick, 2011; White et al., 2015).

Fertilizing the Development of Leaders of Innovation

If we are to continue to fertilize the development of leaders of innovation, we must ensure that innovation education is incorporated into the curricula of academia and into the practice of nurse leaders. There needs to be closer collaboration between the academic and practice settings, and we must be able to differentiate general leadership competencies from innovation competencies when educating nurses to become leaders. This was a finding in our study.

Another important caveat is that innovation capacity development should be interprofessional because innovation is becoming a team sport. The education should be done not in silos but together with other disciplines (Davidson, 2017). This is especially true in most academic settings, where the need for innovation is also evident and where the academic environment can be a barrier to innovation. Melnyk and Davidson (2009) emphasize the need for academia to change from experts providing content that they deem necessary for students to more outcomes-focused curricula that are focused on the synthesis and application of knowledge. The premise here is that knowledge is socially constructed and therefore the process and diffusion of innovation are enhanced and accelerated when students are exposed to more divergent perspectives. Educators must make the shift from content expert to information navigation coach where students and educators are co-learners together (Melnyk & Davidson, 2009, pp. 3–4).

A study by White et al. (2016) gives us also specific pedagogical methods to consider that were preferred by experienced nurse leaders in both academia and practice to educate nurses about becoming innovative leaders. Some of these preferred methods consisted of case studies of failures, project-based exercises, field-based experiences, and case studies of successes (White et al., 2016). In their study, the least-preferred pedagogical methods consisted of traditional lectures such as the sage on the stage sharing his or her knowledge, team-based contests, global experience consisting of exposure to other health-care systems, and interactive learning consisting of simulation and role-playing (White et al., 2016).

It is apparent that nursing leaders must have an opportunity to solve real-world problems in their organizations. Both continuing education programs and graduate programs in nursing leadership or healthcare management must consider introducing the competencies that White et al. (2016) ascertained in their study. These innovative competencies should also begin to be introduced at the undergraduate level.

Lachman et al. (2006) identified four approaches to teaching innovation: case based, problem based, interdisciplinary, and debate. Moreover, the group questioned whether these strategies actually increase innovation or if other strategies are needed. Clearly we are in our infancy in teaching individuals to be leaders of innovation or to be actual innovators, and more research is sorely needed to elucidate optimum methods for educating nurses.

In addition to these pedagogical approaches, innovative leaders should be exposed to innovative approaches so they can plant the seeds of innovation and cultivate them to sprout. One example is Kelley's (2001) deep-dive experiences, which are rapid-cycle processes of brainstorming and building. A deep-dive experience includes observation, storytelling, synthesis, brainstorming, rapid prototyping, and field testing. The innova-tive nurse leader should encourage these deep-dive experiences as part of the innovation process. Another approach is illustrated by Newbold and Stover-Hopkins (2013) where they discuss how to create a culture of innovation in any organization. Both of these authors worked in the healthcare field and have written a book that should be used to educate all healthcare leaders about innovation.

Other innovation methods that can be useful to leaders who wish to facilitate innovation include the Acute Care Innovation Model (Neidlinger, Drews, et al., 1992) and the Maker Nurse program. The latter helps healthcare organizations involved in innovative device or product ideas by offering learning labs where devices or products can be developed, prototyped, and tested. This creates a safe way for nurses to experiment, fail, and try again in a concrete manner (Cianelli et al., 2016, p. 19).

Ensuring That There Is Continuous Blossoming of Innovations

As we have mentioned before, innovation must occur at the point of service, where opportunities abound, and also in academic settings to ensure that we see continuous blossoming of the interventions that are needed to transform healthcare. How does this occur at the patient's side or in the classroom? One example is to have dedicated leaders whose roles are to foster innovation in nursing practice or education. We now see more emphasis on hiring for these specific roles. There are more roles emerging in both academia and the practice setting with "innovation" in the title. One of the authors was involved just recently in employing an associate dean for research and innovation.

The following is a case study of such a leader. One of the authors interviewed this exemplary leader of innovation in a large academic center, and she aptly described how she cultivates innovation among the staff by employing all five of the themes that were validated in our study.

Conclusion

Innovation requires nursing leaders to possess the innovation competencies in order to plant the seeds of innovation, allow these seeds to be fertilized, and then have them blossom into innovative ideas, services, or processes in the leaders' respective cultures. Innovation is evolving into a way of life for those of us in healthcare. We know from our collective experiences that if the leader is not able or willing to value innovation, then neither will the staff. We must educate our current and future leaders to embrace innovation as a way of being for the true benefactors will indeed be patients, their loved ones and our organizations.

CASE STUDY

LD is a PhD-prepared nursing leader who works as a director of nursing research and innovation at a large academic medical center in the Northeast. She has led many innovation projects at her hospital, and we were interested in her perspectives regarding the competencies that we have articulated in our research study. She was interviewed and provided the following comments (italics in brackets indicate related competencies):

As a leader of innovation, I need to help staff either do a research study or think of creative ways to improve nursing care. You must be open yourself to change and be aware that it is never easy to bring about a change when other staff resist change. I try not to be judgmental about any idea that a staff person brings forward. I welcome all ideas no matter how crazy [they sound] at first. [*Disruptive change*]

When approached by a staff [member] with an idea, I often say, "sounds very interesting" [and] "I want to hear more." I suspend judgment regarding the idea and stay open in helping them develop their idea. They and I must be willing to take risks and to keep one's mind open to change. I encourage them to try their innovation in small steps. [*Experimentation, i.e., idea testing*] It is important to provide encouragement and guidance but to also let them know that any innovation project takes time and perseverance. They need to commit to this idea or project for the long haul. [*Risk taking; Innovation and creativity*]

As a leader, I need to think ahead about this innovative idea and to think about how it will function or improve nursing care in our environment. Does it fill a void in nursing care or bring about a novel way of doing a particular thing? [*Design thinking*]

If the innovation involves a new product design, then as a leader I must direct that staff person to the appropriate resources and explore ways of collaborating with an industry partner to bring that design into operation. [*Translating innovation into operations*] We often in nursing give away our ideas but we must rethink our role as a partner with industry to improve the design and application of technology in nursing care delivery. Perhaps a business plan will be needed, and the leader must ensure that all of this is in place to move ahead. [*Translating innovation into operations*]

Any innovation that comes into practice must clearly be communicated to all stakeholders who will encounter or be involved with it. There must be administrative approval when appropriate. The leader must ensure that all concerns are voiced and that there is a willingness to adopt the innovative practice change. [*Translating innovation into operations*] As with any solid innovation, the true benefactor of an innovative product, practice change, or way of delivering nursing care will indeed be our patients and their loved ones.

Chapter Key Points

- Leaders should embrace innovation as a way of being.

- Incorporate innovation education into the curricula of academia and the practice of nurse leaders.

- With the ability to bring about disruptive change, the leader then becomes the change agent for the innovation to take place.

References

Adams, C. E. (1994). Innovative behavior in nurse executives. *Nursing Management, 25*(5), 44–50.

Auerbach, D. I., Staiger, D. O., Muench, U., & Buerhaus, P. I. (2013). The nursing workforce in an era of health reform. *New England Journal of Medicine, 368*(16), 1470–72. DOI: 10.1056/NEJMp1301694

Baregheh, A., Rowley, J., & Sambrook, S. (2009) "Towards a multidisciplinary definition of innovation", *Management Decision, (47)*8, 1323–39. Retrieved from https://doi.org/10.1108/00251740910984578

Blackeney, B. A., Carleton, P. F., McCarthy, C., & Coakley, E. (2009). Unlocking the power of innovation. *Online Journal of Issues in Nursing, 14*(2). DOI: 10.3912/OJIN.Vol14No02Man01

Brown, T. (2008). Design thinking. *Harvard Business Review, 86*(6), 84–2, 141.

Christensen, C. M. (1997). *The innovators dilemma: When new technologies cause great firms to fail.* Boston, MA: Harvard Business School Press.

Christensen, C. M. & Overdorf, M. (2000). Meeting the challenge of disruptive change. *Harvard Business Review, 78*(2), 66–77.

Christensen, C. M. & Raynor, M. (2003). *The innovator's solution: Creating and sustaining successful growth.* Cambridge, MA: Harvard Business School Press.

Cianelli, R., Clipper, B., Freeman, R., Goldstein, J., & Wyatt, T. H. (2016). *The innovation road map: A guide for nurse leaders.* Greensboro, NC: Innovation Works.

Clark, S. P. (2013). Practice-academia collaboration in nursing: Contexts and future directions. *Nursing Administration Quarterly, 37*(3), 184–93.

Clement-O'Brien, K., Polit, D. F. & Fitzpatrick, J.J. (2011). Innovativeness of nurse leaders. *Journal of Nursing Management, 19*(4), 431–38. DOI: 10.1111/j.1365-2834.2010.01199.x

Collins, F. S., & Vamus, H. (2015). A new initiative on precision medicine. *New England Journal of Medicine, 372*(9), 793–95.

Datar, S. M. (2017, June 14). *Design thinking and innovative problem solving.* Paper presented to Newton Wellesley Hospital Board of Trustees.

Davidson, S. (2017). Evidence-based education for healthcare innovation. In S. Davidson, D. Weberg, T. Porter-O'Grady, & K. Malloch (Eds.), *Leadership for evidence-based innovation in nursing and health professions* (pp. 441–75). Burlington, MA: Jones & Bartlett Learning.

Drucker, P. F. (1985). The discipline of innovation. *Harvard Business Review*, 63(3), 67–72.

Fagerburg, J. (2005). Innovation: A guide to the literature. In J. Fagerburg, D.C. Mowery, R. R. Nelson (eds.) *The Oxford handbook of innovation.* (pp.1–26.). Oxford, London: Oxford University Press.

Garcia, V. H., Meek, K. L., & Wilson, K. A. (2011). Advancing innovation in health care: A collaborative experience. *Nursing Administration Quarterly*, 35(3), 242–47.

Horth, D. M. & Buchner, D. (2014). *Innovation leadership: How to use innovation to lead effectively, work collaboratively, and drive results.* Greensboro, NC: Center for Creative Leadership.

Jaramillo, B., Jenkins, C., Kermes, F., Wilson, L., Mazzocco, J., & Longo, T. (2008). Positive deviance: Innovation from the inside out. *Nurse Leader*, 6(2), 30–34.

Jarousse, L. A. (2012). Making innovation a core competency. *Trustee: The Journal for Hospital Governing Boards*, 65(5), 26–27.

Kairisto-Mertanen, L., Penttilä, T., & Nuotio, J. (2011, May). On the definition of innovation competencies. In I. Torniainen, S. Mahlamäki-Kultanen, P. Nokelainen, & P. Ilsley (Eds.), *Series C Articles, reports and other current publications: Vol. 84. Innovations for Competence Management: Conference proceedings*. Lahti, Finland: Esa Print Oy.

Kelley, T. (2001). *The art of innovation.* New York, NY: Doubleday.

Kelley, T. (2005). *Ten faces of innovation: IDEO's strategies for beating the devil's advocate and driving creativity throughout your organization.* New York, NY: Doubleday.

Lachman, V., Smith Glasgow, M. E., & Donnelly, G. F. (2006). Teaching innovation. *Nursing Administration Quarterly*, 33(3), 211–95.

Malloch, K. (2010). Innovation leadership: New perspectives for New York. *Nursing Clinics of North America*, 45, 1–9.

Malloch, K. & Porter-O'Grady, T. (2009). *The quantum leader: Applications for the new world order of work* (2nd ed.). Boston, MA: Jones & Bartlett Learning.

Mauzey, J. & Harriman, R. (2003). *Creativity Inc: Building an inventive organization.* Boston, MA: Harvard Business School Press.

McDonough, K. J. (2009). Leadership in innovation: Life beyond the hospital. *Nursing Administration Quarterly*, 33(4), 325–28.

Melnyk, B. M. & Davidson, S. (2009). Creating a culture of innovation in nursing education through shared vision, leadership, interdisciplinary partnerships and positive deviance. *Nursing Administration Quarterly*, 33(4), 288–95. DOI: 10.1097/ NAQ.0b013e3181b9dcf8

Neidlinger, S. H., Drews, N., Hukari, D., Bartleson, B. J., Abbott, F. K., Harper, R., & Lyon, J. (1992). Components of nurse innovation: A model from acute care hospitals. *Advances in Nursing Science*, 15(2), 39–51.

Newbold, P. A. & Stover-Hopkins, D. S. (2013). *Wake up and smell the innovation! Stirring up a return on imagination* (2nd ed.). CreateSpace Independent Publishing Platform.

Pillay, R. & Morris, M. H. (2016, Summer). Changing healthcare by changing the education of its leaders: An innovation competence model. *Journal of Health Administration Education*, 33(3), 393–410.

Porter-O'Grady, T. (2009) Creating a context for excellence and innovation: Comparing chief nurse executive leadership practices in Magnet and non-Magnet hospitals. *Nursing Administration Quarterly, 33*(3), 198–204.

Porter-O'Grady, T. & Malloch, K. (2017). *Innovation leadership: Creating sustainable value in health care.* Sudbury, MA: Jones & Bartlett Learning.

Seelos, C. & Mair, J. (2012). Innovation is not the holy grail. *Stanford Social Innovation Review, 10*(4), 45–49.

Selman, J. (2002). Leadership and innovation: Relating to circumstances and change. *The Public Sector Innovation Journal, 7*(3), 1–10.

Sitterding, M. C. & Marshall, E. S. (2017). Practice model design, implementation, and evaluation. In. E .S. Marshall & M. E. Broome (Eds.), *Transformational leadership in nursing* (pp. 195–245). New York, NY: Springer.

Weatherford, B., Bower, K. A., & Vitello-Cicciu, J. M. (2018). The CNO and leading innovation: Competencies for the future. *Nursing Administration Quarterly, 42*(1), 76–82. DOI: 10.1097/ NAQ.0000000000000263.

Weberg, D. (2009). Innovation in healthcare: A concept analysis. *Nursing Administration Quarterly, 33*(3), 227–37.

Weberg, D. (2017). Innovation leadership behaviors: Starting the complexity journey. In S. Davidson, D. Weberg, T. Porter-O'Grady, & K. Malloch (Eds.), *Leadership for evidence-based innovation in nursing and health professions* (pp. 43–77). Burlington, MA: Jones and Bartlett Learning.

Weberg, D., Braaten, J., & Gelinas, L. (2013). Enhancing innovation skills: VHA nursing leaders use creative approaches to inspire future thinking. *Nurse Leader, 11*(2), 32–35, 40. DOI: 10.1016/j.mnl.2012.12.008

Weberg, D. & Davidson, S. (2017). Moving to the future of evidence, innovation, and leadership in health care. In S. Davidson, D. Weberg, T. Porter-O'Grady, & K. Malloch (Eds.), *Leadership for evidence-based innovation in nursing and health professions* (pp. 503–24). Burlington, MA: Jones and Bartlett Learning.

White, K. R., Pillay, R., & Huang, X. (2016). Nurse leaders and the innovation competence gap. *Nursing Outlook, 64*(3), 255–61. DOI: 10.1016/j. outlook.2015.12.007

Chapter 10

Leading Evaluation and Research in Nontraditional Settings

Mary Jo Assi, DNP, RN, NEA-BC, FNP-BC, FAAN
Christy Dempsey, MSN, MBA, CNOR, CENP, FAAN
Jaime Murphy Dawson, MPH

Nurses are not just doers. Our work is supported by evidence and guided by theory. We integrate evidence and theory with our knowledge of patients and make important decisions with and for patients and families at the point of care. Research and practice are not separate but integrated. Nursing is a practice discipline with our own theories and research base that we both generate, use, and disseminate to others.

—Antonia Villarruel, PhD, RN, professor &
Margaret Bond Simon, Dean of Nursing
at the University of Pennsylvania

Introduction

In this chapter we explore the attributes of nursing leadership that lead to successful programs or initiatives to impact the health and wellness of patients and caregivers. Utilizing healthcare-focused evaluation, quality improvement, and research, we focus on settings outside those where nurses are typically well represented such as hospitals, healthcare organizations, academic medical centers, and academia. Role definition related to quality improvement, research, and evidence-based practice are often less clear in nontraditional areas where nurses practice such as business and industry. This is important to note because having nursing representation and leadership in all sectors of healthcare provides nurses the opportunity to influence the patient care experience as well as the experience of the caregiver, which are important goals for the profession.

In general, nursing has struggled with its approach to quality improvement, research, and evaluation. Potential barriers include uneven skill sets, challenges with human- and financial-resource support, significant lag from publication of research findings to translation of those findings into practice, and the disconnect that too often occurs between academic and practice settings. How do nurse leaders acquire and maintain the skill set and competencies to conduct appropriate evaluations and participate in research and quality improvement to advance the profession of nursing? And what are the characteristics that nurse leaders must possess to achieve results in leading such programs in nontraditional settings?

This chapter illustrates real-life applications of leadership theory to the practice of leadership in two nontraditional settings: the American Nurses Association (ANA), a professional nursing association, and Press Ganey, an organization that influences patient care and the caregiver experience. Several leaders share their perspectives on significant leadership attributes within their respective roles that resulted in large-scale research and quality-improvement programs designed to reduce suffering and improve the health and wellness of patients and nurses.

There have been so many significant changes in healthcare over the past 20 years that it can be challenging to determine which have generated the greatest impact on the workforce, work environment, and ways in which care is delivered. This chapter provides insights into the forces that shaped the movement to use evidence-based strategies to improve the quality, safety, and experience of care for the patient. This movement also led to an increased awareness that the health and wellness of the caregiver workforce is fundamentally important to both patient and nurse outcomes.

The Move to Quality, Safety, and Evidence-Based Practice: Proving Outcomes

The roots of quality improvement in nursing and health were established in the 19th century by notable leaders such as Florence Nightingale and Ignaz Semmelweis, who were early pioneers of personal antisepsis and cleanliness in the environment of care to reduce and eliminate infection (Chassin & Loeb, 2011). Contemporary models of quality improvement began outside the healthcare industry with productivity experts such as William Deming—an engineer by training and founder of continuous quality improvement and total quality management—who worked with the Japanese in the auto and other industries to rebuild Japan after World War II (Malloch & Porter-O'Grady, 2010).

In the healthcare arena, Avedis Donabedian is credited with creating the first healthcare framework to measure quality improvement. Donabedian's model proposes that the road to quality improvement should be focused on three elements: structure, process, and outcomes. His work has been widely adopted and adapted since the 1960s and is still widely used by both quality-improvement experts and research scientists in the ongoing quest for quality and excellence in healthcare (Chassin & Loeb, 2011).

The field of quality improvement has grown exponentially since these early visionaries laid the groundwork. During the 1990s and 2000s, research conducted by the Institute for Healthcare Improvement and the National Academy of Medicine uncovered and highlighted the growing quality crisis in healthcare (Institute of Medicine, 2001; Whittington, Nolan, Lewis, & Torres, 2015). The need for reform was clearly evident, and many national-level quality-improvement initiatives followed: professional standards review organizations, peer review organizations, and evidence-based practice guidelines were but a few of those early efforts. However, it became clear after no significant improvements were realized that more decisive actions were required to achieve desired outcomes (Chassin & Loeb, 2011). This led to the pay-for-performance model and value-based purchasing initiatives, which gave hospitals, healthcare systems, and providers a financial stake in quality outcomes for the services they provide. While we have seen inroads in areas such as reduction of some hospital-acquired conditions, we have a long way to go to hardwire the structures and processes needed to achieve excellence in quality of care across all health systems in the United States.

Knowledge, Skills, and Abilities: Education and Preparation of Leaders

Nursing has its own unique and rich history with respect to the development of research and practice-focused doctoral nursing programs. Prior to 1970, nurses who wished to study at the doctoral level to obtain a research-focused doctor of philosophy (PhD) degree had to apply to programs outside the discipline of nursing. In the mid-1960s only six universities offered nursing doctorates titled as EdD, PhD, DNS, or DNSc with expansion gaining in the mid-1980s (Ketefian & Redman, 2015). In 2005 the first doctor of nursing practice (DNP) program was instituted to meet the growing need of nurses to be prepared at an advanced level to manage increasingly complex patients and populations. Many of the growing pains with which DNP programs have recently been challenged—particularly around the scope and role of doctoral-prepared nurses—were also experienced by the first PhD nursing-research-science programs in the 1970s. While the professional nursing landscape has shifted with the addition of the DNP role creating some intraprofessional tensions, there are growing opportunities and potential for collaborative practice between DNP-prepared nurses and PhD nurse scientists to positively impact healthcare outcomes and advance the profession of nursing (Murphy, Staffileno, & Carlson, 2015).

The Role of the PhD Leader

Nurses attending PhD nursing programs typically focus on the science of nursing research. The curriculum is rigorous, culminating in a dissertation—a formal research project that adds new and significant information to the existing body of nursing knowledge. The PhD-prepared nurse leader is well positioned to initiate, implement, and lead programs of research that add new knowledge to the field of nursing or challenge or validate existing knowledge in the field, extending to other areas of healthcare in collaboration with other social science disciplines (Rice, 2016).

The Role of the DNP Leader

Over the past 10 years, DNP programs have grown exponentially to meet the demand of both formal and informal nurse leaders to advance their education and preparation to practice in a highly turbulent healthcare arena. The DNP program is an intense program of study that focuses on population health management, advanced education in information technology and quality improvement, and advanced concepts related to evidence-based practice. The final DNP project synthesizes the knowledge gained in the program and involves translating evidence and research into practice. Evaluating programs and services through the lens of quality at both the macro and micro level is a typical area of focus in the DNP curriculum and is often evident in the final project. The DNP-prepared leader most often uses acquired knowledge and skills to lead in both administrative and clinical practice settings (Murphy et al., 2015).

The Role of the Clinical Nurse as Leader

Through licensure, the registered nurse is charged by state boards of nursing across the nation to advocate for patients entrusted to their care to ensure quality outcomes. Leadership, then, is inherent to the role of the professional nurse at every level of practice because "every registered nurse is seen by law as a leader—one who has the opportunity and authority to make changes for his or her patients" (Yoder-Wise, 2011, p. 25). Clinical nurses are the professionals closest to patient and family care. And they, in collaboration with formal leadership, are essential to ensuring that evidence-based structures and processes that lead to best-in-class care are routinely developed and implemented while remaining realistic to contemporary practice settings.

The Role of the Administrative Nurse Leader

The role of the administrative leader, whether unit or system based, is first and foremost to ensure that direct reports have the human and material resources needed to create and maintain a positive and healthy work environment in which exemplary nursing practice can flourish. As a manager, the nurse provides operational oversight and assumes responsibility for budgeting, hiring, orientation, ongoing professional development, and coaching and mentoring of staff (Yoder-Wise, 2011). The leadership competency model of the American Organization of Nurse

Executives includes five competency domains: communication and relationship building, leadership skills, professionalism, knowledge of the healthcare environment, and business skills (Lacasse, 2013). In addition, the nurse manager as leader must inspire staff to join in a collaborative effort that transforms the work environment and continually raises the bar in the pursuit of excellence.

Improving the Patient and Caregiver Experience of Care

As we further our understanding of the factors that drive exemplary quality and safety outcomes in healthcare, we understand that a laser focus on the patient and caregiver experience of care is critically important to achieving these goals. We need to look beyond the old standard, which focused primarily on clinical and technical expertise, to better understand the human component—the connection between patients and caregivers and among care team members—when selecting best practices and designing care delivery (Dempsey, Wojciechowski, McConville, & Drain, 2014).

Leadership Models: Success Factors for Leaders

In addition to leveraging different attributes or characteristics of leaders that might be most helpful in creating, developing, and implementing programs, one can find many different theories and models of leadership that offer valuable perspectives for both formal and informal leaders (Borkowski, 2011). These models can provide a framework on which to develop projects and initiatives. As you learn about the various models out there, here are a few pearls to consider:

- Newer is not necessarily better. There are a number of tried-and-true models that have endured over time because leaders have found them to be practical and useful.

- You don't need to stick with just one. You may use different models for different types of work or apply aspects from disparate models to the work at hand.

- Simplicity is usually best. Whatever model you select should make sense to you and help you organize how you do your work. If it does not, ditch it.

Leadership and Management Characteristics

Healthcare professionals who move into positions of leadership in nontraditional settings often come from education or traditional practice settings such as hospitals, ambulatory care, or community care. One reason that both for-profit and not-for-profit businesses and industries seek these individuals is to facilitate a two-way bridge between the industry, with its work-and-product focus, and the practice environment. The aim is to ensure that current clinical practice and patient care needs inform the work of industry and that the resulting work product is relevant to practice and, ultimately, to quality patient care.

There are numerous contemporary models and theories of leadership in the world, and most include specific characteristics inherent to particular leadership styles (see table 10-1).

TABLE 10-1. Selected leadership models

Leadership Model	Description
Situational leadership	Situational leadership changes based on three dimensions: task behavior, relationship behavior, and maturity of subordinates. The style is ultimately determined by the maturity of the subordinate. The less experienced the subordinate, the greater the focus on task orientation. As the subordinate matures in their role, they need less overt management, and the leader places greater emphasis on the relationship.
Transactional leadership	Transactional leadership tends heavily toward task orientation, accomplishing tasks, and maintaining the status quo. Transactional leaders build and maintain relationships and typically influence performance by rewarding expected and agreed-upon behaviors.
Transformational leadership	Transformational leadership is predicated on vision and inspiration. The transformational leader promotes institutional innovation, vision, values, and change by creating an environment that promotes dialogue and encourages the innate leadership qualities and abilities of all. They inspire followers to go beyond their own interests to meet the needs of the organization.
Visionary leadership	Visionary leadership is all about managing change in an organization. The visionary leader facilitates change by harnessing resources and influencing followers to work together to achieve a vision. Visionary leaders can articulate the vision, adapting as needed to ensure ultimate success.

(continued)

Leadership Model	Description
Servant leadership	Servant leadership highly values individual performance and professional development. The servant leader creates goals and objectives and follows the people by promoting an environment in which each team member can do their best work and realize their full potential.

Borkowski, 2011

Nurse and other healthcare leaders who transition to roles in business and industry will certainly use skills and knowledge acquired while working in leadership roles within healthcare. Ultimately, success in leading and evaluating a large-scale program in a nontraditional setting (or any setting for that matter) requires a leader to possess a number of different characteristics. The leader must be transformational, innovative, and inspirational, have the ability to create a clear vision and align the people and resources needed to support the work, and have the abilities and competencies to lead and successfully execute the work. All are important factors.

Vision, Alignment, and Execution

The Work of Leaders by Straw, Davis, Scullard, and Kukkonen (2013) is a model that ANA leaders have used for several years to frame the work that leaders do. The model proposes that three critical elements should be considered to ensure a 360-degree view of the work at hand and to achieve the best possible outcome.

Vision: Identifying and Engaging Key Leader Stakeholders

It starts with the vision. There are many opinions on how visions are formed and who has the skill set or abilities to lead or craft a vision for an organization's future. But everyone who works in an organization likely impacts the organizational vision in one way or another, and if they don't, then they should. We talk about buy-in so often, but are we doing everything we can to engage participants who are in the early stages of developing a vision?

Alignment: Organizational Buy-In

Alignment is the most people-centered part of the model, and it includes working with all employees to clearly articulate a vision or strategic direction, to answer their questions and concerns, and to align their work through inspiration. Inspiring leaders authentically convey how the work relates to the mission, vision, and values of the organization. In practice, however, alignment may be curtailed or overlooked altogether in the excitement at the start of a new and major initiative. Think about times when you and perhaps several colleagues had come together to create a vision, and seemingly within minutes the group jumped to discussing how to execute the vision. Not taking the time to ensure alignment can be one of the fastest ways to derail a project.

Execution: Working Effectively with Interprofessional Teams Outside Healthcare

Execution is all about realizing the original vision and seeing it come to life. It is how team members "take good ideas and turn them into results" (Straw et al., 2013, p. 108). Those leading a complex project must often juggle multiple aspects of the project at the same time, and it is therefore important to recruit champions early. A champion is a defender and advocate for the project who positively communicates the work to other team members. It is also important that the leader create and sustain momentum until the goals are met by clearly communicating team expectations and setting realistic deadlines. This creates tension, which generates excitement around milestones as they are completed if the tension is well employed.

Creating a structured plan is also an important component. Depending on the project's or initiative's scope, this may require a full, formal project-management plan, allowing for ongoing analysis and feedback as the project develops. Honest feedback and even pushback from team members, particularly those who have subject-matter expertise, should consistently and periodically be invited. The final result may very well be greater than the one originally proposed if leaders course correct based on analyses of the project's status as it evolves.

Innovation Leadership

Nurse leaders in nontraditional settings are often recruited for their ability either to think outside the box or to expand the box in which they practice. Innovation leaders often tap into design thinking to solve complex problems, accelerate their work, and achieve goals. Design thinking is a solution-focused rather than problem-focused framework. It integrates "art, craft, science, business savvy, and an astute understanding of customer needs and the marketplace" (Porter-O'Grady & Malloch, 2010, p. 46).

Exemplars: Leadership in Nontraditional Settings

The following exemplars provide insights into designing, leading, and implementing large-scale health-focused initiatives in two nontraditional settings: a professional nursing association and industry. Leaders share their experience and knowledge and provide various perspectives, both strategic and operational, on what it takes to successfully design, build, and implement major initiatives with the potential to achieve positive impact at the national level. While these exemplars are not all encompassing of the full scope of work that goes into developing and implementing large-scale initiatives, they will provide you with some of the practical considerations that go into such endeavors.

Professional Nursing Association: Healthy Nurse, Healthy Nation Grand Challenge

Mary Jo Assi, DNP, RN, NEA-BC, FNP-BC, FAAN
Jaime Murphy Dawson, MPH

In May 2017, ANA Enterprise launched the Healthy Nurse, Healthy Nation Grand Challenge (HNHN), a social movement aimed at improving the health of the nation's 4 million registered nurses and the health of the nation. This initiative utilizes the collective-impact model, a methodology for bringing together a group of stakeholders from different sectors to solve a specific problem using a structured form of collaboration (Kania & Kramer, 2011). This model emerged from the social sector to address complex problems that require a systems approach. Key elements of the collective-impact model include a common agenda, a backbone support organization, shared measurement systems, mutually reinforcing activities, and continuous communication. The ANA Board of Directors embraced the initiative and framework for development when it was first proposed in 2014, recognizing that the ANA would be the backbone support organization for this grand challenge. Steering and advisory groups composed of thought leaders from diverse areas including nursing, industry, philanthropy, and the US military were convened to work with ANA leaders to create a high-level road map to move this national initiative forward.

In Their Own Words: Leading a Grand Challenge
Vision: Executive Leadership

Marla Weston, PhD, RN, FAAN

If you are the executive sponsor or leader of a large-scale movement, you essentially serve as the visionary. You need to inspire people by creating a compelling view of the desired future state, as unattainable as it may seem. Fundamentally, the leader traverses the tightrope between the current operational complexities and the future state. This navigation involves championing the cause, reminding people of their capabilities, filling the gaps in resources and abilities, and creating the safety for real-time learning. Where traditional leadership of change involves outlining and enacting a detailed sequence of steps or activities, the quantum leadership necessary for large-scale change involves having a facilitative and coaching approach, encouraging and enthusing the group to proceed without having all elements of the change detailed out, and trusting that they will adapt and iterate to meet the ultimate goal. For example, after an inspiring first meeting of the advisory committee for the HNHN, the attendees left stimulated by the exciting prospect while the staff team was overwhelmed by the difficulty of the operational execution. I had to create a safe space for them to acknowledge their legitimate fears and reassure them that they had the essential skills to begin, learn, and—through iteration—achieve the ultimate goal.

Alignment: Strategic Leadership

Mary Jo Assi, DNP, RN, NEA-BC, FNP-BC, FAAN

I transitioned from a career in clinically focused healthcare to a role at a professional nursing association, the ANA, after obtaining my DNP in 2014. When asked by the CEO of the ANA to participate in creating a grand challenge designed to improve the health of nurses, I jumped at the chance. Although I was a seasoned nurse of over 30 years, I had never worked on a project so large in scope. Clearly this was an incredible learning opportunity, and I was also compelled by the chance to co-create a vision for a social movement that could positively impact the health of the nation's 4 million nurses and, by extension, everyone a nurse interacts with. I also recognized, as social connectedness continues to expand, that this was an innovative way of conducting professional-association work that could increase the engagement of nurses from all areas of practice and provide opportunities to use what we were learning in other areas of professional-association work. Over the next 18 months I worked heavily with a core planning team to develop the vision and road map for this work, eventually assuming responsibility for implementation. My primary leadership responsibility as we moved through planning into implementation was to align the work of many different people to achieve a successful launch. This presented challenges, as the concept of a grand challenge was very new to many on the team, and sometimes created anxiety for members when they perceived expectations as unclear. Ongoing communication and clarification were successful tactics in reducing concerns when they arose, and the HNHN was launched during Nurses Week of 2017.

Execution: Operational Leadership

Jaime Murphy Dawson, MPH

My role as the director of program operations was my first leadership position, and I wanted to be intentional about my approach to the work. My first step was to immerse myself in the literature and seek advice from others who had led similar initiatives. More than anything, this exercise shed light on the importance of collaboration and identifying others who would be tirelessly committed to the mission of our work.

Getting organized and establishing communication channels were also important first steps. We worked with our steering committee to develop our road map—the essential components to success. It included things like fundraising and marketing and our plan for using data to measure our impact. The structure of the road map made it possible to move forward in a systematic way. After developing the road map, we identified the key people who would work on each element and put together a work plan and timeline.

For me, the biggest challenge was not getting lost in the many details and demands of the day-to-day work. We needed to execute the tasks to quickly move the initiative forward while staying true to the vision and goals of the grand challenge. To do this, we found it necessary to pause often and consult our steering committee and, most importantly, the nurses and organizations who would be our end users. We held countless conference calls, held focus groups, conducted surveys, did qualitative research, and beta tested elements of the program. From there, we would make the necessary tweaks and sometimes major changes.

This is undoubtedly the greatest lesson—success is possible when we step back, measure impact, and truly listen to our stakeholders.

Collaborative Leadership

In collaboration with ANA leadership and staff, the HNHN Steering Committee and the Advisory Board identified the key road map elements for the initiative, which were ultimately approved by the ANA executive leadership team. The road map elements include:

I. **Strategic Structure:** Convening the Steering Committee, Advisory Board, staff work groups, and partners to achieve collective impact.

II. **Data and Metrics:** Establishing targets and key performance indicators to evaluate success; developing shared measurement systems.

III. **Digital Platform:** Developing a digital platform to engage individual nurses and organizations.

IV. **Beta Phase:** Testing the digital platform to ensure it meets the goals of the initiative.

V. **Communications, Public Relations, and Marketing:** Increasing awareness through the media, creating media partnerships, and engaging stakeholders through social media and other ANA Enterprise communications channels. Creating a logo, branding, and other graphics, developing toolkits and resources for stakeholders, deploying strategies to engage stakeholders to join.

VI.   **Social Media:** Utilizing social media to engage nurses to partic-ipate in HNHN activities and to identify stories and exemplars related to the program's domains.

VII.   **Fundraising:** Raising funds to sustain the initiative and identifying models for generating revenue.

VIII.   **Outreach/Engagement:** Outreach to interested organizational partners; educating stakeholders through webinars and in-person presentations.

IX.   **Business Model Development**

X.   **Budget**

XI.   **Responsibility Assignment Matrix**

Each of the road map elements required a detailed action plan to develop and execute the activities necessary to move the project forward. Several detailed progress reports for selected road map elements follow.

Evaluation and Measurement of a Grand Challenge

The Data and Metrics workgroup of the HNHN Steering and Advisory Committees was formed to develop an HNHN measurement-and-evaluation plan that would capture data to provide leaders with information about achievement of desired goals and aims. In addition to ANA staff, several researchers from prominent universities worked collaboratively with the ANA to develop the core metrics of the plan.

For a period of 12 months, this group worked to refine the current model for the HNHN and provide expert guidance to develop a data-and-metrics evaluation plan. The final plan has two measurement components: engagement and impact metrics.

Engagement metrics necessarily come first and measure the level of engagement of individuals and organizations when they join the HNHN and interact with various social media and web functions. The Data and Metrics workgroup and ANA staff constructed the final draft of a longi-tudinal survey to measure impact on individual participants' health and wellness over time. Virtually every organization that ANA engaged with on the HNHN was interested in having access to organization-specific benchmark data. Staff worked with organizational participants including six early adopter constituent and state nurses' associations and six healthcare organizations to ensure that metrics specific to the safety domain were developed that were important to organizational participants. The final survey included questions to assess both individual and organizational health, wellness, and safety.

Digital Platform

A digital platform was developed to enable participants to socially engage. Communities can be convened around shared topics of interest as well as participation in blogs, discussion boards, and integrated social sharing and gamification. Expanded functionality of the platform will be rolled out over time. This approach provides the ANA with flexibility to develop the platform at a pace congruent with its strategic goals.

ANA staff determined that this technology solution will meet the implementation model of the HNHN, which includes:

- **Registration and Onboarding:** Organizational partners and individual nurses register to join the HNHN.

- **Survey Capabilities:** All users are invited to take a survey; survey responses will be tracked longitudinally to determine HNHN impact over time. This is a critical element because shared measurement is a top priority in the collective-impact model, a key methodology and framing model for HNHN.

- **Making a Commitment to HNHN:** Organizational partners and individuals are prompted to make a commitment related to the five domains to improve health.

- **Relevant Content:** Nurses can access blogs, articles, policy documents, and publications related to their areas of interest.

- **Engage in Activities:** Organizational partners and nurses can act related to the domains of physical activity, rest, nutrition, quality of life, and safety. Participants can also participate in discussion boards and health and wellness challenges.

Communications, Public Relations, and Marketing

The communications, public relations, and marketing plan outlines the promotional tactics to increase awareness about the HNHN and to use key messages (see table 10-2) to educate nurses about HNHN. The goals of this plan include:

- Increase awareness of nurses and the nursing profession regarding the benefits of improving one's health.

- Generate organizational partners.

- Engage individual nurses to interact with HNHN content and activities.

- Encourage nurses to take the online survey.

- Raise visibility of the ANA Enterprise and leadership.

- Reach nonmembers, promote membership interest and activity, and generate leads.

- Educate nurses about the importance of activity, rest, nutrition, and quality of life.

- Continue to promote that nursing is the most honest and ethical profession as rated by the Gallup poll for 14 years straight and therefore the best advocate.

TABLE 10-2. Healthy Nurse, Healthy Nation Grand Challenge key communication messages

◆ The good health of nurses, the largest subset of workers in America's healthcare system, makes a meaningful difference.   ◆ The health of nurses is critical to an effective, safe, and sustainable healthcare system.
Positioning statement
◆ As the largest subset of healthcare workers, nurses are critical to America's healthcare system.   ◆ Nurses have the fourth-highest rate of injuries and illnesses that result in days away from work.   ◆ Join nurses around the nation on their personal journey to becoming healthier nurses to create a healthier nation.

Anticipated audiences include:

- ANA members

- Nonmember nurses

- SNAs, CNSAs, and OAs

- Hospitals and healthcare systems

- Sponsors and partners

- National, trade, and health media

- State and local media

Ownership and Accountability: Using Responsibility Charting as an Organizing Framework

The RACI (responsible, accountable, consulted, and informed) model is an organizing framework that clarifies collaborative work relationships regarding role responsibilities, role expectations, and communication between project stakeholders. When applied consistently, this model can mitigate duplication of effort or, conversely, lack of follow-through due to confusion about who is responsible and accountable for ensuring work is completed (Smith, Erwin, & Diaferio, 2005). We used the RACI model to delineate and communicate responsibility and accountability because HNHN has many moving parts, each with its own project plan and staff (see table 10–3).

TABLE 10–3. HNHN responsibility grid

Roadmap Element	Responsible	Accountable	Consult	Inform
Program Operations (day-to-day direction to coordinate all road map elements)	Director of Program Operations	Director of Program Operations	VP Nursing Practice & Innovation, ANA Executive Director	CEO (strategic updates)
Budget/Finance	VP Nursing Practice & Innovation, Director of Program Operations	VP Nursing Practice & Innovation	CFO	ANA Executive Director

(continued)

Roadmap Element	Responsible	Accountable	Consult	Inform
Business Model	Director of Program Operations	VP Nursing Practice & Innovation	Executive Director of Marketing & Products, VP Marketing & Products, COO	ANA Executive Director
Communications	VP Communications, PR Director, Manager of Social Media and Outreach	VP Communications, PR Director, Manager of Social Media and Outreach	Director of Program Operations, VP Nursing Practice & Innovation	ANA Executive Director
PR	PR Director	PR Director	Director of Program Operations, VP Nursing Practice & Innovation	VP Communications, ANA Executive Director
Social Media	Manager of Social Media and Outreach	Manager of Social Media and Outreach	Director of Program Operations, VP Nursing Practice & Innovation	VP Communications
Data/Metrics	VP Nursing Practice & Innovation, Director of Program Operations	VP Nursing Practice & Innovation	ANA Executive Director	Executive Director, Foundation
Digital Platform (IT project manager)	IT Project Manager, IT Director	IT Project Manager, IT Director	VP Information Technology, Director of Project Management, Director of Program Operations, VP Nursing Practice & Innovation	
Fundraising	Director of Charitable Giving	Executive Director, Foundation	Director of Program Operations, VP Nursing Practice & Innovation,	ANA Executive Director, CEO
Marketing	Director of Marketing	Director of Marketing	Director of Program Operations, VP Nursing Practice & Innovation	

Roadmap Element	Responsible	Accountable	Consult	Inform
Products	VP Marketing & Products	VP Marketing & Products	VP Nursing Practice & Innovation, Director of Program Operations	Executive Director of Marketing & Products;
Strategic Structure (Steering Committee, Advisory Board, consultants, internal work groups)	Director of Program Operations, VP Nursing Practice & Innovation	Director of Program Operations	ANA Executive Director, VP Nursing Practice & Innovation	CEO

(Smith, Erwin, & Diaferio, 2005)

THE RACI ACRONYM DEFINED

The acronym RACI stands for

R—Responsible: the person who completes the task

A—Accountable: the person who is ultimately responsible for ensuring the task is completed

C—Consultant: a person who acts as a consultant to the group before the final decision is made

I—Informed: a person who is kept apprised of progress but does not need to be informed about decisions before they are made

Industry: Compassionate Connected Care

Christy Dempsey, MSN, MBA, RN, CNOR, CENP, FAAN

After I graduated from a nursing program with an associate's degree in in 1985, the acute hospital environment—particularly the ICU—was the first step in my career. I began in the neuro/trauma ICU after working as a burn technician throughout school. I loved the adrenaline-pumping, think-on-your-feet kind of work. I continued my education throughout my career in the hospital, earning a bachelor's degree and master's degrees in nursing and business. I sought out opportunities to grow both my career and my role in healthcare. I became the liaison to a consulting company that was working with my hospital to redesign periopera-tive services in the late 1990s. This work gave me experience with the inner workings of administration and navigating multiple stakeholders and agendas.

I became the OR manager in 1996 and then in 2004 was promoted to vice president responsible for all perioperative services, emergency services, two service lines (trauma and senior), and "other duties as assigned." As both director and VP, I worked to create an environment in which staff and physicians worked together to achieve quality, operational, and financial goals. As a part of the Institute for Healthcare Improvement (IHI) flow collaborative, we operationalized separation of scheduled and unscheduled volumes, smoothed the flow of elective volume in the ED, reduced waiting times in the OR and ED, improved physician–hospital collaboration, and improved quality indicators (Dempsey, 2017).

In 2007, after 23 years in the hospital going from staff nurse to the administrative suite, I had the opportunity to join a startup company led by Dr. Eugene Litvak of IHI and Boston University and Rick Seigrist of Harvard, an entrepreneur. This company, PatientFlow Technology, provided consultation to healthcare organizations to improve the flow of patients throughout the continuum of care using the scientific methods of queuing theory and simulation modeling. We worked with hospitals, ambulatory surgery centers, and medical practices that succeeded in reducing waiting times by up to 70%, improving patient satisfaction by double-digit percentiles, developing and enhancing teamwork and leadership, and improving operations through scheduling, staffing, and data integration.

In 2009, Press Ganey Associates acquired PatientFlow Technology. As the leader of clinical and operational consulting, Press Ganey was becoming increasingly aware that the patient experience encompasses much more that patient satisfaction—a superficial notion that implies making patients happy and wowing them. To that end, Press Ganey leader Patrick Ryan, CEO, reinforced the impact of nursing on the totality of the patient experience: clinically, operationally, culturally, and behaviorally. It was an epiphany that led to the creation of a chief nursing officer (CNO) role at Press Ganey. This role was to be the voice of nursing to Press Ganey and the voice of Press Ganey to nursing. It was the first time that this role had appeared in the patient-experience-measurement space, and it was one of the first CNO roles in industry. Some organizations had nurses in leadership roles, and many nurses were involved in product development, sales, service, and consulting. However, with a nurse as a part of the C-suite with the role of partnering with client organizations around strategy, product, and innovation, Press Ganey was on the cutting edge and they were on to something. Press Ganey understood that nurses are in every part of the healthcare continuum and will continue to be integral to population health management. Nurses are at the bedside, in the home, in the clinic, in post-acute care, and in the community providing preventive care. Nurses are key to health promotion and care.

Evidence-based practice begins with identifying an opportunity for improvement, collecting data to understand the current state, and monitoring data throughout any improvement effort. Surveying patients regarding their perception of care began in 1985 when Drs. Irwin Press and Rod Ganey, both professors at Notre Dame, developed their survey. It was widely used by hospitals to understand their specific patient populations and to target improvement efforts.

Then in 2006, hospitals had an additional survey to utilize. This survey, the Hospital Consumer Assessment of Healthcare Providers and Services (HCAHPS) was part of an overall strategy sponsored by the Agency for Healthcare Research and Quality (AHRQ). The Centers for Medicare & Medicaid Services (CMS) had also requested a survey that provided for public reporting and a uniform evaluation of patients' perceptions on the care they received at hospitals. In 2012, CMS required that all hospitals implement the HCAHPS survey as part of its Inpatient Quality Reporting Program. To that end, CMS tied Medicare reimbursements to survey scores in order to drive accountability and improvement. CMS approved Press Ganey as a vendor to administer the HCAHPS survey and also stated that HCAHPS should complement rather than compete with quality-improvement instruments such as Press Ganey's that hospitals were already using (CMS, n.d.).

There are key differences between the HCAHPS survey and surveys like the Press Ganey survey. HCAHPS uses a frequency scale that provides a score based on patients' perceptions of how *often* certain behaviors are demonstrated, while the Press Ganey survey provides scores based on how *well* certain behaviors are exhibited. For example, one HCAHPS question asks how often nurses treated you with quality and respect: never, sometimes, usually, or always. The Press Ganey survey asks, using a 5-point Likert scale from very poor to very good, how courteous the nurse was during your hospital stay. The key difference and reason to ensure that both frequency and competency are measured is illustrated in nurse hourly rounding. Measurement of frequency may provide a good score demonstrating that the nurse was in the room hourly. However, there may be poor scores for overall rating and likelihood to recommend because every time the nurse enters the room, they are stressed and distracted. The additional Press Ganey questions also ask for a patient's perception about the nurses' attitudes to requests, the amount of attention they paid to special or personal needs, and how well the nurses kept the patient informed. This provides much deeper insight into where to focus improvement efforts.

The large amount of data allows healthcare organizations to benchmark their results with other like organizations and, as required by CMS, all hospitals with the exception of critical access hospitals. Benchmarking provides the ability to identify where other organizations are performing better on certain items and where there are key opportunities for improvement. Since CMS linked reimbursement to the patient experience, there has been a concerted effort to improve it. As such, this tightening of the scores has resulted in a very narrow distribution of scores. This means that it is difficult to obtain top decile performance and even harder still to stay there. Figure 10–1 demonstrates that the score necessary to achieve the 50th percentile on "Rate the Hospital 0–10" in 2013 was 70.3. However, the score required to achieve the 50th percentile in 2017 was 71.3. Further, over the past five years, the percentage of patients giving their hospital top-box scores for Overall Rating has increased steadily.

From 2015 to 2016, providers overall improved on nearly every HCAHPS measure. During this period, most health systems stayed in the same quartile of performance for Overall Rating from one year to the next, and approximately 15% moved up to a higher quartile. The top drivers of performance on the Overall Rating measure included patients' perceptions of nurse courtesy and teamwork. Of the health systems that showed improved performance on all three top drivers from 2015 to 2016, 86% also increased their Overall Rating top-box scores. Striving to maintain the status quo in the patient experience is no longer an option. Standing still actually means going backward—a problem that results in reduced reimbursement and declining patient loyalty.

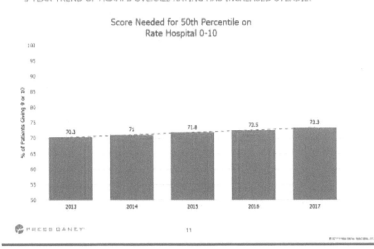

FIGURE 10–1. Five-year trend of HCAHPS scores

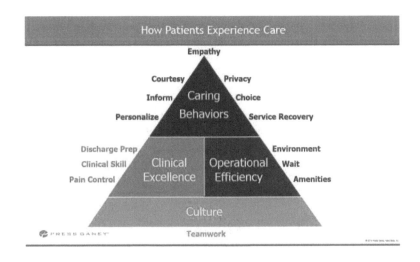

FIGURE 10–2. Compassionate Connected Care for the patient

As thinking evolved, it became evident to Press Ganey and the healthcare market that patient satisfaction was not, in fact, what was actually being measured. The survey questions provided a window into the met and unmet needs of patients. In addition, rather than superficially measuring satisfaction, surveys were actually measuring the suffering encountered by patients.

Suffering, as measured by met and unmet needs, may be divided into inherent suffering and avoidable suffering. Inherent suffering is experienced with the diagnosis and treatment of disease, even when healthcare is perfect. Consider a diagnosis of cancer; just the diagnosis and treatment itself causes a measure of suffering in terms of pain, fear, physical symptoms, and body image. These would exist regardless of the way that healthcare is provided. Although providers can mitigate this suffering with medications and communication, it cannot be eliminated. However, there is a great deal of avoidable suffering that patients experience as a result of the dysfunction in our healthcare systems and processes. When patients must wait for appointments, procedures, or results; when providers do not share information or work well together as a team; when the environment is not clean; when we do not listen and respect our patients—these are all ways in which healthcare providers actually impose suffering upon the people who come to them for care.

However, it is not enough to measure met and unmet needs or to discuss patient suffering; caregivers must understand and address it. The scores and percentile ranks provide a window into where effort is needed, but much like an x-ray provides a picture of what may be wrong with a patient, it does not provide the treatment plan to address it. In 2013, after a great deal of listening and observing both data and operations in healthcare organizations, the Compassionate Connected Care framework was developed. This framework recognizes the totality of the experience that connects clinical excellence with outcomes, quality with efficiency, engagement with action, and mission, vision, and value with engagement of caregivers. Viewed in its totality, the patient experience links to safety and clinical quality and, in fact, is indistinguishable from them. Figure 10-2 shows the Compassionate Connected Care framework and how the survey questions fit into the domains.

An affinity diagram was utilized to understand what compassionate and connected care looks and feels like. Hundreds of clinicians, nonclinicians, and patients were asked to provide a specific image and 117 images were analyzed and distilled into six themes:

- **Acknowledge Suffering:** We should acknowledge that our patients are suffering and show them that we understand.

- **Body Language Matters:** Nonverbal communication skills are as important as the words we use.

- **Anxiety Is Suffering:** Anxiety and uncertainty are negative outcomes that must be addressed.

- **Coordinate Care:** We should show patients that their care is coordinated and continuous, and that *we* are always there for them.

- **Caring Transcends Diagnosis:** Real caring goes beyond delivery of medical interventions to the patient.

- **Autonomy Reduces Suffering:** Autonomy helps preserve dignity for patients.

For each theme, actions along with very specific tangible and tactical strategies to demonstrate those actions were provided (see table 10–4).

TABLE 10–4. Tactics and strategies to reduce patient suffering

Anxiety and uncertainty are negative outcomes that must be addressed.	
Actions	Images
Reducing uncertainty and anxiety for patients and families acknowledges that they are in a stressful situation.	Caregivers do rounds with patients frequently in a way that is purposeful and meaningful to the patient, inquiring about pain, positioning, toileting, and at least one non-disease- or non-treatment-oriented discussion topic.
	The employee notices a "lost guest" and personally escorts the person to their destination.
	Staff members describe what will happen next when the patient arrives at the exam room.
	Clinicians tell patients when they will be in to see them again.
	Caregivers greet patients warmly (e.g., "We've been expecting you, Mrs. Smith").
	Caregivers provide reassuring phrases (e.g., "Mrs. Smith, I am going to be with you every step of the way"; "Mrs. Smith, we are going to take very good care of you"; "Mrs. Smith, we are going to do this together").
	Volunteers escort patients and families to their destinations (e.g., surgery area, tests and treatment areas).

(*continued*)

Reducing waits shows we understand patients' suffering and respect their time.	There is no lag time in response when a patient presses the call light.
	Staff members provide an estimate of wait times.
	Staff members do not pass call lights without inquiring if they can help.
	Staff members work together to reduce waiting time for bed placement, transfers, and testing.

We should show patients that their care is coordinated and continuous, and that we are always there for them.

Actions	Images
Showing patients that the relationship doesn't end when they are not directly in contact deepens the relationship.	The clinician calls the patient for follow-up within 48 hours.
	Clinicians follow up appropriately when information is received on the discharge phone call.
	Clinicians show that they are concerned about what will happen when the patient goes home and provide instructions to make them successful in their recovery.
	Caregivers "manage up" each other, complimenting the caregivers on the care team.
	The nurse explains who will be taking care of the patient after shift change.
	The clinician uses good handoff techniques and is accountable for communicating the patient's condition and needs.
Showing patients that the relationship doesn't end when they are not directly in contact deepens the relationship. (continued)	Caregivers use the teach-back method to ensure patients understand discharge instructions. Patients are provided with written instructions for home care prior to the day of discharge with an opportunity to read and ask questions.
	Clinicians use data to improve patient care processes.

Real caring goes beyond delivery of medical interventions to the patient.

Actions	Images
Personal touches outside medical care strengthens relationships.	The nursing assistant brings a patient their favorite dish from the cafeteria as they awaken from surgery.
	The director of service excellence walks a patient's service dog outside the hospital to give a stressed family member time to grab lunch.
	The nurse talks with a patient about their children.
	The nurse is simply silent while touching the patient or family during a difficult time.

Caring for the patient means caring for the family.	The nurse gives a warm blanket to a family member who is cold.
	On a nightly basis, the nurse holds the phone to the ear of a terminally ill patient so his daughter can say goodnight.
	Caregivers provide instructions to the family prior to discharge to ensure they are comfortable with caring for the patient at home.

Dempsey, Wojciechowski, McConville, & Drain, 2014; Press Ganey Associates, 2017

The understanding that the patient experience is more than patient satisfaction and more than a score or percentile rank helps galvanize caregivers toward a meaningful improvement effort—that of reducing suffering.

Engagement of caregivers is critically important in providing an optimal patient experience. Measuring caregiver engagement helps identify areas of improvement as well. Organizations with high employee and physician engagement receive higher scores on every HCAHPS dimension. And those hospitals scoring in the top 10% of employee engagement average 61 percentile points higher on the HCAHPS Overall Hospital Rating item than hospitals in the bottom 10% (figure 10-3).

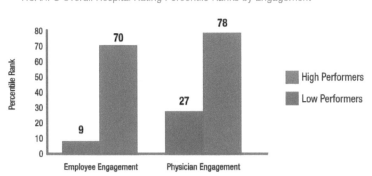

FIGURE 10-3. HCAHPS hospital rating of engagement

Engaged workers are committed to their employers, satisfied with their work, and willing to work harder to achieve the organization's goals, remain in their jobs, perform better, and have lower absenteeism. Hospitals and health systems with highly engaged employees perform better on safety, quality, and experience measures and find it easier to recruit top talent (Press Ganey Associates, 2017). Figure 10-4 demonstrates how the measures of caregiver engagement fall into the domains of Compassionate Connected Care for the caregiver.

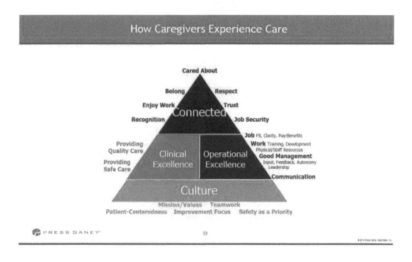

FIGURE 10-4. Compassionate Connected Care for the caregiver

Again, it is not enough to talk about the stress and distress that caregivers experience or to measure it in engagement surveys. Although both are important, addressing opportunities to reduce stress and distress and build resilience is more important. A similar affinity diagram elicited six themes for caregivers:

- Management should acknowledge the complexity and gravity of the work provided by caregivers

- Management has a duty to provide support in the form of material, human, and emotional resources

- Teamwork is a vital component for success

- Empathy and trust must be fostered and modeled

- Caregivers' perception of a positive work/life balance reduces compassion fatigue

- Communication at all levels is foundational

Similarly, actions and strategies demonstrate how to address each theme (see table 10–5).

From an industry perspective, there is a risk of becoming isolated and insulated since industry personnel rarely take care of patients or provide operational leadership in healthcare organizations, except in some cases at the board level. That makes listening, reading, and attending meetings where healthcare providers and leaders are present all the more important. As CNO, one of my first orders of business was to talk with CNOs from multiple organizations and across the country to hear thoughts, concerns, and platforms that were important to them. It is particularly important that industry organizations actually look like the client organizations they serve. If the industry partner serves healthcare organizations, where arguably nurses have the biggest impact, there must be nursing representation in leadership on the industry side mirroring the nursing-leadership representation on the client side. As the Institute of Medicine (IOM) report *The Future of Nursing: Leading Change, Advancing Health* states, "Eventually, to transform the way health care is delivered in the United States, nurses will have to move not just out of the hospital, but also out of health care organizations entirely" (IOM, 2011). In order to fully transform healthcare delivery, nurses must be relevant and outspoken in industry partnerships as well. To that end, after extensively listening to nursing leaders and observing the healthcare landscape, Press Ganey formed a CNO advisory council consisting of CNOs from small, medium, large, academic, community, pediatric, ambulatory, and oncology organizations. This group meets face to face annually and virtually every quarter for two hours. By partnering with these nursing leaders, Press Ganey is able to ask questions and solicit information regarding potential products and services and also gain invaluable information about the leaders' needs and challenges. In this way, healthcare and industry are true partners and not simply a vendor–client interactional relationship. This can only be accomplished with nurse leadership in both industry and healthcare.

TABLE 10–5. Tactics and strategies to reduce caregiver suffering

Actions	Images
We should acknowledge the complexity and gravity of the work provided by caregivers.	
Caregivers need to receive recognition from leaders and colleagues for the work they do. Rewards may be tangible or intangible. Leaders voice their understanding of and appreciation for the work of caregivers.	Managers recognize good work (not just pointing out what the unit is doing wrong). Managers work side by side with me. I receive positive feedback from coworkers and patients. Provide small doses of appreciation: thank-yous, thank-you notes, managing up, positive approaches. Managers ask me, "What can I do to help you and support you as a caregiver?" There is caring and true support from nurse managers that order food or bring in other treats for the staff on occasions. Provide positive praise daily! Use liberally for coworkers and as a nurse manager to subordinates. Leadership provides resources for dealing with difficult situations and establishing a safe and standard (daily) practice to decompress (being able to talk about the situation, sharing what went well, what needed to go better, and how you felt about what was happening).
It is the responsibility of management to provide support in the form of material, human, and emotional resources.	
Leaders create a positive work environment. Appropriate staffing is ensured and well communicated. Material resources necessary for care are available and in good working order.	Managers invest in the staff and let them know they care and support them. Managers understand the hurt, stress, or grief that I am going through. Managers see that a staff member is going through something and would communicate and put themselves in my shoes. Management provides training and exposure to new ways to care and communicate with others. Adequate staffing is available to allow me the time needed to connect with my patients. Necessary lunch breaks or a quick break to take a walk off the unit to recollect are provided. Management addresses clinical competence concerns. Leadership provides resources for dealing with difficult situations and establishing a safe and standard (daily) practice to decompress (being able to talk about the situation, sharing what went well, what needed to go better, and how you felt about what was happening). You are able to cry with the family and know that you are also supported. Create an environment that is safe, nonjudgmental, supportive, empathetic, and healthy so that the caregiver feels comfortable and encouraged to share concerns, questions, and suggestions for improvement and so that the caregiver can thrive in their role.

Actions	Images
Teamwork is a vital component for success.	
Multidisciplinary teams work together with patients and are organized around patient needs. Team members support one another.	Team building, holding each other accountable and working together, is active and fostered. Staff is aligned with the mission of the organization. Everyone works together as a team to meet one common goal: patient care. There are employee assistance programs for teammates dealing with difficult situations. We engage in mutual relationships with patients, families, and colleagues to foster physical and spiritual healing while honoring human dignity, values, and beliefs. There is pastoral care and pet therapy at huddles for teammates when there is a difficult loss of a patient or loved one. 360-degree communication regarding the plan of care allows the team to present a unified approach and promotes a feeling of safety for our patients.
Empathy and trust must be fostered and modeled.	
Caregivers demonstrate empathy to each other and patients. Trust is built on accountability, integrity, and fidelity at levels of the organization.	We treat one another with respect, anticipating others' needs. Staff are capable of putting themselves in their patient's position (empathy) and being nonjudgmental. Staff are people oriented rather than task oriented. There is an environment of mutual respect and support—standing behind me and not just beside me. Know me on a personal level. After losing a patient in an exhausting code, my sense of failure melted away when a respected colleague hugged me tightly and said: "You did a great job. I am so sorry." The first people on my doorstep after my brother died were my coworkers.
Caregivers' perception of a positive work/life balance reduces compassion fatigue.	
Caregivers feel that their work is meaningful. Leaders identify caregivers who exhibit burnout and intervene appropriately.	Support is available to prevent and to treat burnout. Choices are provided; offer a selection of incentives to choose from. Flexibility in shift assignments is provided. I protect my own health and healing as a whole being of body, mind, and spirit with as much enthusiasm and dexterity as I give to others. One has quality downtime on days off, doing something the healthcare provider enjoys, which is important to recharge one's batteries. Debriefing sessions occur after a traumatic patient or family event for therapeutic talk and support. Caregivers leave work a good tired—that is, they may be tired from a long day, but they know that they gave their patients excellent care and feel good about that care when they leave.

(continued)

Actions	Images
Communication at all levels is foundational.	
Communication and transparency are fundamental to demonstrate empathy and trust.	I listen to my patients and other staff members to understand their needs.
	Managers and coworkers listen and hear your worries and physical needs.
	We need to be alert because things can change so quickly and life can change instantly; communication and response is key.
Listening is a key component of communication.	There is clear, direct, timely communication of clinical impressions and plans between all members of the team to align our focus and messaging to our patient.

Reflective Questions

Think about your involvement in a major initiative or project either as a leader or participant.

- What leadership characteristics were most impactful on the outcome of that project? What leadership characteristics would have improved the structure, process, or outcomes of that project?

- What was the vision for the project?

- Was there alignment on this project across all stakeholders and departments? If not, why not? And how would you do it differently on a future project?

- How well was the project executed? Were the desired goals and aims met or unmet?

- Take a few minutes to develop a RACI model for the project. Are you able to easily identify the R, A, C, and Is for the project? If not, why not?

Chapter Key Points

- The voice and influence of professional nursing on policy and practice is important for all sectors of healthcare.

- While we have made progress on the journey to consistently achieve exemplary patient and nurse outcomes with quality and safety, significant gaps in knowledge and skills among nurses remain.

- Leader preparation and training and contemporary leadership models provide insights into the most influential leader characteristics that promote change and support best nursing practice in all practice settings.

- Examples of leadership in two nontraditional settings—a professional association and industry—provide insights into the leadership qualities and practices that are successful in driving large-scale initiatives and change.

References

Borkowski, N. (2011). *Organizational behavior in health care* (2nd ed.). Burlington, MA: Jones & Bartlett Learning.

Chassin, M. & Loeb, J. (2011). The ongoing quality improvement journey: Next stop, high reliability. *Health Affairs, 30*(4), 559–68.

Centers for Medicare & Medicaid Services. (n.d.). *The HCAHPS survey: Frequently asked questions.* Retrieved from https://www.cms.gov/medicare/quality-initiatives-patient-assessment-instruments/hospitalqualityinits/downloads/hospitalhcahpsfactsheet201007.pdf

Dempsey C. (2017). *The Antidote to suffering: How compassionate connected care can improve safety, quality, and experience.* New York, NY: McGraw-Hill Education.

Dempsey, C., Wojciechowski, S., McConville, E., & Drain, M. (2014). Reducing patient suffering through compassionate connected care. *The Journal of Nursing Administration, 44*(10), 517–24.

Institute of Medicine. (2001). *Crossing the quality chasm: A new health system for the 21st century.* Washington, DC: National Academies Press.

Institute of Medicine. (2011). *The future of nursing: Leading change, advancing health.* Washington, DC: National Academies Press.

Kania, J. & Kramer, M. (2011). Collective impact. *Stanford Social Innovation Review.* Retrieved from https://ssir.org/articles/entry/collective_impact

Lacasse, C. (2013). Developing nursing leaders for the future: Achieving competency for transformational leadership. *Oncology Nursing Forum, 40*(5), 431–33.

Malloch, K. & Porter-O'Grady, T. (2010). *Introduction to evidence-based practice in nursing and health care* (2nd ed.). Burlington, MA: Jones & Bartlett Learning.

Murphy, M. P., Staffileno, B. A., & Carlson, E. (2015). Collaboration among DNP- and PhD-prepared nurses: Opportunity to drive positive change. *Journal of Professional Nursing, 31*(5), 388–94.

Ketefian, S., & Redman, R. W. (2015). A critical examination of developments in nursing doctoral education in the United States. *Revista Latino-Americana de Enfermagem, 23*(3), 363–71. http://doi.org/10.1590/0104-1169.0797.2566

Porter-O'Grady, T. & Malloch, K. (2010). *Innovation leadership: Creating the landscape of health care.* Sudbury, MA: Jones & Bartlett.

Rice, D. (2016, March). The research doctorate in nursing: The PhD. *Oncology Nursing Forum, 43*(2), 146–48.

Smith, M. L., Erwin, J., & Diaferio, S. (2005). *Role & responsibility charting (RACI)*. Retrieved from https://pmicie.starchapter.com/images/downloads/raci_r_web3_1.pdf

Straw, J., Davis, B., Scullard, M., & Kukkonen, S. (2013). *The work of leaders: How vision, alignment, and execution will change the way you lead*. New York, NY: Wiley & Sons.

Whittington, J. W., Nolan, K., Lewis, N., & Torres, T. (2015). Pursuing the triple aim: the first 7 years. *The Milbank Quarterly, 93*(2), 263–300.

Yoder-Wise, P. (2011). *Leading and managing in nursing* (5th ed.). St. Louis, MO: Mosby.

Chapter 11

Academic Practice Partnerships: Key to the Future of Our Profession

Judy A. Beal, DNSc, RN, FNAP, FAAN
Marsha L. Maurer, MS, RN
Cecilia McVey, MS, RN, FAAN

It is all about relationships . . . relationships that start at the top and transcend all levels of the partnering organizations. Mutual trust and respect are the cornerstones of this relationship.

Introduction

As stated in the 2010 report *The Future of Nursing: Leading Change, Advancing Health* published by the Institute of Medicine (IOM; now the National Academy of Medicine), nurses are in a key position to transform healthcare delivery (IOM, 2010). This landmark report is the most cited report ever published by the National Academy of Medicine. Its four key messages recommend that nurses, having achieved higher levels of education, must be able practice to their full scope of education and practice as full partners with physicians and other healthcare providers to transform the American healthcare delivery system. Regardless of the political landscape and the future of the Affordable Care Act, it is clear that our healthcare system needs redesign. Nurses today—more than seven years later—remain pivotal as leaders of healthcare transformation.

Originally defined by Merriam-Webster's Dictionary within a mathematical construct, *transformation* is "the operation of changing . . . one configuration or expression into another; a change of variables or coordinates in which a function of new variables or coordinates in substituted for each original variable or coordinate" ("Transformation," 2018). In our case, transformation refers to the variables of healthcare redesign and an antecedent variable, specifically the educational level of nurses. *The Future of Nursing* report specifically recommends that 80% of all nurses be educated at the baccalaureate level by 2020 and that the number of doctorally prepared nurses increase by 50% in that time. Anticipated consequences of this transformation include removing scope-of-practice barriers and achieving nursing's full participation with other healthcare providers. Nurse executives in both academic and service (practice) settings are the leaders critical to this transformation.

Transformational leadership has been defined as "a leadership approach that causes change in individuals and social systems" (Bass, 1985) was originally introduced in 1978 by James McGregor Burns and later extended by Bernard M. Bass (1985). Bass focused on the individual traits of transformational leaders, which can clearly be extrapolated to today's nursing leaders. These leadership competencies include:

- Individualized consideration to followers' needs,

- Intellectual stimulation during which the leader challenges assumptions and develops independent followers,

- Inspirational motivation whereby the leader inspires a shared and exciting new vision, and

- Idealized influence through which the leader commands and receives trust and respect (Bass, 1985).

More recently, Scott and Schwartz (2017) identified the top ten S&P 500 companies that ranked highest in new-growth transformation. They then identified common characteristics and strategies of the companies' CEOs. Common themes included a dual-transformation approach in which leaders repositioned core business while actively pursuing new opportunities for growth, leveraged core values of the business, used narrative storytelling to describe the vision for the future, and developed a road map or strategy early on before the disruptive innovation took hold.

In this chapter, we share our stories of how three Boston-based nurse leaders—one academic dean and two chief nursing officers—transformed academic–practice partnerships to address the recommendations of the 2010 *The Future of Nursing* report. We highlight critical work that has been done at the national level as well as specific exemplars from Boston. We specifically address the transformational leadership strategies we have shared.

Academic–Practice Partnerships Redefined

When we first became leaders in Boston in the late 1990s, it was a rare-but-nice collegial gesture for us to share what we were each doing at our respective institutions. We were however completely siloed, and academic–practice partnerships were viewed as purely clinical placements. We had a partnership because the school of nursing had asked for a number of clinical placements, which the hospital gladly provided and where students and faculty were viewed as guests in the service arena. Even before the landmark 2010 report published by the National Academy of Medicine, we were beginning to realize that this was not an effective approach to getting our work done or to preparing the nurses of the future. Joint faculty–clinical appointments, partnerships on clinical and research projects, and some minimal consultation began to spring forth.

Shortly after *The Future of Nursing* report, national leaders began to realize that the only significant approach to meeting the recommendations by 2020 was to bring the dialogue to the national stage. In 2012, the American Organization of Nurse Executives (AONE) joined together with the American Association of Colleges in Nursing (AACN) to establish a task force on academic–practice partnerships. Based on earlier work during a Robert Wood Johnson Executive Nurse Fellowship (Beal et al., 2011), the task force developed a series of guiding principles for developing and sustaining such partnerships. These guidelines included: (1) mutual trust and respect; (2) a shared vision, mission and goals; (3) a formalized relationship that begins with senior leadership and cascades through all levels of the organizations; (4) systematic evaluation of goals; (5) shared responsibility and resources; and (6) frequent engagement, ongoing commitment, and transparency (Beal et al., 2012). These guiding principles were applied to strategies that aligned with *The Future of Nursing*'s recommendations.

Early work by this task force included a survey of members of the AACN, AONE, and the Association of State and Territorial Directors. The top partnership activity identified by the 455 participants was clinical-affiliation agreements. While participants met anywhere from monthly to once or twice a year with their partners, more than 50% did not have a formalized partnership agreement beyond clinical-affiliation agreements and more than 60% never evaluated outcomes against goals. The task force subsequently conducted eight focus groups with volunteers from these member associations; the results were similar (Beal et al., 2012).

Recognizing that there was monumental work to be done to accomplish the goals put forth in *The Future of Nursing* report, the AACN and AONE partnered further. Both committed to institutionalizing the work within their respective missions and goals by establishing the AACN-AONE Steering Committee. The work of this committee has included a tool kit of best practices that includes an extensive literature review on academic–practice partnerships; guiding principles of academic–practice partnerships; a step-by-step guideline of best practices to build, sustain, and evaluate partnerships; and exemplars of AACN-AONE Award recipients for Best Academic-Practice Partnerships. Additionally, the AACN continues to host webinars and an internet-based collaboration community (https://www.aacnnursing.org/Academic-Practice-Partnerships/Webinars).

In 2015 the AACN commissioned Manatt Health to conduct a study on how academic nursing can thrive in an era of healthcare transformation. The final report, *Advancing Healthcare Transformation: A New Era for Academic Nursing,* was published in 2016 and deeply examines the potential for enhanced partnerships between academic and service institutions. While the report was originally commissioned to address gaps in academic health centers and affiliated schools of nursing, as is the case in Boston, the majority of AACN member schools are not housed in an academic health center. While AACN is currently commissioning a similar report more related to schools of nursing like Simmons, the findings of this report hold significant weight for all schools and their practice partners. The major findings of the report include:

- Academic nursing is not positioned as a partner in healthcare transformation;

- Institutional leaders recognized the missed opportunity for alignment with academic nursing and are seeking a new approach; and

- Insufficient resources are a barrier to supporting a significantly enhanced role for academic nursing (AACN, 2016).

Recommendations from this report focus on how to "embrace a new vision for academic nursing" and include:

- Enhance the clinical practice of academic nursing;

- Partner in preparing the nurses of the future;

- Partner in the implementation of the Affordable Care Act;

- Invest in nursing research program and better integrate research into clinical practice; and

- Implement an advocacy agenda to support a new era for academic nursing (AACN, 2106).

This chapter highlights how two innovative partnerships have worked to specifically implement several of these recommendations.

In 2017 the boards of both the AACN and the AONE committed to further this important work during a day of dialogue in April. We agreed to strengthen our collaboration by convening the AACN-AONE Advisory Committee to discuss issues and opportunities for collaboration between academic and service leadership, focusing on emerging workforce issues that impact our profession and healthcare delivery. A key component of this work will focus on innovative strategies to prepare a better-educated professional nursing workforce to lead healthcare transformation—and that is our story from Boston.

Exemplars from Boston
Simmons College School of Nursing and Health Sciences
Judy A. Beal, DNSc, RN, FNAP, FAAN

Simmons College has been educating nurses since 1902 and nurse practitioners since 1978. Simmons has an exceptionally strong reputation for preparing nurses with expertise in clinical and leadership competencies, as documented by preceptors, patients, employers, and practice partners. Located in the heart of the Longwood Medical Area, Simmons is one of more than twenty-two baccalaureate and graduate programs in Massachusetts and one of six in Boston. This richness creates both a challenge and an opportunity. In many cities there is a clear alignment of an academic institution's nursing and medical schools with a particular academic medical center. In Boston there is no such alignment of academic nursing, academic medicine, and the medical center. This lack of alignment offered us the opportunity to create an innovative academic–practice partnership but also challenged us as leaders to work collaboratively in a competitive environment.

When I first became chair of nursing in 2000, I invited every chief nursing officer (CNO) to participate on my advisory board. At these meetings we discuss future trends in professional nursing and how we can best partner to meet the needs for the future workforce in Boston.

As a leader of one of the largest schools of nursing in Massachusetts, I envision my role as one that must transform professional nursing education for the Commonwealth. As an individual, nurse, educator, and chief academic officer, I have always predicated my work around the values of relationships, trust, and respect. Having had a long tenure in Boston, I have had long-term relationships with most of my practice colleagues. I believe that a personal relationship is just as important as a professional relationship and can solidify and strengthen it. I have strong personal and professional relationships with my colleagues Marsha Mauer, at Beth Israel Deaconess, and Cecilia McVey, at the Boston-Bedford Veteran's Administration Hospital System. I know that I can call them up and ask a favor and that I can count on a helpful and prompt response—and they can count on me as well. This mutual trust, deep respect, and friendship greatly enhances our professional partnership. It allows us to have the difficult conversations around mission and goals, strategy, resources, and accountability. This strong foundation allows us to take risks, make mistakes, start over, and make bold changes that are so necessary to transform how we can prepare nurses of the future. The following sections highlight successful academic–practice partnerships between Simmons College and the Veteran's Administration Boston Medical Center and between Simmons College and Beth Israel Deaconess Medical Center (BIDMC).

Veteran's Administration Boston Medical Center

Cecilia McVey, MS, RN, FAAN

As the associate director of nursing and patient care at the Department of Veterans Affairs (VA) Boston Medical Center, I led the initiative to develop an academic–practice partnership between the VA Boston Medical Center and six prestigious schools of nursing in 2007. The Northeast Region Veteran Administration Nursing Alliance (NERVANA) consists of Boston College, Northeastern University, Regis College, Simmons College, UMass Boston, and UMass Lowell. The relationships and commitment of the alliance have forged the development of leaders from administration to staff nurses.

NERVANA's mission statement was derived from the VA's parent mission:

> To employ an innovative educational model to expand and enrich nursing students and faculty, to educate nursing students in the care of veterans, and to expose nursing students to the advanced model of medical informatics, patient safety, quality improvement and integrated systems of care employed by the VA's National Health Care System.

The goals of NERVANA were developed and agreed upon as follows:

- To improve the recruitment and retention of VA nurses,

- To strengthen the faculty infrastructure for nursing education,

- To promote the entry of veterans into the nursing profession, and

- To enhance the nursing care of veterans within the VA healthcare system and the private sector.

Because we all share the same passion and excitement for the future of nursing and the importance of collaboration, the alliance continues to meet regularly to share, brainstorm, and discuss innovative educational nursing models. As a result, a significant increase in nursing research studies, publications, and presentations has emerged.

One of my first initiatives was to establish a nurse scientist role at the VA Boston. Two doctorally prepared nurse researchers from the academic partners were appointed to the VA. Under their expertise, nursing research studies were conducted. The nurse scientists are available as mentors to the VA staff nurses who are pursuing advanced nursing degrees. The nurse scientists serve on doctoral committees and mentor the next generation of nurse researchers. Current research includes new models of nursing education (dedicated educational units), patient-centered care, NP residency programs, heart-failure research, and evidence-based-practice projects.

Many VA Boston nurses are now seeking advanced degrees because of the addition of the nurse scientists from the NERVANA partnership. VA nurses are enrolled in programs including Doctorate of Nursing Practice, PhD, Masters in Nursing Education, and RN–BSN. The NERVANA partnership has provided advanced-degree opportunities for the staff nurses with several programs housed at the VA Boston Medical Center.

Of equal importance to the nurse scientist role is the VA associate chief of nursing service/academic affiliations. This position is pivotal to ensure timely communication between key stakeholders with the academic partners and with the practice site. This communication provides guidance and support to the variety of educational initiatives meeting the oversight qualifications and criteria. Guidance includes undergraduate clinical nursing placements in traditional and dedicated-education models as well as graduate-nursing clinical placements. The creation of this position was instrumental in providing the high-quality leadership that has contributed to the successful on-site survey visit and subsequent accreditation by the Commission of Collegiate Nursing Education (CCNE). Both the federally funded RN residency training program and the RN residency employee-based program at the VA Boston Healthcare System were accredited. The VA Boston Healthcare System Post Baccalaureate Nurse Residency program continues to maintain and excel in achieving its mission, goals, and expected outcomes because of the ongoing collaboration and support of the NERVANA academic partnership.

The addition of the nurse scientist has allowed more and expanded novel clinical rotations. The VA Boston is a leader in the development of dedicated nursing educational units (DEUs). This model of clinical education depends on the relationship between the academic and practice partners. It is based on the concept of the staff nurses educating the nursing students and the academic partners working with the staff nurses to develop their clinical teaching skills. The VA Boston currently has DEUs on medical-surgical, spinal cord injury, and long-term care units. Many staff nurses have adjunct faculty appointments and serve as clinical faculty for the nursing schools. With the shortage of nursing faculty, our academic–practice partnership has developed the next generation of nursing faculty and has tripled the number of nursing student clinical rotations and preceptor experiences.

Because of our DEUs with Simmons College, Boston College, Northeastern University, and Regis College, VA staff nurses have received vital training and education. These opportunities opened up new vistas for the staff, who are thrilled to help shape the nursing workforce of the future. It added variety and challenges not seen in the everyday staff-nurse roles, invigorated the nurses to advance their educations, and enhanced their employment satisfaction as nurses. The embedded academic faculty educate the VA staff on becoming clinical instructors and on the evaluation process, among other skills. The benefits of this additional education not only bolstered morale but made the VA rotation for students highly desired. Although DEUs have existed now for several years, I foresee them continuing to grow in popularity as they benefit all students, all staff, and the schools, and they are not cost prohibitive for the Medical Center. Nursing student rotations serve as a prime recruitment tool as nursing staff and unit managers know the graduates who are familiar with the VA and the mission. Many of the nursing students upon graduation apply to the CCNE-accredited VA Boston Nurse Residency Program.

In the newest publication from the AACN, *Advancing Healthcare Transformation: A New Era for Academic Nursing*, one of the main goals is to embrace a new vision for academic nursing. NERVANA accomplished this goal more than 10 years ago when we first sat at the extended table and agreed to work together for our academic partners. We became full partners in healthcare delivery, education, and research. By participating in one another's advisory boards and partnering together in enhancing the clinical practice of academic nursing, we discuss this goal at our NERVANA Steering and Advisory Board meetings over the course of each year. We established a VA colloquia series in 2009. Known as Care of the American Veteran Colloquia Series, this program is hosted by one school in the spring and one in the fall to present issues related to the specialized healthcare needs of the veteran population. These take place on campus so that the information available can be presented to all members of the college community, on such topics as military sexual trauma, post-traumatic stress, spinal cord injury, and myriad others. Attending and presenting at these series as a VA leader have exposed me to the views of the academic community and given me an opportunity to market the VA in a different light than is portrayed by the press.

In *Advancing Healthcare Transformation: A New Era for Academic Nursing*, the emphasis is on the shared vision of academic nursing and practice. I have found that embracing this shared partnership breeds only success for both. Transformational leaders in both areas need to declare the shared mission and values. They must lead by example on a new path for all in improvement of health outcomes and educating our future workforce—those already working and those about to graduate—with emphasis on the enhanced integration between the reality of practice and the preparation of academics.

Two successful NERVANA programs developed directly from the vision of the academic–practice partnership are the Care of the American Veteran Colloquia Series and the Growing as a Mentor Educational Series. Each has representation from the VA and six of the partnering schools.

Care of the American Veteran Colloquia was established during the first year of the partnership to meet the learning needs of the public and the nursing community at large. This would be the forum used by both clinical practice and academic partners to share insights about care of veterans and to generate ideas for advancing nursing and interprofessional practice, education, and research. A committee was established to identify topics, select content experts, and coordinate the programs. The academic partners agreed to rotate as the host for the program. The VA Boston agreed to provide the expert speakers to meet the proposed programs objectives. Several of the veteran-specific topics that have been presented at this biannual event at the schools have included traumatic brain injury, spinal cord injury, women veterans' healthcare needs, homelessness, care of the aging patient, and military sexual trauma. All programs have been interprofessional. The NERVANA colloquia series has excited the partnership's students and staff, and the programs are very well received and attended.

Growing as a Mentor Educational Series has been developed by the NERVANA partners to assist in developing competent staff nurses from novice nursing faculty to confident, competent adjunct faculty members. This biannual programing helps network the VA staff with both NERVANA partners' students and faculty. The educational series provides specific topics such as legal and ethical issues, the importance of reflection, patient-centered care, leadership, and evaluation.

At VA Boston, my role was to envision that shared vision and mission with the deans of the six schools and inventory our assets and liabilities in order to maximize our partnership. From the beginning, we explored ways to integrate our aspiring leaders into each setting. I initially thought that this would require a change in culture, but it was really as simple as providing opportunities for the VA nurses to sit on academic advisory boards, precept nursing students in the clinical practice site, participate in educational classes at the academic schools, listen to professional career goals, and respond with the programing to achieve the goals. Hiring nurse scientists at VA Boston cost little to the organization but has reaped benefits far beyond my expectations. Their participation in establishing our DEUs with Simmons (our sentinel partner) and training and educating our staff opened up new vistas for the staff, who were just thrilled to be help shape the nursing workforce of the future. It added variety and challenges not seen in their everyday staff nurse roles and invigorated them to advance their educations as well as enhanced their satisfaction as nurses. We were frequently oversubscribed with willing preceptors to participate in the Simmons DEU and oftentimes had to rely on a rotation system so that all of the staff could have an opportunity to participate as an instructor! The exposure to academic professional nursing staff, whether at the college or at the healthcare organization, served to educate the VA staff on becoming clinical instructors and how to provide constructive feedback to learners and evaluate the process, among other skills. The benefits of this additional education not only bolstered morale (which was already good) but made the VA rotation for students at Simmons one of the most highly desired. Simmons faculty provided on-site support and ongoing education for our staff and constantly provided feedback and guidance.

Having a successful academic–practice partnership that has grown and flourished during the past 10 years with no signs of weakening is evidence that bridging academic and clinical practice is feasible when the key leadership team allows and supports an environment for creative ideas in educating professional nurses of the future. The time invested and money is minimal; the outcomes and benefits are measurable and substantial. I have been so fortunate to have surrounded myself with transformational deans and faculty that it has enhanced my own satisfaction and that of my staff in ways I never envisioned. NERVANA was recipient of the 2017 AACN-AONE Academic-Practice Award and all deans and staff attended this momentous occasion. We recently learned that we are recipients of the 2017 New Era Award as well by AACN, another exciting affirmation of our success.

Beth Israel Deaconess Medical Center (BIDMC)

Marsha L. Maurer, MS, RN

I have been the CNO at Beth Israel Deaconess Medical Center (BIDMC) in Boston for over a decade. BIDMC is a Level I trauma center with 657 adult and 111 newborn licensed beds. It is an academic medical center affiliated with Harvard University and situated in what is known as the Longwood Medical Area, which houses not only BIDMC but several other Harvard-affiliated teaching hospitals, including Boston Children's Hospital, the Dana Farber Cancer Institute, and the Brigham and Women's Hospital. Both the Harvard Medical School and Simmons

College are also located in the Longwood Medical Area. The greater Boston area is also home to a number of other medical centers and hospitals, making for a rich learning and clinical care environment.

This richness creates both a challenge and an opportunity. The proximity of Simmons College, with its large and highly esteemed school of nursing, made it a natural partner and convening entity for multiple hospitals. Executing on this opportunity required us to come together to define a partnership vision. We were able to build on our history of shared work, including long-standing clinical placements of Simmons students in our institutions and the participation of local CNOs in the Simmons School of Nursing Advisory Board. This history had brought us together many times for shared work and discussion and was foundational to our working together to build shared programming. Through these historic relationships we had built the level of trust required to jointly develop a long-range strategic vision for an academic–practice partnership with the potential to transform nursing-leadership development.

The work of both AONE and IOM *The Future of Nursing* reports provided a starting place to develop our vision. In 2005 the AONE described the competencies required for effective nursing leadership. These include communication, relationship management, knowledge of the health-care environment, professionalism, and business skills and principles (American Organization of Nurse Executives, 2005). As previously noted, in 2010 the National Academy of Medicine published *The Future of Nursing: Leading Change, Advancing Health* report, which set the goal of preparing nurses to advance educational preparation and work to the full scope of their license in order to transform healthcare (IOM, 2010).

As the CNO of an academic medical center, I was keenly aware of the needs described by both the AONE and National Academy of Medicine and aware of the gap between BIDMC nursing leaders' level of skill and those competencies. This gap was rooted in the natural history of nursing-leader advancement in hospitals. Typically, new nurse leaders were pulled from the ranks of the clinical staff, always with excellent clinical skills but rarely formally prepared for the demands of a healthcare management position. It was also frequently the case that few clinical nurses aspired to be nurse leaders. The posting of a new entry-level nursing-leader position often yielded no internal applicants despite a candidate pool of clinical nurses numbering in the thousands. Clinical nurses often saw their local leaders struggling in the domains highlighted by AONE, such as establishing professionalism within their units, managing relationships across department lines, and managing finances. What clinical nurses saw was not drawing them to a leadership path. It was clear to me that we had a structural problem in the ways we developed nursing leaders, which required a long-range solution to address. Our transformational challenge was to understand the clinical nurses' needs and perceptions of nursing leadership, create an inspiring vision for their future as leaders, and develop and support the educational and practice paths that would prepare them to successfully transform healthcare.

The shared work of BIDMC and Simmons has focused on developing both the aspiring and the experienced nurse leader. For the aspiring leaders, we developed a Master's in Nursing Administration program. For the experienced leader, we developed an executive-track Doctorate of Nursing Practice program. Taken collectively, these two programs have created a clear path supporting nurses from direct clinical practice, into early management, and ultimately to executive-level healthcare leadership positions.

We initially focused on preparing the frontline nurse leader, the nurse manager. The CNOs and professional-development staff from each hospital worked collaboratively with Simmons College to tailor a curriculum that would prepare nurse leaders to meet the demands of healthcare management roles. Since all of our staff were in full-time management roles, we needed to structure the program to balance work, class, and study time and to ease the financial burden for participants. Careful joint planning led to a curriculum and program that integrated well with participants' work responsibilities, supported optimization of hospital tuition reimbursement and ease of payment through payroll deduction, and leveraged multiple organizations' opportunities for challenging clinical placements. BIDMC is now recruiting for its fourth class of MSN participants. While the first classes included primarily nurses who were already in management roles, more recent classes are recruiting aspiring future leaders.

The MSN program addressed the issue of academic preparation for more junior leaders but did not address the needs of our more experienced nurse leaders, who were already prepared at the master's level. For this group, and for our profession, the DNP was the next frontier. Hospital

CNOs and Simmons began to discuss how to develop a program that would meet the learning needs of very busy nurse leaders. In spring 2016 we launched our first Executive DNP cohort, with 31 students from five participating hospitals. BIDMC had 15 of the 31 students. The two-year program is largely online, with two face-to-face weekend sessions each semester. Anticipated graduation for this cohort is spring 2018.

By spring 2018, these two programs will have graduated a total of 53 BIDMC nursing leaders, 38 MSNs and 15 DNPs. Of the 38 MSN participants, 36 are still working at BIDMC, and more than half have moved into new, higher-level leadership roles within the organization. With each subsequent cohort, we are identifying clinical nurses with leadership potential at an earlier point, creating a continuous pipeline of future nursing leaders. This supports not only BIDMC but also the nursing profession more generally. Program graduates are supported to present and publish their program projects in healthcare journals and national conferences. They are likewise supported to become actively involved in professional organizations, such as the Organization of Nurse Leaders of Massachusetts, New Hampshire, Rhode Island, Connecticut and Vermont (ONL) and the AONE.

The academic–practice partnership between BIDMC and Simmons College has clearly brought enormous benefit to BIDMC. It has helped us establish a pipeline of nursing leaders who are well prepared to face the challenges of healthcare management. None of this would have been possible without the history of a strong and trusting working relationship between our institutions. This history allowed us to bring together the recommendations of the AACN *Advancing Healthcare Transformation* report, the IOM report on *The Future of Nursing*, and the AONE recommendations for nurse executive competencies to create a strategic vision for a partnership. This partnership would not only serve our respective institutions and our shared profession but ultimately form the underpinnings for nurses to lead healthcare into the future.

The benefits to Simmons, our students, and our faculty have been impressive as well. In addition to the expected increase in enrollment and revenues, Simmons and the School of Nursing and Health Sciences benefits by strengthening of both of our reputations with the practice community and in turn our ability to recruit preceptors and clinical faculty. Benefits to the cohort model for students include shared learning through group study, shared best practices, additional support for students by students, networking, and strengthening of work relationships within and outside of the practice environment. For faculty, the mutual learning and sharing of best practices that goes on in the classroom has led to increased faculty engagement and excitement. As the program director stated: "I feel like I work at BIDMC. I feel that I am intimately involved with the issues that healthcare organizations are facing every day and as a result I am a better teacher."

The outcome that this collaboration has produced so far—dozens of nurses prepared to lead both healthcare and professional organizations and to develop the evidence base for clinical and administrative nursing practice—reflects a truly transformative leadership process. This transformation required both CNO and Simmons College leaders to develop a long-range vision for nursing practice and to inspire, engage, and persuade not only program participants but the leaders of our respective institutions to support these initiatives. We needed to convince both participants and organizational leaders that their commitment of time and money would be a worthwhile investment. We accomplished this in two ways. First, we were able to describe a compelling long-range vision for the future of nursing leadership and the value it would bring to individuals and organizations. Additionally, we had a strong collective track record of credible and effective leadership within our respective organizations, which has been critical to our success.

Conclusions

In reflecting upon our partnerships, we all shared the vision for a more educated workforce for Boston. We have strategically advanced initiatives that respond to the IOM and *Advancing Healthcare Transformation* reports. We have partnered together in preparing the nurses of the future and in turn to transform healthcare delivery at both practice and academic settings. Specifically, through our successful academic–practice partnerships, we have:

- Increased the numbers of employees at both the VA and BIDMC who have advanced their education at baccalaureate, master's, and doctoral levels;

- Created an innovative succession plan for clinical and academic partners;

- Enhanced the clinical practice of our faculty at Simmons;

- Invested in nursing research programs and effectively integrated research findings into practice; and

- Enhanced the quality of patient care by advancing the education of the nursing workforce.

We have learned from each other and grown from our shared lived experiences. Our relationships both personally and professionally have been transformed. What's next in Boston for us? Who knows? But as Seth Godin (2012)—an entrepreneur, blogger, and former CEO of Yoyodyne, the industry's leading interactive direct-marketing company, which Yahoo acquired in 1998—has been credited with saying, "Transformational leaders don't start by denying the world around them. Instead, they describe a future they'd like to create instead."

Questions for Reflection

1. What are the values that shape your organization? What are the values that shape you as a leader? What is important to you? Think about these before you have your first meeting with a potential partner.

2. What are the major or emerging issues facing nursing in your locale?

3. What goals do you have for your organization? With whom might you partner to realize these goals more efficiently and effectively?

4. What are the benefits and barriers to partnering around these goals? With this potential partner? How might you work together to eliminate these barriers?

5. What kind of institutional resources do you have to bring to the partnership table?

6. How as a leader will you build a relationship with the leader(s) of your potential partnership?

7. What do you need help with? Who is a good resource for you as you begin your partnership journey? We would suggest that you link to the *AACN-AONE Academic-Practice Partnership Toolkit* (https://www.aacnnursing.org/Academic-Practice-Partnerships/Implementation-Tool-Kit).

Chapter Key Points

- It is all about relationships.

- Successful academic–practice partnerships are possible when the environment for creative ideas in educating professional nurses of the future can flourish.

- Communicate a shared vision to build momentum for change.

Key Points	Lessons Learned
We cannot transform nursing and healthcare in our traditional silos.	Academic–practice partnerships are the key to advancing the nursing profession and transforming healthcare.
Leaders have the responsibility of building and sustaining relationships.	Mutual trust and respect are the cornerstones of any academic–practice partnership.
There are several key components of an academic–practice partnership.	Shared vision and goals.
	A formalized relationship that begins with senior leaders and cascades through all levels.
	Systematic and regular evaluation of goals.
	Shared responsibility and resources.
	Frequent engagement, ongoing commitment, and transparency.
Academic nursing is not positioned as a partner in healthcare transformation.	There must be a commitment on the part of academia and service to change this paradigm. The 2016 AACN report *Advancing Healthcare Transformation: A New Era for Academic Nursing* provides suggestions for making this happen!
Sustaining academic–practice partnerships during leadership transformation is difficult.	But it is doable with institutional support and willingness on the part of leaders
Developing academic practice partnerships can be transformational for the profession and its leaders.	While it is not easy, the rewards far outweigh the barriers. Academic–practice partnerships are critical to the legacy and advancement of the profession as well as to leadership development.
Several transformational leadership strategies were used in Boston.	A long-range shared vision for the future of nursing.
	Long-standing mutual respect and trust for each other.
	Ability to inspire, engage, and persuade key stakeholders of the value of our partnership and initiatives.
	An understanding of the business of nursing.
	Tolerance for risk.
	Ability to procure institutional support and resources.
	Shared accountability for resources as well as our successes and failures.
	Commitment to life-long learning.
	Having fun!

References

American Association of Colleges of Nursing (2016). *Advancing healthcare transformation: A new era for academic nursing.* Washington, DC: Author.

American Organization of Nurse Executives (2005). AONE nurse executive competencies. *Nurse Leader, 3*(1), 15–21.

Bass, B. M. (1985). *Leadership and performance.* New York, NY: Free Press.

Beal, J. A., Breslin, E., Austin, T., Brower, L., Bullard, K., Light, K., . . . Ray, N. (2011). Hallmarks of best practice in academic-service partnerships: Lessons learned from San Antonio. *Journal of Professional Nursing, 27*(6), E90–E95. DOI: 10.1016/j.profnurs.2011.07.006

Beal, J. A., Alt-White, A., Erickson, J., Everett, L. Q., Fleshner, I., Karshmer, J., . . . Gale, S. (2012). Academic practice partnerships: A national dialogue. *Journal of Professional Nursing, 28*(6), 327–332. DOI: 10.1016/j.profnurs.2012.09.001

Institute of Medicine. (2010). *The future of nursing: Leading change, advancing health.* Washington, DC: National Academies Press.

Godin, S. (2012, October 2). Deny facts you don't like [blog post]. Retrieved from https://seths.blog/2012/10/denying-facts-you-dont-like-doesnt-make-them-not-facts/

Nagy, B. & Edelman, D. (2014). Transformation leadership in planning curricula. *Current Urban Studies, 2*(3), 198–211. DOI: 10.4236/cus.2014.23020

Scott, A. & Schwartz, E. I. (2017, May 8). What the best transformational leaders do. *Harvard Business Review.* Retrieved from https://hbr.org/2017/05/what-the-best-transformational-leaders-do

Transformation. (2018). In *Merriam-Webster online.* Retrieved from https://www.merriam-webster.com/dictionary/transformation

Additional Resources

American Association of Colleges of Nursing (2012). *AACN-AONE academic-practice partnership toolkit.* Washington, DC: Author.

Burns, J. M. (1978). *Leadership.* New York, NY: Harper and Row.

Chapter 12

Geriatric Leadership

Susan M. Lee, PhD, RN, CNP, ACHPN, FAAN
Teri Tipton, MSN, RN-BC, CNE
Deborah Marks Conley, MSN, APRN-CNS, GCNS-BC, FNGNA

What motivates me even more is that—as a nation— we didn't do well with taking care of our older population. From a nursing perspective, competencies did not adequately focus on the special needs of the older adult. The nursing process may be the same, but understanding of the goals, outcomes, and interventions varies widely. Who influences patient outcomes the most? Nurses. We had a long way to go.

—Teri Tipton

During my 31 years in nursing, most of my experience has been in the care of the geriatric patient. Two days after graduating from college, I started working the evening shift in the largest skilled nursing facility in Nebraska. I had other choices, but geriatrics interested me the most. My relationship as an adolescent with two mentors who were five to six times my age could have been what led me to my passion for older adults.

Or perhaps it is the state of healthcare. Unless you work in labor and delivery, pediatrics, or neonatal ICU, your predominant "clients" are older adults seeking health services. All I know is that it was a connection! I got my gerontological certification as soon as I had acquired the practice hours. I also had some amazing work mentors in my formative professional years who shared the same passion. I had the opportunity early in my career to become an Eden Alternative Associate, and I soon came to understand geriatric-friendly concepts.

—Teri Tipton

How nurse leaders get things done, particularly in times of shrinking resources, is of great interest to others. Influence plays a central role in helping stakeholders resource, adopt, and sustain new initiatives. As a core competency of nursing leadership, influence is defined as "the ability of an individual to sway or affect another person or group" (Adams & Ives Erickson, 2011, p. 186).

In this chapter, I (Susan) reflect with my coauthors on their extraordinary abilities to develop the gerontological nursing workforce and program at Omaha's Methodist Hospital (MH). Over the course of six years, MH ascended to Exemplar status, the highest of four levels of designation, as a member organization of Nurses Improving Care to Healthsystem Elders (NICHE), which recognizes the overall geriatric capacity of a health system. Because of their influence and efforts, Teri and Deborah have managed to integrate and sustain all major geriatric care models into the interprofessional practice environment, uniquely and expertly meeting the needs of older adults and their families. We frame these accomplishments through the lens of the Adams Influence Model (AIM) to demonstrate the effects of influence evident in their work (Adams & Ives Erickson, 2011).

Author Connections

In 2009 I issued a competitive call to US Magnet-designated hospitals inviting them to participate in AgeWISE, a geropalliative care nurse-residency program that was being piloted as a train-the-trainer program in Boston, Massachusetts. AgeWISE was made possible with financial and visionary support from Brenda Cleary, PhD, RN, FAAN, inaugural executive director of the Center to Champion Nursing in America, and Jeanette Ives Erickson, DNP, RN, FAAN, chief nursing officer and senior vice president of patient care services at Massachusetts General Hospital. The national selection committee chose MH as one of the first six pilot sites because of its demonstrated ability to enact and sustain geriatric initiatives. I still continue to be thoroughly impressed with the nurses at MH under the leadership of Teri Tipton, chief nursing officer and vice president for patient care, and Deborah Marks Conley, director of the geriatric service line, as they continue to evolve one of the most progressive general hospitals in the country that excels in geriatric care. Their achievements are impressive and difficult to obtain. I invited them to tell their story with me in this chapter—a story of influence that stems from their commitment to geriatrics.

The Setting

Methodist Hospital is a 420-bed community hospital serving the greater metropolitan community of Omaha, Nebraska. A Magnet hospital since 2004, and the first in the state of Nebraska, MH provides comprehensive tertiary inpatient services for diagnosis, treatment, and supportive care of medical-surgical patients and provides 22 beds in the licensed rehabilitation unit within the facility. The parent company of MH is Methodist Health Systems, which also runs the Methodist Women's Hospital, Methodist Jennie Edmundson Hospital, and Methodist Physician's Clinic. The RN–BSN and RN–MSN program at Nebraska Methodist College, which is affiliated with the health system, provides tuition-free education to registered nurses (RNs) who work at MH and its affiliates. In return, RNs agree to stay within the system a minimum of five years following graduation. The purpose of the RN–BSN program is to increase the number of BSN nurses, to improve retention, and to fulfill the goals of the Institute of Medicine's (2011) *Future of Nursing* report. The combined percentage of nurses with a BSN or higher at Methodist Hospital and Methodist Women's Hospital is 85%.

Geriatric Milestones at Methodist Hospital

In 2012, MH earned the highest level of NICHE designation, indicating an exceptional level of geriatric integration throughout the organization. In fact, MH has adopted every evidence-based geriatric model of care across the spectrum of care delivery. Our aim here is to focus on the implementation of each of these programs. The timeline (figure 12–1) gives an overview of geriatric milestones at MH and provides context as to when Teri (CNO) and Deborah (Gero CNS) joined MH.

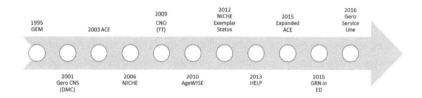

FIGURE 12–1. Timeline of geriatric initiatives at Methodist Hospital

1995: Geriatric Evaluation and Management Clinic

The Geriatric Evaluation and Management (GEM) Clinic, established in 1995, is the first milestone of geriatric specialty care at MH. It is staffed by an interprofessional team of geriatricians and other experts who conduct comprehensive geriatric assessments, resulting in plans of treatment that incorporate medical, functional, and psychosocial aspects of care to older adults, over one-half of whom have cognitive impairment. The goal is to improve quality of life for older adults and to provide support to family caregivers. Since its inception, the GEM Clinic has expanded services to include visits by an advanced practice nurse and geriatrician to retirement centers, long-term care facilities, and assisted-living facilities. Geriatric models of care strive to engage patients in their plan of care, assist them with living safely in the least restrictive environment, and focus on prevention strategies that optimize their functional status and quality of life. Although the GEM Clinic was not an initiative of the patient care division and it preceded the arrival of Teri and Deborah at MH, it was an important first step in setting MH's agenda of specialty geriatric care.

2001: Clinical Nurse Specialist

Methodist Hospital did not have any geriatric inpatient models of care prior to 2001, when Deborah Marks Conley was hired as the geriatric clinical nurse specialist (GCNS). She brought extensive community experience in implementing geriatric models of care as well as a strong national presence as a gerontological nursing leader. The clinical nurse specialist (CNS) is an advanced practice registered nurse prepared at the graduate level with expertise in a particular specialty, population, type of problem, setting, or type of care (National Association of Clinical Nurse Specialists, 2017). Deborah's specialty is geriatrics, most recently in the acute care setting.

It is interesting to note that the role of the CNS is described in terms of influence, the theoretical framework of this chapter. The National Association of Clinical Nurse Specialists (NACNS) defines the role of the CNS in terms of three spheres of influence: (1) patients, (2) nurses and nursing practice, and (3) organizations and systems (NACNS, 2010). According to the NACNS (2010), CNSs directly interact with patients and families "to promote health or well-being and improve quality of life" (p. 15). CNSs advance "nursing practice and improve patient outcomes by updating and improving norms of care and by using standards of care that direct actions of nurses and nursing personnel" (NACNS, 2010, p. 16). And they "influence systems changes that facilitate improvement of quality cost-effective patient outcomes" (NACNS, 2010, p. 16).

The GCNS is an expert in current geriatrics evidence and actively participates in geriatric professional organizations, joins committees, and leads teams and projects all while developing relationships that promote consensus around geriatric issues. Notably, the GCNS uses implementation science to teach and disseminate geriatric evidence across institutions. Implementing the GCNS role in organizations is an essential, cost-effective method to support nursing practice at the point of care (Conley et al., 2012a).

Deborah began by engaging staff nurses in best practices and by improving patient outcomes, along with encouraging and enabling nurses to achieve gerontological nursing certification (Conley et al., 2012a). She notes that less than 1% of US nurses are certified in gerontological nursing despite the growing population of older adults, which is estimated to nearly double by 2050 to 83.7 million (U.S. Census Bureau, 2014). Deborah formed collaborative relationships with many stakeholders to improve safety, quality, and fiscal responsibility and to facilitate care transitions for patients and families across the system.

She has developed, implemented, and evaluated the geriatric programs described below.

2003: Acute Care for Elders (ACE) Unit

Methodist Hospital's first inpatient geriatric program was a 14-bed acute care for elders (ACE) unit added in 2003. The ACE model is a proven, function-focused, prehabilitation, and restorative approach to hospitalized care (Fox et al., 2013). During hospitalization for an acute illness or injury, older adults are at risk of iatrogenic complications and functional decline. These complications have been associated with increased costs, institutionalization, and mortality in this population. Studies have documented, however, that the ACE model of care has benefits including improved processes of care; fewer complications common to older adults, such as delirium; improved patient, family, provider, and nurse satisfaction with care; reduced length of stay and 30-day readmissions; and lower per capita cost of care (Ahmed, Taylor, McDaniel, & Dyer, 2012; Barnes et al., 2012; Fox et al., 2013).

The original ACE unit at MH was formed from a skilled nursing and transitional care unit where the culture of care promoted patient function and a restorative approach. Staff development included education in the acute care of older adults and geriatric-focused interdisciplinary rounds. A geriatrician, a social worker, and the advanced practice GCNS (Deborah) led the development of this program and trialed and refined various geriatric practices. The motto on the ACE unit is that "the bed is not your friend" (Conley et al., 2012a). The four fundamental principles of the ACE unit include an environment prepared for older adults' patient-centered care, medication prescribing optimized by multidimensional assessment, and interdisciplinary team rounds linked with early, comprehensive discharge planning. In 2015 the initial ACE unit moved to a larger 32-bed medical unit where geriatric medical patients who do not need a higher level of care or disease specialty are admitted. After evidence is translated into practice on the ACE unit, these successful ACE protocols are disseminated to staff on all units to manage geriatric syndromes and prevent complications. Therefore, it continues to serve as an incubator for new geriatric protocols.

One lesson learned is that extensive geriatric education was needed to equip all staff with the knowledge and skills necessary to implement concepts of the ACE model. When MH implemented the model, it was not a NICHE hospital and was thus without access to the NICHE Knowledge Center educational resources. In addition, the inpatient acute physical therapist was accustomed to treating disease or injury rather than focusing on maintaining or promoting function in their absence. Once the interprofessional staff understood the concepts, they were all on board. The ACE unit was a pivotal jump start to implementing other geriatric models of care at MH. The outcomes of the ACE unit showed a decreased average length of stay by 0.5 days, decreased overall cost for specific medical diagnoses, and increased staff satisfaction.

2006: Nurses Improving Care for Healthsystem Elders (NICHE)

In 2006, MH began its membership in NICHE, an organization located at New York University that provides evidence-based knowledge, implementation resources, and leadership that helps drive change in geriatric systems among its 700-plus member hospitals and healthcare facilities in the United States and other countries (NICHE, n.d.). The goal of NICHE is to ensure that older adults receive sensitive care that aligns with patient preferences and promotes autonomy, function, and dignity. NICHE member sites improve care by addressing workplace needs, promoting leadership skills in nursing staff, promoting geriatric staff competence, and encouraging interprofessional processes. Member sites employ patient- and family-centered approaches in an environment that is safe for older adults. NICHE has expanded outside of acute care to include assisted-living, long-term care, and post-acute care facilities.

Methodist Hospital began its NICHE program in 2006. Since that time, multiple departments and interprofessional staff have enrolled in the NICHE Knowledge Center for online continuing education. The hallmark of NICHE is the geriatric resource nurse (GRN) model, which is a 21-hour online (or live classroom) training that results in the designation of GRN. Nurses who complete this advanced geriatric training become resources for their units in the care of older adults and implement geriatric best practices across the hospital (Conley et al., 2012a). The NICHE Steering Committee is composed of interprofessional and interdepartmental staff, including Teri, and serves as the overall structure from which geriatric models of care are implemented.

The success of NICHE at MH has been impressive. Since its NICHE affil-
iation began in 2006, MH ascended in six years to the highest level of
NICHE designation, that of Exemplar Hospital, demonstrating an impressive commitment to geriatrics. The hospital boasts a complement of 220
GRNs individualizing the comfort, care, and safety of geriatric patients.

One lesson learned was that the success of NICHE relies on its being
interprofessional and interdepartmental. Furthermore, Teri remains a
member of the NICHE Steering Committee, which signals the importance
of NICHE to the organization. Annually setting goals keeps the program
on a steady course and includes fun celebrations, like promoting older
adult awareness each year in May.

2010: AgeWISE

In 2010, just one year after Teri became the CNO, MH was selected as
one of the original six national pilot sites for AgeWISE (Lee et al., 2012).
This was Teri and Deborah's first joint geriatric initiative. AgeWISE is a
model of implementation for geropalliative care in the acute setting with
the goal of increasing nurses' effectiveness in caring for older persons in
the last two years of life. Six nurses from MH attended a train-the-trainer
program at Massachusetts General Hospital in Boston, where AgeWISE
was developed by one author (Susan). After the nurses returned, MH
committed significant resources in terms of faculty and indirect time to
AgeWISE, which was offered to 20 nurses in the first year as 12 classroom
days of eight hours each over the course of six months.

Since the initial implementation, MH has developed, refined, and transformed the AgeWISE nurse residency. It is a collaborative effort with
the Nebraska Methodist College Department of Nursing. The college
provides a faculty member who is an End-of-Life Nursing Education
Consortium (ELNEC) trainer and who has been with the program since
its development.

Both experts (more experienced nurses) and novices (less experienced
nurses) are invited by their managers and leaders to participate in the
six-month residency, which meets twice per month for eight hours.
Nurses from all levels of practice in multiple units and departments
participate, and there is a waiting list to enroll. Most AgeWISE residents
are staff nurses, but nurse directors, house supervisors, care managers,

nurse managers, charge nurses, staff-development nurses, and emergency nurses have also completed the residency. Two cohorts are implemented per year with an average of 21 nurses in each. The residency is treated as a work day for which staff are paid. It is rare that AgeWISE residents miss seminars, as the commitment is recognized and valued. Coursework is both within the residency and on the nurses' own time. The curriculum is based on modified components from ELNEC along with the Conley Gerontological Nursing Course and Palliative Care Clinical Practice Guidelines. Seminars, using transformational learning methods, include presentations from the hospital staff and from experts in the community. AgeWISE residents go to community clinical sites to learn about the continuum of care. They are required to obtain certification in either gerontological nursing, hospice and palliative care nursing, or their own specialty. Over 220 nurses at MH have completed the AgeWISE residency—more than at any other hospital in the country. AgeWISE is the expected norm of geropalliative nursing practice at Methodist Hospital.

Nurse-level outcomes of AgeWISE include providing better patient-centered geriatric care that focuses on the preferences, values, and beliefs expressed by older adults. AgeWISE nurses express feeling passionate about caring for this population and about being equipped to assess and manage the complexities of aging. They report becoming self-reflective in their nursing practice. They also report a feeling of pride with their new knowledge and skills, such as being able to initiate discussions about palliative care and the end of life. Professional growth occurs in other ways as well. AgeWISE nurses chair shared-governance councils and committees, are preceptors for new nurses, lead unit-based councils, and participate in quality-improvement and evidence-based practice projects. These same nurses are often selected by their peers for nurse-excellence awards each spring. Over one-third of AgeWISE participants continue their studies in graduate school, many selecting adult–gerontological nursing. An estimated 80% have maintained employment at Methodist throughout the past seven years.

By preparing nurses in primary palliative care, AgeWISE readied the hospital for the advent of its palliative care consult service, which ramped up more quickly than anticipated because the culture had been socialized to palliative care. In fact, the Pause for PEG initiative was started by AgeWISE nurses along with the speech and language pathologist who serves as a faculty member in AgeWISE. The initiative is a protocol that requires specific education to patients and families prior to the insertion of percutaneous enterostomal gastric (PEG) feeding tubes when the patient has advanced dementia. Evidence demonstrates that PEG feeding tubes are ineffective in these cases (Aparanji & Dharmarajan, 2010). Since starting this required education, no PEGs have been inserted for treatment of adult failure to thrive in advanced dementia, which represents a significant change in culture across disciplines at MH.

The implementation of AgeWISE did required a substantial financial commitment by the health system. Teri collaborated with the dean of the College of Nursing at Methodist College to have AgeWISE offered as a for-credit course. Staff nurses who are enrolled in the RN–BSN program at Methodist College obtain college credit for AgeWISE in lieu of taking the Complexity in Aging course.

2013: Hospital Elder Life Program (HELP)

The Hospital Elder Life Program (HELP) was adopted by MH in 2013 and is coordinated by the hospital's Volunteers in Partnership Program. Developed at Yale University, HELP aims to prevent delirium and functional decline by using volunteers who provide orienting visits, diversional therapies, and opportunities for ambulation and sleep hygiene (Inouye, Bogardus, Baker, Leo-Summers, & Cooney, 2000). Multicomponent strategies to address known risk factors are used by the HELP volunteers— college students in MH's case—many of whom are premedicine, nursing, and rehabilitative therapy majors. HELP education and training is conducted by certified gerontological nurses and a multidisciplinary team of geriatric experts who serve on the NICHE Steering Committee. The model we developed is unique because we did not employ an elder life specialist to assess patients prior to intervention by a HELP volunteer. Staff nurses at the point of care on each unit identify patients who would benefit from the program. HELP volunteers are specifically assigned to the ACE unit, a progressive care unit, or the emergency department. Additional HELP volunteers make rounds during the day on each unit to determine patient needs.

Core HELP interventions include orienting communication, engaging in therapeutic activities, promoting mobilization, assisting with vision and hearing adaptations, and developing strategies to address pain and comfort. Nurses refer to the HELP volunteers as "walkers and talkers." A DREAM team (which are HELP volunteers at night) was implemented on the ACE unit in 2015 and on the progressive care unit in 2017. The role of this team is to promote sleep hygiene and assist patients in night-time routines.

Deborah notes, "We learned to work around budget constraints by teaching and empowering nurses and nursing assistants to be able to identify patients appropriate for HELP." The program, which depends on volunteers, engages students, asking them to commit at least three hours a week for six months. This volunteer experience has a positive impact on students, who report that they love working with older adults and will consider practicing in geriatrics in the future. The HELP program raises the commitment and understanding of geriatric principles in the community one HELP volunteer at a time.

2016: Geriatric Resource Nurse in the Emergency Department

In 2015, we considered a GRN model of care in our emergency department (ED) to meet the nonemergency needs of older adults while minimizing delays or inefficient care and without disrupting ED throughput (Deschodt, Flamaing, Rock, Boland, Booen, & Milisen, 2012). Accordingly, we conducted a six-month feasibility study in which the GRNs coordinated geriatric-specific assessment and multidisciplinary care into routine ED care for older adults, who represent more than 40% of MH's ED patients. More than 30% of the overall ED population are admitted to the hospital. The GRNs in the ED are AgeWISE graduates and certified in gerontological nursing. In the pilot, an ED nurse screened older patients with the Identification of Seniors at Risk tool; 65% of seniors screened positive. For each of their patients, a GRN completes an assessment and collaborates with the dedicated social worker or an RN care manager in the ED. The GRN can consult a pharmacist or physical therapist per patient needs. The GRN makes two postdischarge phone calls at 24–48 hours and 10–14 days to improve patient outcomes. The outcome measures, currently being collected, are healthcare costs, 30-day ED readmissions, and patient and staff satisfaction. During the six-month pilot, 972 older patients with an average age of 79.4 were screened. Among those who presented with pain, falls, or weakness, 61% were female and 65% scored positively on the Identification of Seniors at Risk tool. The importance of multidisciplinary care coordination for older adults in the ED was evident. The pilot confirmed that the GRN model in the ED can successfully address nonemergency needs without disrupting ED throughput. Ongoing evaluation is in progress.

2016: Geriatric Service Line

In 2016, Teri advocated to create a geriatric service line to organize the existing geriatrics models of care and to provide leadership for continued program growth and development. This would also help fully integrate our geriatric-friendly services with other service lines in the hospital (e.g., women's health, orthopedics, cardiovascular, oncology, surgical services). Deborah was named the first director of the geriatric service line, which is reflected on MH's organizational chart, symbolic of and influential to the future growth of geriatric services.

About Influence

Teri Tipton, MSN, RN-BC, CNE

On November 23, 2009, I joined the Methodist family as the chief nursing officer and vice president of patient care services. CNOs have great influence: the preceding one had taken the organization to two consecutive Magnet designations—the highest level of nursing excellence—as the first in Nebraska to do so. Even more, we are NICHE designated—again the first in Nebraska. Therefore, much of the heavy groundwork was in place. We continued the journey of nursing excellence, developing a nurse residency, a new-graduate mentor program, a Professional Advancement Clinical Excellence Recognition, DAISY awards, and the AgeWISE nurse residency. We achieved a third Magnet designation, with a fourth designation planned in 2018.

To demonstrate the challenges and the parity, we finished construction of the new Women's Hospital in 2010 about 10 miles west of what is now the main campus, which was continually at capacity and still operating with double-capacity rooms. All women's services were relocated to the new location. We had robust labor and delivery services and mother-baby services, but we didn't have a neonatal intensive care unit (NICU).

Although this highly complex and specialized service was new to us, as change agents we included a 28-bed NICU in the construction plans.

So, while preparing for the silver tsunami, we were recruiting NICU nurses, developing NICU services such as competencies and education, recruiting perinatologists and neonatologists, and purchasing ventilators, special lighting, sound minimization, and so on.

I observed that others perceived the NICU as more glamorous than geriatrics. The NICU is a great cause and the board was all in. So was the community. Fundraising for the NICU strategic initiative had lots of support. Leading a culture change to fully integrate geriatric concepts at every encounter would take effective communication, relationship building, advocacy, and change management.

Therefore, advocating for MH to be geriatric friendly and nurses to become AgeWISE was sometimes a challenge, though not rocket science. The facts and statistics speak volumes. We are a community hospital in the heart of Omaha with a reputation of excellence in many service lines, along with our primary care clinics and internal medicine clinics located throughout the community; the volumes were strong. The three patient units that were vacated by women's services at MH were full, mostly with patients over the age of 65. Methodist has greater than a 30% market share in many Omaha-area zip codes, and the baby boomer population is much of that market share.

For the CNO to influence the CEO and board of directors in order to gain support, it takes a fiscal, business mindset. Translating clinical perspectives to business plans, constructing a business case, and determining the return on investment are essential.

The most impactful statement was one word: Medicare. Every health-care management journal attests to the shrinking of reimbursements that was, is, and will continue to be the case for Medicare patients. The CMS's direction to transition from fee-for-service to quality outcomes and patient experience was in my corner.

When the CEO and CFO hear that market-share is increasing—the light goes on. But when it is mostly Medicare patients—the light dulls. Pro forma statements demonstrated what we call soft dollars. The CEO said he has a whole drawer of soft dollars. Nevertheless, we did not run from the transition; we embraced it.

My shared-leadership philosophy is to assess the staff and patient needs and appropriately provide resources, training, and education. The interprofessional NICHE team members were supported with education, training, time, and a budget to trial ideas to improve patient care. The team worked with other councils and committees for things like patient rights and ethics and end of life to promote their geriatric clinical perspective to all disciplines.

The CNO has to take a systems perspective while emulating the voice of the nurse from the bedside and must never ever take their eye off the patient experience and patient-centered care delivery. I looked beyond the walls of MH and reached out to a sister hospital in Iowa, inviting them to join our NICHE meetings to help them start the journey to becoming geriatric friendly.

The ED plays a key role in acute care of illness and injury. It needs to be a safety net for our patients. Integrating emergency medicine with geriatric principles in a cost-constrained environment where consumers have high expectations seemed to this CNO to be crystal clear. The goal was to quickly identify physical and psychosocial needs, ensure the correct inpatient placement and services when needed, identify community resources, and prevent readmissions. I knew this age-appropriate care delivery model was crucial to the care of our geriatric patients and services.

However, when developing the GRN role in the ED, we met with resistance, as happens with most change. We educated and trained. We educated and trained again. We had discussions and conversations. We had support of managers, providers, and nursing executives, leaders, and support staff to attend the NICHE conference but adoption was slow. We pushed instead of pulled.

Then in 2016, the CNO strategically advocated to attend the NICHE conference with an ED nurse, a nurse leader of care transitions who was our NICHE coordinator to speed up adoption. The excellent agenda and breakout sessions facilitated the firsthand knowledge and experience for these nurses and the CNO. The relationship building and the CNO role modeling the priority of this care delivery model was a change maker. Today our GRNs in the ED make a difference every day.

Nursing leaders know the importance of nurse certification. Methodist's nurse certification percentage was good—but not great and certainly not excellent—hovering around 24%. And although our AgeWISE nurse residency was certainly improving patient care and professional advancement, we weren't maximizing this investment.

We wanted patient outcomes to improve as well as nurse satisfaction. Nurses are very proud to say, "I am an AgeWISE nurse." We asked, "Shouldn't gerontological nursing or hospice and palliative care nursing certification be a part of this investment in our RNs' professional development?" Therefore, we created the expectation that those not already holding a nursing certification would achieve one, either in gerontological nursing, hospice and palliative nursing, or in their own specialty.

One barrier our nurses reported was the financial cost of the certification test. Although the Methodist Foundation reimbursed RNs after they completed certification, many nurses shared financial constraints paying for the test at the time of registration. In 2015, I secured participation in the ANCC Success Pays program, providing financial support for certification at the time an RN registered for the certification test. Having the resource of time to attend AgeWISE, and the financial support to test, is an example of nurse excellence at MH.

RN retention on our medical unit was like that of other medical inpatient units, with higher turnover. After a few years of experience, nurses wanted to transfer to a specialty unit. Meanwhile, the scattering of our geriatric medical patients throughout the hospital was ineffective and inefficient. While discussing the annual performance appraisal with the service executive, I established the goal of relocating the existing ACE unit to the larger medical unit. With NICHE and AgeWISE, the soil was warmed on that unit, the seed planted, and all we needed to do was feed and water it—which was a lot of work, but it happened!

This delivery model has benefited not only the patients and their families but also the nurse practice environment. The turnover has quieted down. Employee engagement is on the rise! And this unit had the participation of all 76 full-time employees in the 2017 employee Caring Campaign, the system's annual fundraising appeal.

Providers are also key. Every month, I attend a Medical Executive Committee meeting and provide an operational update to its members. Frequently, that update highlights geriatric-friendly initiatives, keeping patient-centered care front and center. This influence tactic is critically important to our focus on geriatrics. Almost 100% of our physicians and providers rate the quality of nursing care as being very high, contributing to their satisfaction working at MH.

Quantifying Leadership

Perhaps the most difficult aspect of this work is to quantify these accomplishments further than measuring the number of nurses educated, nurses certified, patients who avoided harm, or unplanned nursing home admissions and further than measuring metrics like length of stay. One of my (Susan's) mentors is Marita Titler, PhD, RN, FAAN, and author of the Iowa Model of Evidence-Based Practice to Promote Quality Care. She told me about the guiding principle behind her impressive evidence-based-practice program at the University of Iowa Hospitals and Clinics. She said, "You just have to do the right thing for patients" (personal communication, 2009). I am certain that doing the right thing for patients is also what motivates Teri and Deborah.

Gerontological nurses understand that hospitalization is a sentinel event for older adults. Geriatric knowledge and expertise is fundamental to identifying and mitigating risk. The fact that every nurse leader is a certified gerontological nurse on the unit is important to understanding why this extensive geriatric programming occurred.

While the evidence for ACE and HELP is convincing (Fox et al., 2013; Inouye et al., 2000), evidence for the GRN model is still in its infancy. There is some evidence that higher rates of nursing certification are associated with lower rates of total patient falls, hospital-acquired pressure injuries, selected hospital-acquired infections, failure to rescue, and mortality, but there is also contradictory evidence (Boyle, 2017). Biel et al. (2014) reviewed eight studies of nursing certification and patient outcomes, concluding that there are methodological limitations in the current research, all of which considers certification as a nominal demographic variable (yes or no) in descriptive research. The authors make a compelling argument that current research methods may fail to capture what constitutes certified nursing practice. In other words, it's complicated.

Kendall-Gallagher, Aiken, Sloane, and Cimiotti (2011) found that certification had no effect on patient outcomes for nurses with less than baccalaureate education. They concluded that a 10% increase in baccalaureate nurses who are certified is associated with lower mortality and less failure to rescue among surgical patients. This supports Teri's strategy of increasing the number of baccalaureate-prepared and baccalaureate-certified nurses at MH.

While acknowledging that research methods are insufficient to explain the benefits of certification and even some models of care, we must still forge ahead, requiring and supporting advanced training in geriatrics, a population that faces exceptional vulnerability in today's hospitals.

Final Words of Influence

The AIM recognizes five tactics of influence: knowledge-based competence, authority, status, communication traits, and the use of time and timing, within personal, interpersonal, and social systems. Two certified gerontological nurses have successfully advocated for education, committees, for-credit courses, personnel, free tuition, indirect time, certification fees reimbursement, and several geriatric models of care including the pioneering work in the ED to bring this 420-bed hospital to the forefront of geriatric-centered care in the United States.

Deborah, as a leading authority in gerontological nursing, has used each of the AIM influence tactics in her roles at MH. Her guiding values have always been upholding function, dignity, and choice of older persons by identifying risk and preventing harm and functional decline.

Teri also has a laser focus on geriatrics in her role at MH. Enabled by influence, she has broad support across disciplines to enact a bold vision. These remarkable nurse leaders and how they built geriatric capacity is a most unusual story that deserves attention and replication everywhere.

Chapter Key Points

- The challenges of the aging population will continue to require more resources in the coming years as 20% of the population reaches age 65 and above.

- Those over the age of 65 have been called the core business of hospitals and are the primary population affected by hospital-related harms, such as falls, pressure ulcers, hospital-associated disabilities, infections, delirium, and other geriatric syndromes.

- The geriatric population requires and deserves a nursing workforce that can care well for their specific needs.

References

Adams, J. M. & Ives Erickson, J. (2011). Applying the Adams Influence Model in nurse executive practice. *The Journal of Nursing Administration, 41*(4), 186-92.

Ahmed, N., Taylor, K., McDaniel, Y., & Dyer, C. B. (2012). The role of an acute care for the elderly unit in achieving hospital quality indicators while caring for frail hospitalized elders. *Population Health Management, 15*(4), 236-40.

Aparanji, K.P. & Dharmarajan, T.S. (2010). Pause before a PEG: A feeding tube may not be necessary in every candidate! *Journal of American Medical Director Association. 11*(6), 453-56.

Barnes, D. E., Palmer, R. M., Kresevic, D. M., Fortinksy, R. H., Kowal, J., Chren, M., & Landefeld, C. S. (2012). Acute care for elders units produced shorter hospital stays at lower cost while maintaining patients' functional status. *Health Affairs, 31*(6), 1227-36.

Biel, M., Grief, L., Patry, L. A., Ponto, J., & Shirey, M. (2014). *The relationship between nursing certification and patient outcomes: A review of the literature.* Retrieved from American Board of Nursing Specialties: http://www.nursingcertification.org/research

Boyle, D. K. (2017). Nursing specialty certification and patient outcomes: What we know in acute care hospitals and future directions. *Journal of the Association of Vascular Access, 22*(3), 137-42.

Conley, D. M., Burket, T. L., Schumacher, S., Lyons, D., DeRosa, S. E., & Schirm, V. (2012a). Implementing geriatric models of care: A role of the gerontological clinical nurse specialist—part I. *Geriatric Nursing, 33*(3), 229-34.

Deschodt, M., Flamaing, J., Rock, G., Boland, B., Boonen, S., & Milisen, K. (2012). Implementation of inpatient geriatric consultation teams and geriatric resource nurses in acute care hospitals: A national survey study. *International Journal of Nursing Studies. 49*, 842-49.

Fox, M. T., Sidani, S., Persaud, M., Tregunno, D., Maimets, I., Brooks, D., & O'Brien, K. (2013). Acute care for elders components of acute geriatric unit care: Systematic descriptive review. *Journal of the American Geriatrics Society, 61*(6), 939–46.

Inouye, S. K, Bogardus, S. T., Jr., Baker, D. I., Leo-Summers, L., & Cooney, L. M., Jr. (2000). The Hospital Elder Life Program: A model of care to prevent cognitive and functional decline in older hospitalized patients. Hospital Elder Life Program. *Journal of the American Geriatrics Society, 48*(12), 1697–1706.

Institute of Medicine. (2011). *The future of nursing: Leading change, advancing health.* Washington, DC: National Academies Press.

Kendall-Gallagher, D., Aiken, L. H., Sloane, D. M., & Cimiotti, J. P. (2011). Nurse specialty certification, inpatient mortality, and failure to rescue. *Journal of Nursing Scholarship, 43*(2), 188–94.

Lee, S. M., Coakley, E. E, Blakeney, B. A., Brandt, L. K., Rideout, M. L., & Dahlin, C. (2012). The national AgeWISE pilot. *The Journal of Nursing Administration, 42*(7/8), 356–60.

Lee, S. M., Coakley, E. E., Dahlin, C., & Ford-Carleton, P. (2009). An evidence-based nurse residency program in geropalliative care. *Journal of Continuing Education in Nursing, 40*(12), 536–42.

National Association of Clinical Nurse Specialists. (2010). *Clinical nurse specialist core competencies: Executive summary 2006–2008.* Retrieved from https://nacns.org/wp-content/uploads/2016/11/CNSCoreCompetenciesBroch.pdf

National Association of Clinical Nurse Specialists. (2018). *Statement on clinical nurse specialist practice and education* (Draft 3rd ed.). Retrieved from http://nacns.org/wp-content/uploads/2018/05/3rd-Edition-Statement-on-Clinical-Nurse-Specialist-Practice-and-Education-2018-line-numbers.pdf

Nurses Improving Care to Healthsystem Elders. (n.d.). *Our story.* Retrieved from https://www.nicheprogram.org

U.S. Census Bureau. (2014, May 6). *Fueled by aging baby boomers, nation's older population to nearly double in the next 20 years, Census Bureau reports* [press release, no. CB14-84]. Retrieved from http://www.census.gov/newsroom/press-releases/2014/cb14-84.html

Additional Resources

American Organization of Nurse Executives. (2015). *AONE nurse executive competencies.* Chicago, IL: Author. Retrieved from http://www.aone.org/resources/nec.pdf

Chapter 13

Mindfulness and Leadership

Teri Pipe, PhD, RN

Work is love made visible. . . . When you work,
you fulfill a part of earth's fondest dream
assigned to you when that dream is born.

—Kahlil Gibran

How do we make compassion a regenerative force for our patients, colleagues, organizations, students, and ourselves? How can we identify and learn to appreciate our sources of strength so that they are available to serve us and others? How do we develop the skills that will help us become more conscious of our thoughts and choices in the present moment, allowing us to put the endlessly noisy and demanding world into perspective?

We start with ourselves. We give ourselves the important opportunity to reflect and find better, more restorative, and less reactive ways to care for ourselves and thus the world around us. This opportunity presents itself many times every day; in fact, in every moment an opportunity resides anew (Pipe, 2015).

This chapter explores the intersections of mindfulness and leadership from a pragmatic view that can be applied immediately if that suits the reader. It provides practical tips, guided practices, and resources along with questions for self-discovery.

Reflection Question

What intrigues you most about mindful leadership? How are you already using mindfulness as you understand it right now?

Context for Mindfulness and Leadership

The concepts of mindfulness and leadership are nested in the larger context of health policy, caring theory, and national nursing initiatives. The Institute for Healthcare Improvement's Triple Aim includes goals to produce healthcare value, including better health for populations, better care for individuals, and lower per capita healthcare costs. Recently, healthcare leaders added a fourth aim of restoring joy and satisfaction to the employees delivering healthcare. A resilient, compassionate, and present nursing workforce is critical to delivering healthcare value. *Human Caring Science* (Watson, 2012) guides this exploration of the importance of mindfulness for leaders. Likewise, the Healthy Nurse, Healthy Nation program of the American Nurses Association highlights the importance of well-being for the nursing workforce and is particularly applicable to the mindful leadership journey.

In our fast-paced, overcommitted world, our habitual first response is often the automatic strategy of multitasking, working harder or longer, and problem solving on the fly. However, when used chronically and simply out of habit, this pattern can lead to increased stress, decreased productivity, and the sense that something is missing in life. The effects of these automatic, habitual reactions include physical illnesses, such as heart disease, hyperlipidemia, hypertension, chronic inflammation, anxiety, depression, insomnia, general malaise, and an overall sense of missing out on what is good in life. Intentionally focusing on mindful leadership practice may reduce and actually reverse these processes.

As leaders in the high-stakes, constantly changing, uncertain landscape of healthcare, we focus our attention outward on the health and well-being of others and of our organizations. We face changing and competing priorities, interruptions, distractions, and massive information loads that often threaten to get the best of us, despite our attempts to work harder or better or faster. Sometimes it seems the noisy world has taken up residence within us.

And yet often we yearn for that quiet center we know still exists somewhere within us. It might be a small, nagging feeling that we have lost touch with something essential to our selfhood or it might be a sense that we are missing out on something we can't quite name. This pang of awareness can signal that it is time to turn inward, even if only for a short time, to once again find what is unique and true for us individually. This is the chance to explore as leaders what being authentic means for us, personally, over and over again.

Reflection Question

Think for a moment about the elements of your personality and your life that you enjoy the most. Are these parts of yourself easy for you to access and share with others in your role as leader?

The chaotic, unrelenting traffic of mental activity and the associated physiological responses have previously been viewed as an impetus for creativity, productivity, and success. This creativity, productivity, and extended high energy are apt to result not from prolonged engagement with stressful mental frameworks but rather from a more balanced, caring approach to managing personal energy and responding to one's environment and situation. Most importantly, individuals and groups can learn to process their responses to stressful conditions in productive ways that support well-being, resilience, and long-term health (Tugade & Fredirckson, 2004). One of the approaches capturing the imagination of many researchers, business leaders, educators, athletes, and health professionals is that of mindfulness.

> *In our present culture silence is something like an endangered species . . . an endangered fundamental. We need it badly. Silence brings us back to basics, to our senses, to ourselves. It locates us. Without that return we go so far away from our true natures that we end up, quite literally, beside ourselves. We live blindly and act thoughtlessly. We endanger the delicate balance which sustains our lives, our communities and our planet.*
>
> —Gunilla Norris

What Exactly Is Mindfulness?

As the research and practice of mindfulness have grown immensely in the past two decades, many definitions have emerged. This section includes several definitions so that you may get a broader view of what most appeals to your leadership style and personal preference.

Perhaps the simplest definition of mindfulness is a present heart. A nuance of this definition is that it brings us away from considering that mindfulness is only within the purview of the brain and toward thinking that it resides within the whole being. Janice Marturano (2015) approaches mindful leadership as follows:

> *When you are mindful of this moment, you are present for your life and your experience just as it is . . . not as you hoped it would be, not as you expected it to be, not seeing more or less than what is here, not with judgments that can lead you to a conditioned reaction . . . but for exactly what is here, as it unfolds, meeting each moment with equanimity.* (p. 16)

Exercise

Right now, stop reading and take a few deep breaths, and maybe even close your eyes. Bring yourself into a more present state with yourself. Simply focus on how you feel this very minute, physically, mentally, and emotionally. Don't try to change anything; just be present with whatever is real for you right now. Stay in that state of focused, relaxed awareness as long as you like before continuing with your reading. Notice what it feels like to be both relaxed and awake at the same time.

Mindfulness has also been explained as a state of kind and benevolent attention to everything that arises into the mind's awareness by Jon Kabat-Zinn (2005). Kabat-Zinn also described attitudinal foundations of mindfulness practice including nonjudging, patience, having a beginner's mind (a mind that is willing to see everything for the first time), trust, nonstriving, acceptance, and letting go. Mindfulness is a way of paying attention, with intention, to the present moment. It allows an individual to transform from a habitual way of responding to a more awake and informed approach.

When we approach our daily lives through a lens of nonjudgment and self-awareness, we experience our world in a whole new way. Becoming more mindful and in the moment provides us with the skills of authentic presence and compassion. These are sorely needed skills to lead at any level. Having a beginner's mind allows us to experience each moment of our day with great clarity, empathy and renewal; good leaders are good beginners (Pipe, 2015).

The operational definition of mindfulness has two components. The first involves regulating one's attention to maintain it in the present experience, allowing one to better recognize mental events in the immediate present. The second aspect is adopting a particular attitude toward one's experiences in the present moment that is characterized as curious, open, and accepting (Bishop et al., 2004).

Mindfulness also refers to learning skills and practices that focus on paying careful attention. Once you have learned the skills of mindfulness in a practice setting, you can apply them to everyday activities like speaking, listening, emailing, consuming social media, eating, studying, physical activity, and creative pursuits. While mindfulness often involves slowing down to pay attention to what is happening, slowing the pace is not always necessary. The essential component is focusing your attention, which is possible even at a fast pace.

And as you learn and practice the skills of mindfulness, you can bring their benefits to bear when high-intensity, time-pressured issues emerge that demand clarity of focus and direction.

The essence of mindfulness is focusing on the present-moment experience rather than dwelling in either the past or future. This can be challenging for leaders to learn and to practice, particularly since many leaders rose to their positions through accomplishment, effort, and hard work. Learning to be present in the moment and accept things as they are without trying to change anything may be a relatively new skill set. Note, however, that mindfulness skills do not diminish one's ability to be goal-oriented, highly achieving, or performance oriented; in fact, a mindfulness practice can actually enhance leadership impact and effectiveness (Wasylkiw, Holton, Azar, & Cook, 2015). Setting aside time to practice mindfulness builds a reservoir of the ability to focus on what is important in the real world.

Mindfulness is *not*:

- **A religion.** Most of the world's wisdom and faiths place a high value on setting aside time and attention for silence and reflection. The way we use mindfulness here does not rely on any one tradition of faith and can be used regardless of the presence or absence of a personal belief system.

- **Having an empty mind or zoning out.** The brain is actually quite active during mindfulness activities, building new connections and changing structures with the practice. It is normal and expected for thoughts to arise during mindfulness practice; the instruction is to bring your attention back to the object of focus. Being aware of distraction is a key signal in identifying the need to refresh focus, and thus your ability to focus becomes stronger each time this is repeated.

- **Stress relief.** While you may feel relaxed and less tense during and between practices, this is a side effect rather than a goal of practice. The situation does not change; the response to the situation changes.

- **Deep breathing.** Breath is often used as an anchor for attention since breathing is free, portable, and familiar and presents a clear connection between the body and mind, but it is the quality of attention that is important and not simply the breath. Sometimes the target of attention is movement, food, body awareness, communication, and so on. The breath is just one possible recipient of focused attention.

- **The same as meditation.** While sitting meditation is often a very helpful way to experience mindfulness, mindfulness is aptly applied to a variety of activities including but not limited to meditation. For instance, mindful ways of movement like yoga, tai chi, qi gong, walking, and running can also involve mindfulness.

Learning Mindfulness Practices

Mindfulness as it is described here is a skill set. There are many courses, workshops, books, and audio and video teachings as well as executive leadership courses on mindfulness. The classic, standardized approach is mindfulness-based stress reduction (MBSR), which is a structured educational program founded in 1979 by Jon Kabat-Zinn at the University of Massachusetts Medical Center. The initial program was designed for patients with chronic health conditions and was intended to teach individuals a means of enriching their lives through adaptive coping, focused attention, and cognitive restructuring. MBSR education focuses on teaching mindfulness meditation to enhance one's ability to cope with stress, pain, and illness. Its benefits have since been extended to healthy individuals, professional organizations, business leaders, elementary schools, and healthcare professionals.

The practice is safe, effective, and cheap and has a growing appeal to many audiences. Learning the practice involves tuning one's attention to simple, automatic behaviors (breathing, eating, walking, stretching, conversing, and other everyday activities) in order to make them less automatic, which requires the participant to be engaged and attentive. With time and repeated use, the practiced engagement and attention begin to spill over into other areas of life, effectively "waking up" the participant. The awareness is not always pleasant, but it does make one genuine and alert to the reality of the situation rather than respond out of habit or dulled sensation.

Compassion toward self and others is often a byproduct, if not an intentional effect, of mindfulness practice. As the participant becomes more accustomed to accepting the present moment as it is, this nonjudgmental acceptance often extends to the self and then to others. This type of acceptance is not meant to negate ambition, goal achievement, or productivity but rather to build a realistic picture of the present, which can then be used to propel performance if that is the context of the practice (often the case in athletics, academic test performance, or endurance of some personal challenge). In this sense, mindfulness and compassion are often interrelated. Projected outcomes for students include increased ability to focus on academic content, reduced test anxiety, reduced overall stress, engagement with learning, academic success, retention, improved sleep, mindful eating and consumption of media, improved communication, and an overall stronger community-of-care culture.

Mindfulness meditation specifically deepens one's capacity for attention and strengthens present-moment awareness. Its underlying precepts are perhaps best described in this way:

> *Each moment missed is a moment unlived . . . [and] makes it more likely I will miss the next moment . . . cloaked in mindless habits of automaticity of thinking, feeling, and doing rather than living in, out of, and through awareness.* (Kabat-Zinn, 2005, p. 52)

Thus the ultimate goal of MBSR is to empower individuals to respond consciously (i.e., with full attention) rather than automatically to both internal and external circumstances. Such responses are useful whether an event is associated with urgent or routine matters, pain, or stress or with positive experiences such as joy, self-efficacy, and caring. Strengthening skills that focus one's attention cultivates conscious responses to stressful or otherwise meaningful events.

A number of academic medical centers currently employ MBSR training, producing an ever-expanding body of empirical research as well as clinical services with considerable patient demand. The growing list of institutions supporting formal MBSR programs includes Arizona State University, Stanford University Medical Center, Duke University Medical

Center, UCSF Medical Center, Brigham and Women's Hospital, and MD Andersen Cancer Center. Classes are offered free of charge at Columbia University Medical Center to patients and family members within inpatient cardiac units. Insurance carriers have similarly recognized the value of program participation; Aetna, Kaiser Permanente, and Cigna Healthcare, among others, offer MBSR training as a covered benefit for subscribers. And because the benefits of stress reduction and heightened attention go beyond those sustained in patient populations, an increasing number of healthy individuals, professional organizations, business leaders, and championship athletic teams have participated in or implemented MBSR programs.

Empirical Findings of Interventions and Education for Mindfulness-Based Stress Reduction

Mindfulness-based stress reduction has been found to successfully reduce stress and its symptoms in people with breast and prostate cancer, cardiovascular disease, chronic pain, fibromyalgia, rheumatoid arthritis, diabetes, insomnia, and other stress-related conditions. Similarly, numerous studies have shown significant improvements in coping skills, immune function, and depression and reductions in the disabling symptoms of stress among clinical and healthy populations completing MBSR programs.

The following is a very brief overview of research on the health-related impacts of mindfulness as found in the literature. These impacts are just a few of the growing number of evidence-based outcomes that are emerging from studies from multiple disciplines across many different populations:

- Decreased severity of depression.

- Decreased severity of anxiety.

- Increased performance (e.g., academic, athletics, military).

- Symptom management for conditions such as irritable bowel syndrome, cancer, and HIV.

- Changes in brain structure and function:

  - The amygdala—the brain's fight/flight/freeze center—shrinks.

  - The prefrontal cortex—related to higher-order cognitive functions such as awareness, concentration, and decision-making—thickens.

- Connectivity within the brain changes. The connectivity between the amygdala and the rest of the brain weakens and the connections between areas associated with attention and concentration strengthen.

- Reduced markers of inflammation such as C-reactive proteins, interleukin 6, and cortisol.

- Increased ability to manage pain, even when not actively meditating.

- Increased immune cell telomerase activity (a predictor of long term cellular viability).

Why Is Mindfulness Relevant for Leaders?

Leaders benefit from focusing on self-nurturing behaviors and thoughts because doing so cultivates stamina, resilience, and sustained energy to lead others. Leaders play an important role in caring for one another and in modeling courageous self-compassion in the service of others. How can leaders and aspiring leaders cultivate mindfulness practices?

Leadership, just like direct patient care, is an art and a science. Like direct care, excellent leadership has at its core a focus on healing, nurturing and bringing about optimal states of healing for individuals and organizations. Leadership can be defined as behaviors and ways of being that inspire a positive, enduring influence on those whose lives are impacted by one's leadership presence. When guided by caring science, leadership has the possibly and responsibility to bring about healing through the power of transpersonal caring relationship. In caritas-focused leadership, regard for the one being led is enlivened with a spirit of dignity, respect and compassion (Nyberg, 1998; Pipe, 2008, Watson, 1999, 2006a, 2006b, 2008).

The healing influence of the leaders may be directed at self, other, organization, community—truly limitless is the scope. Yet, no matter the breadth or scope of influence, much of the healing potential of leadership is rooted in a deep sense of authenticity and personal integrity. Strong and resilient leaders have the ability to be guided by what they believe is valuable, meaningful and true. Leaders stay focused on their inner compass, so they can inspire and direct others with clarity, compassion and purpose.

Two of the key relationships that require constant attention and nurturing form leaders are the relationship with self and the relationship with source. Source in this context means the leader's source(s) of strength, meaning and joy. The relationship with self and source are often intertwined. By knowing the self, one can accurately identify and access sources of strength. By nurturing and developing the relationships with self and source, the leader can, by extension, have inspirational and enduring influence on those they lead. Showing loving kindness and equanimity to one's self leads to transcendent leadership, so that loving kindness and equanimity are extended to others (Nyberg, 1998; Pipe, 2008; Watson, 2008). Watson (2008) stated:

Preparing for any worthwhile endeavor requires the cultivation of skills to engage in doing the chosen work. One cannot enter into and sustain Caritas practices for caring-healing without being personally prepared. It is ironic that nursing education and practice require so much skill to do the job, but very little effort is directed toward developing how to Be while doing the real work of the job. (p. 47)

Personal Preparation for Leadership: Authenticity and Self-Reflection

Authentic presence is a key leadership skill. It builds on the foundation of knowing oneself by presenting that genuine self to others. In order to convey a sincere sense of self, authentic leaders take the time, courage, and energy to be present for themselves. They conduct ongoing self-reflection with a spirit of gentle curiosity and kindness. Cultivating self-knowledge is an ongoing, dynamic navigational practice that helps a leader remain grounded in their vision and purpose and provides the strength necessary for high performance. Since the self is continually developing and changing, self-reflection practices vary based on the dynamic nature of oneself and others. The same strategies will not work for every person, and some approaches may be more effective than others at certain times. Effective leaders continually evaluate the changes in themselves, looking for opportunities to learn more about their personal sources of strength and how to leverage their strengths in the service of others.

Leaders might start with answering questions such as:

- How do I feel cared for?

- How do I express my care for others?

- What are the signs that I am not feeling well nurtured?

- How do I replenish myself?

- How does self-replenishment relate to the leadership of others?

- What makes me happy?

- What are my personal rituals to let go of work and obligations at the end of the day?

- Am I growing?

- Am I helping others grow professionally?

The caritas process of practicing loving-kindness and equanimity within the context of a caring consciousness supports the leader approaching self-nurture as preparation for leading others (Pipe, 2008; Watson, 2008). These practices are ideally woven into practical routines, preferably throughout the day, and integrated with the flow of activities that typify a life of leadership. Boyatzis and McKee (2005) describe resonant leadership as living in a state of full conscious awareness of one's whole self, other people and the context in which we live and work (p. 73).

Mindfulness impacts leadership skills by fortifying and nurturing the self in service of others. It counters the compelling momentum to operate on autopilot and encourages full and conscious experience. Mindfulness also helps one more astutely assess what one is experiencing; mindful leaders are better able to appreciate and understand their people, environment, and situation. Mindfulness reduces stress-related symptoms such as anxiety and depression, thus contributing to the overall resiliency and hardiness of a leader over time. Lastly, mindfulness can also help one cultivate a genuine sense of appreciation for the relationships with oneself and others along with gratitude for the opportunity to effect positive change.

Case Study

After learning about mindfulness at a professional conference, Sam decided to learn the skills by taking an online seminar focused on mindfulness skills for executives. Sam realized during the seminar that in order to fully realize the benefits, he needed to set aside at least 20 minutes a day for formal practice. For Sam, setting his alarm a bit earlier was the best way to ensure that he practiced before the uncertainties of the day took hold. After only a few days, Sam noticed a slight difference: a willingness to be curious and explore rather than jumping to habitual conclusions. Sam decided to use a 20-second breathing space between phone calls, meetings, and emails—just to briefly reset by pausing to center himself in the midst of the day. His sleep gradually improved and his tendency to overeat to numb the stress of the day slowly decreased. In terms of leadership, Sam became more comfortable really connecting with people and sincerely listening to them when they told him of their work situations and issues. Sam's problem solving became more effective because he understood the issues before rushing to solutions. It is a work in progress and of course setbacks happen, but like any behavior change, the important thing is to keep trying and to use the lapses as opportunities to learn. Sam's next step is to teach his executive team the basic centering skills so they can use them to start meetings or to create a pause when they arrive at an impasse.

Case Study

Angie is a nurse manager on a busy medical-surgical unit. She has improved patient experience scores and financial outcomes over the past three years and her staff turnover rate is well below the hospital average. For the most part staff morale is good, but she has started to notice more sick-time requests, more-frequent staff conflicts, and staff beginning to complain about patients and families. Angie has a personal mindfulness practice, which helps her pick up on these clues very early, and she begins to listen and watch even more carefully as she makes walking rounds. She decides to have a conversation with a few key opinion leaders on the unit to explore what is happening and how she can help. She gets immediate feedback that staff are feeling even more pressured for time and constrained by resources. During the feedback session, Angie takes a few concrete steps to intervene using her mindfulness skills:

- Acknowledging the situation and the impact on staff

- Providing quick, practical strategies for becoming more present and focused (such as taking a moment before and after each patient encounter to breathe, reset focus, and let go of what just happened to prepare for what is happening presently)

- Role modeling behaviors of deep listening, personal presence, and nonjudgment

- Reiterating that the staff are encouraged to find ways to become more centered and to help each other do so as part of the unit culture

- Creating tangible, physical reminders that it is OK to take quick time-outs to refresh and center personal attention as a pathway to patient safety and personal/professional resilience

- Providing access to articles, apps, and a physical space where staff can regroup and recharge, especially after a challenging clinical experience

- Enlisting help from staff to present stories about times the clinical care they delivered was enhanced by mindful presence and compassion

Angie recognizes that reenergizing staff is an ongoing process and not just a one-time initiative and that to be sustainable, she needs to cultivate a group of champions that will keep the culture of mindfulness and resilience alive and growing into the future.

Mindfulness Practice Exercises

Focusing on the Breath

Set a timer for the desired amount of time. Sit in a comfortable, upright, and dignified posture. Rest your feet on the floor and your hands open in your lap. Close your eyes or soften your gaze, and gently turn your attention inward. Slowly notice your breath, each inhale and exhale, as it happens. Please don't try to change anything. Simply notice where your breath meets your body, in your nose, throat, chest, or maybe all the way in your abdomen. Just breathe, and notice the breath. When thoughts or distractions happen (and they will), simply notice them, set them to the side, and come back to the breath. Let go of the past. Let go of the future. You are exactly where you are to be. Just rest in the present moment. Notice when distractions arise and begin again. When the timer rings, gently bring your attention back to your environment, maybe wiggling your fingers and toes and slowly scanning your body, mind, and overall energy to note any response to the breath-awareness exercise. You may want to write a few words in a journal or notebook about your experience.

If your circumstances don't allow you to set aside 5–30 minutes to do this breathing practice every day, there are alternatives. One is simply to notice your breath throughout the day, whenever you think to do so. Regardless, when you remember to focus your attention and awareness, you are making this muscle of focus stronger for other things in your life as well. Just notice.

Paying Attention to the Body

Set a timer for the desired amount of time. Sit upright or lie comfortably, allowing your eyes to close. Turn your attention inward. Notice your breath, perhaps letting the breath become deeper and slower if this feels right to you. Next, starting at the very tips of your toes and slowly working your way up through your entire body, bring a nonjudgmental and perhaps even appreciative awareness to every part of your body. Notice and remember how each part of your body supports you in your life, most of the time without your awareness or intentional control.

The bottoms of your feet meet the ground and support your weight, moving you through life every day. Your muscles work together to coordinate motion and create activity. Your heart beats on and on, and it has since before you were born. Your abdominal organs take care of their work on their own, balancing chemicals and nutrients without your awareness most of the time. Your shoulders support your head, your brain, and your amazing face that provides a window between you and the world. Bring awareness to every part of your face, your scalp, and your entire head. As you move through your body, release any areas of tension or tightness that are not needed. Finally, bring awareness and appreciation to the whole of your body. Rest in that awareness, feeling what it is like to be fully embodied, alive, awake, and yet serene. Carry that awareness forward as long as you can, even as you move into your regular daily round.

Intentional Awareness of Eating

Select a small, simple food to eat, perhaps a raisin, grape, tangerine, or a piece of dark chocolate. Wash your hands, intentionally noticing the feel of soap and warm water as you cleanse your skin and the feel of the towel as you dry your hands. Sit in an upright, dignified posture with the morsel of food in front of you. Take a few relaxing deep breaths. Be grateful for the food in front of you, maybe offering a blessing if that is within your belief system. Use your eyes to take in every detail of the piece, noting how the light hits it and the colors and textures you see. Take the morsel in your hand, noticing the texture of it. If the item requires peeling or unwrapping, do so carefully, noticing any texture or sensation as you open the object.

Now bring your food up to your nose and deeply inhale the aroma. Note any memories that arise, and just enjoy the act of breathing in the aroma of your food. Notice any other sensations or activities in your body as you are aware of the smell and sight of your food. Place your morsel on your lips for a moment, noting the texture of your food on your lip. Place the morsel on your tongue but don't bite in just yet. Feel the sensation of food on your tongue, noting the taste and any memories that arise. After a moment or so, let your teeth chew the item very slowly and carefully, fully chewing prior to swallowing.

Remember what the food looked like, and consider for a moment what it was like as a seed planted carefully in the soil. Imagine the sunlight and the moonlight shining on the seed and the plant as it grew. Think about the ripened food harvested by people you do not know, packaged carefully, and transported to the store where you selected it. Think of the grocery clerk who stocked the shelves and the one who helped you buy it. Consider how the food was stored awaiting your hunger. Consider all the people, energy, and connections the food represents as it becomes part of your body, giving you energy to care for yourself and others. Cultivate gratitude and awareness for this experience. Reflect on how food is usually consumed and consider what it would be like to be more fully present with food as it is chosen, prepared, and eaten. This is mindful eating, and it can be practiced with every meal and snack, at least to some extent.

Mindful Movement

Select an activity you enjoy, like walking, stretching, swimming, yoga, or gardening. As you prepare for this activity, take a few deep breaths, noticing how your mind and body prepare for movement. Bring your intentional, nonjudgmental focus to your motion, maybe even slowing down a bit to be aware of every part your body as it moves through space. Continue to pull your attention and focus back to your body any time your thoughts wander. Give your thoughts a break and simply be in your body totally. Use your senses to notice everything around you, not judging or making up stories but rather noticing how your body reacts to the sunlight or the movement of air across your skin or the feel of the earth beneath you. Notice your breathing, not trying to change it but just noticing it.

Try to keep this level of mindfulness and intentional attention to your movement for as long as you can. As you finish your activity, notice how your body feels compared to how you felt at first and when you were moving. Mentally scan through your body and note any sensations that arise. Perhaps even create a feeling of gratitude for the ability to move your body in this way. You can bring mindfulness to literally any movement, even simple things like walking to the mailbox or opening the refrigerator, just by bringing awareness to the way your body moves and letting go of any distractions or other thoughts you have. Maybe notice what it is like to be more fully present with your entire body rather than being caught up in your thoughts or emotions. Perhaps this provides a respite for you.

Communication

Select a time that you plan to talk with someone face to face. As the conversation begins, create an intention for how you want to be as the interaction unfolds, perhaps neutral, supportive, or loving. Take a few deep breaths as the conversation starts. Remove any potential distractions such as a TV, phone, and other noise. Focus on the other person and silently appreciate something about them, even if you don't agree with what they are saying. Listen deeply, not planning what you will say but rather really listening to the other person. Sometimes you can note meaning that goes beyond the words they are saying. Try to get a grasp on what they are actually feeling, which may lie deeper than their words.

As it is your turn to talk, carefully choose your words. As you are talking, notice the tone of your voice, any gestures you are using, and any emotions that are coming through in the dialogue. Continue to be fully present in the conversation, keeping your focus on the other person despite any distractions that arise. Notice how it feels to be fully attentive and appreciative of the other person, even if you may not agree with or fully understand what they are saying. Mentally scan through your body as the conversation takes place, noticing if you are unnecessarily tensing up or holding any areas of your body. When the conversation is over, remind yourself to be grateful for the interaction if you can. If it was a difficult conversation for you, perhaps extend gratitude to yourself and the other person for having the courage to have the discussion. Notice what it was like to be fully present and listening to the other person rather than being distracted by the TV, phone, or other interruptions. What would it be like to communicate this way more often? Would it work over the phone or when you are reading and writing emails?

Awareness of Senses

Select a time when you decide to intentionally draw your attention to your senses. It is nice to do this outdoors if possible, but it works anywhere. Hone into your vision by noticing everything you can about the colors, lighting, shapes, and visual textures of your environment. Work from the area close to your body, and as you take in everything close to you, move your gaze gradually further away, again taking in all the visual images and noting objects that you may have grown so accustomed to that you no longer notice them. Eventually move your gaze all the way to the farthest point out, perhaps the horizon if you are outdoors. Notice everything you can about what you are seeing. Take a moment to note what it is like to have filled your eyes with all of these images. Another way to practice mindfulness of sight is to look at a photo, painting, sculpture, physical object, or the face of someone you care about. Look for a long time. Really see everything you can.

With the other senses (touch, hearing, taste, the sense of moving with your body), likewise select what you want to pay attention to, and spend the time diving as deep into that sensory experience as you can. For example, mindfully listen to a piece of music or to birdsong, closing your eyes and filling your ears with every part of the sound that comes your way. Try not to grasp but rather to let the sound come to you gently so you can receive it. Or use your hands to notice the way something feels, maybe something as ordinary as an orange or pencil or as amazing as a loved one's hand. Notice everything you can about the sensation of touch, perhaps again closing your eyes so you can delve deeper into the sensation. Try being aware of your senses in this way as you go about your daily round, bringing awareness to things that might otherwise be unnoticed or automatic.

Mindfulness of Everyday Routines

In much the same way as cultivating sensory awareness, experiment with bringing your attention to the things you do regularly, like brushing your teeth, paying bills, or washing the dishes. Slow down and wash just one dish, noticing everything you can about the feel of the soapy water, the dishcloth, the texture of the dish, the color of the dish, and the way it looks when it is clean. As with the other practices, if distracting thoughts interrupt your focus, simply bring your full attention back to what you are doing. This creates a mental break from worrying about the past or future and brings you back to the present moment. Also, it is a wonderful reminder that in other areas of our life we can pause to choose how we want to respond rather than respond by habit; all we have to do is bring our attention to what we often do automatically.

Gratitude Practices

Upon awakening, and at any transition throughout the day, take a moment to notice something you are grateful for. This may be something large and profound, like life itself, or it may be something quite ordinary, like your morning cup of coffee or tea. Leaving home and coming back are good signals to trigger practicing gratitude. Sometimes this may feel artificial until the real feeling of appreciation comes along, but the important thing is to make an effort toward being grateful.

Communicate gratitude to others. When you consider all of the kindness and help that others have shown to you over your lifetime, it may inspire you to get in touch with one or many of these people. It may be a wonderful teacher, a friend, a neighbor, your postal carrier, or maybe even that person at the grocery store who is always cheerful. There is much in the world to be grateful for when we take the time to focus our attention on it, even in the midst of hardship or pain. Sending a card or email or calling someone to express your gratitude can be very life affirming for both of you. You can even express your gratitude anonymously.

Another strategy is to write down five things every day that you are grateful for. Put the date on the paper and start the list. It can be big or small, full of humor or deeply felt; the important thing is to draw your attention to what you are grateful for by writing it down. After several entries you can read back over what you've written and consider whether there are any patterns. Gratitude practices often help us tune our attention to what is good in our lives.

Chapter Key Points

- Mindfulness is an important skill for leaders.

- Science on mindfulness is growing in terms of personal health and well-being as well as performance.

- The skills of mindfulness, once learned and practiced, can be applied to everyday life experiences.

References

Bishop, S. R., Lau, M., Shapiro, S. L., Carlson, L., Anderson, N. D., Carmody, J., Segal, Z. V., et al. (2004). Mindfulness: A proposed operational definition. *Clinical Psychology Science and Practice, 11*(3), 230–41.

Bohlmeijer, E., Prenger, R., Taal, E., & Cuijper P. (2010). The effects of mindfulness-based stress reduction therapy on mental health of adults with a chronic medical disease: A meta-analysis. *Journal of Psychosomatic Research, 68*(6), 539–44.

Boyatzis, R. & McKee, A. (2005). *Resonant leadership: Renewing yourself and connecting with others through mindfulness, hope, and compassion.* Boston, MA: Harvard Business Press.

Chiesa, A. & Serretti, A. (2009). Mindfulness-based stress reduction for stress management in healthy people: A review and meta-analysis. *Journal of Alternative and Complementary Medicine, 15*(5), 593–600.

Chiesa, A. & Serretti, A. (2011). Mindfulness based cognitive therapy for psychiatric disorders: A systematic review and meta-analysis. *Psychiatry Research, 187*(3), 441–53.

Congleton, C., Holzel, B. K., & Lazar, S. W. (2015). Mindfulness can literally change your brain. *Harvard Business Review.* Retrieved from https://hbr.org/2015/01/mindfulness-can-literally-change-your-brain

Dekeyser, M., Raes, F., Leijssen, M., Leysen, S., & Dewulf, D. (2008). Mindfulness skills and interpersonal behaviour. *Personality and Individual Differences, 44*(5), 1235–45.

Carlson, L. E., Speca, M., Patel, K. D., & Goodey, E. (2003). Mindfulness-based stress reduction in relation to quality of life, mood, symptoms of stress, and immune parameters in breast and prostate cancer outpatients. *Psychosomatic Medicine, 65*(4), 571–81.

Gotnick, R. A., Chu, P., Busschbach, J. J., Benson, H., Fricchione, G. L., & Hunink, M. (2015). Standardised mindfulness-based interventions in healthcare: An overview of systematic reviews and meta-analyses of RCTs. *PLOS One, 10*(4), e0124344.

Greater Good Science Center. (2017). *Explore the Greater Good Science Center.* Retrieved from https://ggsc.berkeley.edu/

Gross, C. R., Kreitzer, M. J., Reilly-Spong, M., Wall, M., Winbush, N. Y., Patterson R., . . . Cramer-Bornemann, M. (2011). Mindfulness-based stress reduction versus pharmacotherapy for chronic primary insomnia: A randomized controlled clinical trial. *Explore, 7*(2), 76–87.

Grossman, P., Niemann, L., Schmidt, S., & Walach, H. (2004). Mindfulness-based stress reduction and health benefits: A meta-analysis. *Journal of Psychosomatic Research, 57*(1), 35–43.

Grossman, P., Tiefenthaler-Gilmer, U., Raysz, A., & Kesper, U. (2007). Mindfulness training as an intervention for fibromyalgia: Evidence of postintervention and 3-year follow-up benefits in well-being. *Psychotherapy and Psychosomatics, 76*(4), 226–33.

Hanson, R. (2016). *Key scientific papers.* Retrieved from http://www.rickhanson.net/key-papers/

Jacobs, T. L., Epel, E. S., Lin, J., Blackburn, E. H., Wolkowitz, O. M., Bridwell, D. A., . . . Saron, C. D. (2011). Intensive mindfulness training, immune cell telomerase activity and psychological mediators. *Psychoneuroendocrinology, 36*(5), 664–81.

Kabat-Zinn, J. (1990). *Full catastrophe living: Using the wisdom of your body and mind to face stress, pain and illness.* New York, NY: Delacorte.

Kabat-Zinn, J. (2005). *Wherever you go, there you are: Mindfulness meditation in everyday life.* New York, NY: Hyperion.

Kluepfel, L., Ward, T., Yehuda, R., Dimoulas, E., & Smith, A. (2013). The evaluation of mindfulness-based stress reduction for veterans with mental health conditions. *Journal of Holistic Nursing, 31*(4), 248–55.

Ledesma, D. & Kumano, H. (2008). Mindfulness-based stress reduction and cancer: A meta-analysis. *Psycho-Oncology, 18*(6), 571–79.

Lengacher, C. A., Johnson-Mallard, V., Post-White, J., Moscoso, M. S., Jacobsen, P. B., Klein, T. W., . . . Kip, K. E. (2009). Randomized controlled trial of mindfulness-based stress reduction (MBSR) for survivors of breast cancer. *Psycho-Oncology, 18*(12), 1261–72.

Marchand, W. R. (2012). Mindfulness-based stress reduction, mindfulness-based cognitive therapy, and zen meditation for depression, anxiety, pain, and psychological distress. *Journal of Psychiatric Practice, 18*(4), 233–52.

McCracken, L. M., Gauntlett-Gilbert, J., & Vowles, K. E. (2007). The role of mindfulness in a contextual cognitive-behavioral analysis of chronic pain-related suffering and disability. *Pain, 131*(1/2), 63–69.

Marturano, J. (2014). Finding the space to lead: A practical guide to mindful leadership. Bloomsburg Press: New York, NY.

Pipe, T. (2015, February 2). Journey towards becoming a mindful leader [blog post]. Retrieved from https://www.rwjf.org/en/blog/2015/02/journey_towards_beco.html

Pipe, T. & Bortz, J. (2009). Mindful leadership as healing practice: Nurturing self to serve others. *International Journal for Human Caring, 13*(2), 34–38.

Pradhan, E. K., Baumgarten, M., Langenberg, P., Handwerger, B., Gilpin, A.K., Magyari, T., . . . Berman, B. M. (2007). Effect of mindfulness-based stress reduction in rheumatoid arthritis patients. *Arthritis and Rheumatism, 57*(7), 1134–42.

Santorelli, S. (1999). *Heal thy self: Lessons on mindfulness in medicine.* New York, NY: Random House.

Shapiro, S. L., Bootzin, R. R., Figueredo, A. J., Lopez, A. M., & Schwartz, G. E. (2003). The efficacy of mindfulness-based stress reduction in the treatment of sleep disturbance in women with breast cancer: An exploratory study. *Journal of Psychosomatic Research, 54*(1), 85–91.

Speca, M., Carlson, L. E., Goodey, E., & Angen, N. (2002). A randomized, wait-list controlled clinical trial: The effect of a mindfulness meditation-based stress reduction program on mood and symptoms of stress in cancer outpatients. *Psychosomatic Medicine, 62*(5), 613–22.

Tacon, A. M., McComb, J., Caldera, Y., & Randolph, P. (2003). Mindfulness meditation, anxiety reduction, and heart disease: A pilot study. *Family Community Health, 26*(1), 25–33.

Tugade, M.M. & Fredrickson, B.L. (2004). Resilient individuals use positive emotions to bounce back from negative emotion experiences. *Journal of Personality and Social Psychology. 86*(2), 320–33.

Vago, D. R. & Nakamura, Y. (2011). Selective attentional bias towards pain-related threat in fibromyalgia: Preliminary evidence for effects of mindfulness meditation training. *Cognitive Therapy Research, 35*(6), 581–594.

Wasylkiw, L., Holton, J., Azar, R., & Cook, W. (2015). The impact of mindfulness on leadership effectiveness in a health care setting: a pilot study. *Journal of Health Organization and Management. 29*(7), 893–911

Whitebird, R. R., Kreitzer, M. J., & O'Connor, P. J. (2009). Mindfulness-based stress reduction and diabetes. *Diabetes Spectrum, 22*(4), 226–30.

Winbush, N. Y., Gross, C. R., & Kreitzer, M. J. (2007). The effects of mindfulness-based stress reduction on sleep disturbance: A systematic review. *Explore, 3*(6), 585–91.

Wong S. S. & Nahin, R. L. (2003) National Center for Complementary and Alternative Medicine perspectives for complementary and alternative medicine research in cardiovascular diseases. *Cardiology in Review, 11*(2), 94–98.

Zgierska, A., Rabago, D., Chawla, N., Kushner, K., Koehler, R., & Marlatt, A. (2009). Mindfulness meditation for substance use disorders: A systematic review. *Substance Abuse, 30*(4), 266–94.

Chapter 14

Leading Relational Care: Ensuring That Patients Feel Known by Their Nurses

Jacqueline G. Somerville, PhD, RN, FAAN

Leaders of a revolution, in contrast to a rebellion, must make a philosophical leap and become more human human beings.

—Grace Lee Boggs

As nurse leaders, we must balance the executive responsibilities that we hold in common with our administrative colleagues along with the responsibility and privilege of serving and leading as chief of a clinical discipline—a discipline that has tremendous impact on the advancement of health and patient outcomes (Clifford, 1998). We recognize that co-creating a professional practice environment with nurses and for nurses advances the outcomes of patients, families, and communities including the human experience of health and illness. As a discipline, all nursing actions are based in the context of relational care. This chapter explores the impact of this approach from the unique perspective of patients. Theory-infused practice that grounds nurses in this unique, holistic perspective ensures that nurses remain connected to the meaning and purpose of their work, supporting their engagement in the current healthcare environment, whose focus may not always be consistent with nursing's worldview.

> *There is a real danger that measurable tasks and procedures can be misconstrued for nursing practice in contemporary healthcare organizations focused on the measurement of quality, safety and productivity.* (Cathcart, 2008, p. 87)

Our current healthcare system is broken, and some would say it has lost its humanity under the yoke of administrative burdens, cost pressures, and its mechanistic focus. As a doctoral candidate, when I had the privilege of asking patients what it meant to feel known by their nurses, their responses underscored so much of what we as human beings are looking for from the healthcare system. Although my study was specific to patient perceptions of feeling known by their nurses, after presenting my research to many interprofessional audiences, I have received much anecdotal feedback that this may be a transprofessional phenomenon.

Patients Perceptions of Feeling Known by Their Nurses

As described by Jones (2007) and others (Newman, 2008; Willis, Grace, & Roy, 2008), the phenomenon of feeling known is grounded in the perspective of knowledge as process; it's a reflective, relational process in which knowledge emerges or unfolds through genuine, dynamic partnership of the patient and their nurse. The nurse comes to know the person, the patient's story and not just their medical history, through dialogue. The nurse "seeks to embody a mutual process, guiding the person through a journey of self-discovery, meaning, choice and activities to promote the human experience" (Jones, 2007, p. 167). Knowledge as problem solving may be complementary during an acute episode, but it cannot be a substitute for knowledge as process for nurses. Health as transformation is the intent of the relationship (Newman, 2008).

Within the current healthcare environment, nursing care is often driven by task-oriented activities with little time for nurses to respond fully to the experience of patients, families, and communities. Charles Kunkle (2016) in his book *No Time to Care* was told by one caregiver that "she felt like a task oriented zombie" (p. ii). Each time a system or safety issue emerges, we generate yet another checklist for clinicians rather than strategically leverage the power of evidence-based tools for each specific situations in which they have proven to provide the highest yield. Although nurses have long articulated the value and professional meaning in knowing their patients and the fact that this knowledge leads to skilled clinical judgment and individualized nursing interventions (Horvath, Secatore, & Reilly, 1990; Minick & Harvey, 2003, Radwin & Alister, 2002; Tanner, Benner, Chesla, & Gordon, 1993), the patient perspective of feeling known by their nurses had yet to be explored.

A qualitative, descriptive study (Somerville, 2009) was first completed and then guided item development for a scale that quantifies how well patients feel known by their nurses. A convenience sample of 17 surgical inpatients were asked to describe the experience of being known by their nurses and how this knowledge did or did not impact the care that they received. Interviews continued until saturation occurred and then the data were analyzed. Four themes emerged. When patients felt known by their nurses, they felt recognized as a unique human being; they felt safe; they experienced a meaningful, mutual, personal connection with their nurses; and they felt empowered by their nurses to participate in their care.

Feeling recognized as a unique human being is defined as a patient's experience of nurses who through purposeful interaction gained insight into the people, events, history, and experiences that were meaningful in shaping the patient's life. Nurses used this knowledge to deliver care that was respectful of patient preferences and values. Within the sample, patients most frequently identified "their" nurses as "knowing" them best. When participants experienced a feeling of being known, they described their care as being individualized and responsive to their unique needs. A participant stated, "They treat me like a person, not like a patient. Nobody wants to be a number or a person without a name."

Feeling safe is defined as patients' having confidence in their nurses' intentions and abilities to act upon patient concerns and advocate for their well-being based upon the nurses' unique knowledge of the patient as person. A consistent theme was the importance of having a voice and feeling heard. Most patients were not prepared for the sense of isolation during hospitalization and the experience of being dependent upon others who may or may not choose to hear their concerns and act on them. Patients described the importance of having access to clinicians who were emotionally available and who communicated interest in their well-being. New encounters with clinicians and changes in routine were perceived as threats to being known and causing possible miscommunication, which created a sense of vulnerability and uncertainty. Patients felt the burden of telling their story once again to ensure that their unique needs were known and to ensure their safety. A lack of feeling known gave patients the perception of being viewed as a task or a diagnosis, which led to a feeling of anxiety. A patient described being ordered a medication to which she had experienced a previous reaction: "The nurse listened to my concern, stopped, and double-checked."

Experiencing a meaningful, mutual, personal connection with their nurses is defined as a shared consciousness and mutual partnership between the patient and their nurses. In this relationship, nurses are willing to share of themselves, changing the dynamic from one of dependency to one of partnership. Patients felt that nurses did not simply provide care but actually cared about them as a person. One participant stated, "She goes the extra mile . . . she picked up on things like my anxiety without me telling her."

Feeling empowered to participate in their care is defined as patients' experience of nurses who valued patients as knowledgeable partners in their care. Nurses helped the patient gain insight into their life pattern and recognize new choices and opportunities in their lives. One participant stated, "When I knew that I had to get up and walk, they [the nurses] gave me choices about when and how much."

Discussion and Implications: The Role of the Leader

Nurses have an ethical imperative as defined by the American Nurses Association (ANA; 2015) *Code of Ethics* to advance the "good" on behalf of each patient, ensuring that their unique needs are honored. This requires that the nurse understand what the good is, as defined by each unique, human being in the context of their life. How do nurse leaders create space for this knowing in our current fast-paced healthcare environment? How can we ensure that this knowing is not lost in the endless tasks that increasingly fall to the clinical nurse? Knowing the patient is a relational process that does not fit into a check box on a task list. It requires the ability to center, take a breath, and be fully present as the nurse enters each encounter.

When I had the privilege of serving as the chief nurse at Brigham and Women's Hospital, I decided to begin my leadership journey by witnessing the nurses' practice. I spent time with clinical nurses in each area where nurses practice, observing the environment and their contribution to patient care. What I witnessed was both breathtaking and variable. The acuity was staggering, the cutting-edge technology and practice were technically expert, but the attention paid to the person and family experiencing the health event was variable, both setting and nurse dependent. I began to think about how to systematize expectations and support related to relational care in the same way expectations and systems had been systematized related to quality, safety, technical care, and evidence-based practice. What appeared to be missing was theory-infused care, grounding nurses in why they serve and balancing the humanity with the technical and state-of-the-art, scientific innovations. Enter, Watson's (2008) Theory of Human Caring.

Jean Watson's Theory of Human Caring is based on 10 Caritas processes or professional competencies and grounds nurses in their ability to create, with clear intention, a healing space. The competencies are as follows:

- Sustaining humanistic-altruistic values by practicing loving kindness, compassion, and equanimity for self and others. Please note that she calls us to care for self. Recall that the *ANA Code of Ethics* (2015) states that the nurse has a *duty*—not a right—to self as much as to others to promote health and safety.

- Being authentically present, enabling faith and hope, and honoring the subjective inner-life world of self and others.

- Being sensitive to self and others by cultivating one's own spiritual practices.

- Developing and sustaining loving, trusting, caring relationships.

- Allowing for expression of positive and negative feelings by authentically listening to another's story.

- Creatively problem solving. Use all ways of knowing, being, doing, or becoming.

- Engaging in transpersonal teaching and learning within the context of another's frame of reference. Shift toward coaching model for expanded health and wellness.

- Creating a healing environment.

- Opening to spiritual awareness. Allowing for miracles.

- Reverentially assisting with basic needs as sacred acts. (Watson, 2017)

I will never forget the story shared with me by a patient care assistant at Brigham and Women's Hospital. She talked about a Muslim woman for whom she cared. When she entered the patient's room, the patient appeared sweaty and uncomfortable. The assistant learned that the patient had refused to allow others to bathe her for cultural reasons. The assistant said to the patient that she understood and committed to honoring her wishes and would bathe her in such a way as to ensure her privacy and dignity. The assistant told her that if at any point she felt that the assistant violated this promise, then she should ask the assistant to stop and the assistant would stop immediately. The woman agreed. The assistant then left the room and came back with a pile of face cloths and towels. What she then described appeared to be a sacred dance, and visualizing the scene as the assistant spoke brought tears to my eyes. She described placing a washcloth over a small section of the patient and removing the section of clothing under it, repeating this until the woman was covered only in cloths. She bathed and dried sequentially under each section and then finally dressed the woman in the same manner. At the end of the bath the woman cried.

When embraced, the above 10 competencies become a way for nurses, clinicians, and support staff to ground their practice, first working on a relationship with and loving kindness for self, which creates the foundation for practicing loving kindness for others. It is through authentic presence and immersion in each patient's story and what holds meaning for each patient that a healing environment emerges.

So where should we begin to breathe life into these competencies at Brigham and Women's Hospital? How do we make them a values-based lived experience, one that every patient, family, and staff member could expect from every person they encountered at any Brigham and Women's Hospital location?

In partnership with a clinical nurse, I attended the intensive six-month journey to becoming a certified Caritas coach, a true immersion into caring science. The foundation of the theory is loving kindness for self and others, which include patient, family, community, and coworkers. How would a clinical environment steeped in a tradition of research that calls one to be a detached observer respond to the call for loving kindness for self and others? How could we create reflective time and space in a reactive environment to advance relational care? With our challenge defined, we developed a strategic plan to infuse caring science throughout the organization. We took a multipronged approach, integrating caring intention as the foundation of our professional practice model, leveraging the talent and expertise of our shared-governance committees to integrate caring science into their practice and to begin meetings by setting a caring intention. We sent a nurse leader with a clinical nurse every six months to attend the Caritas coach program, charging the pair with implementing caring practices at the local level upon their return. Our patient and family advisory councils became our expert guides. What did loving kindness look like from their perspective?

Things began to change. Caritas rooms, or reflection rooms, began to sprout up across the campus. Caring intentions were established at the beginning of a shift or day on many of the units and ambulatory practice settings. We began to offer Heart Math, a quick heart-centered breathing technique, and acupressure classes to staff to help center themselves in the midst of a dynamic clinical environment. Almost every class was oversubscribed. And most palpable was the focus and discussion about the personhood of patients. During a Joint Commission visit, I was most struck by a comment from one of the surveyors who said that she expected expert clinical care and cutting-edge innovation and technology during her visit, but what surprised and impressed her was the kindness she witnessed, kindness of staff to patients, families, and each other.

This brief case exemplar is shared as just that, not as a road map for others, because just as people are unique, so is each organizational culture at any point in time. The major messages are to:

- Openly acknowledge that nursing care is relational care;

- Meet each person, unit, or clinic where they are and extend an invitation to explore caring science and theory-infused care; and

- Acknowledge that as leaders if we do not care for those we serve, we cannot expect them to care for self or others.

Being intentional about expectations and supporting infrastructures is key. We expect leaders to practice loving kindness for themselves, their staff, and their interprofessional and administrative peers. We provide staff the space and skills and we expect them to practice loving kindness for self and all others. When any of the above does not occur, we have dialogue to understand how the system did not serve stakeholders. Loving kindness is not about self-sacrifice. It occurs in the context of an intentional environment. Many nurses felt that they had to be kind to others despite the obstacles or an uncaring environment. This dichotomy often created internal conflict and led them to describe symptoms of compassion fatigue. As leaders it is our responsibility to remove those barriers and create a caring environment that makes compassion for self and others a part of the fabric of every workday.

Reflective Questions

1. If staff and clinicians are the environment of care, how can leaders in the current healthcare environment support them to be more present and loving to themselves, patients, families, communities, and one another?

2. How can nurse leaders co-create a greater daily connection for nurses:

    a. To relational care?

    b. To the meaning and purpose that nurses and others are seeking in the current healthcare system?

    c. To knowing their patients, which advances the humanity of those who are served as well as those who serve?

Summary

When patients feel known by their nurses, they feel recognized as a unique human being; they feel safe; they feel a meaningful, personal, and mutual connection with their nurses; and they feel empowered to participate in their care (Somerville, 2009). At the heart of relational care, patients feel known. In order to preserve relational care—arguably the essence of nursing—it is essential for nurse leaders to balance evidence-based care with theory-infused practice. The path to this culture must be intentional, the goal being to create common expectations for all to stay in right relationship with self and all others. If we believe that clinicians are the environment of care as experienced by patients and families, then it is our challenge as nurse leaders to systematize relational expectations and intentions to meet the ultimate goal of greater staff engagement. This will transform the human experience of health and illness for all those we touch. Maybe our staff are looking to their leaders for the same things that patients experience when they feel known by their nurses? Perhaps staff are looking to feel recognized as unique human beings; to feel safe; to feel a meaningful, mutual, personal connection with their leaders; and to feel empowered to participate in shaping their practice.

As we move into a new chapter in healthcare where the value equation (cost over quality) will define our success, nursing's contribution to advancing health for our patients, families, and communities is more critical than ever. In our clinical practice and service to others, we have all witnessed patients who have been healed and not cured and inversely patients who have been cured and not healed, remaining traumatized by the experience of illness and treatment. As members and leaders of interprofessional teams across the continuum of care, nurses enjoy a rich history of meeting patients and communities where they are, gaining insight into their unique patterns of health and illness, and partnering with patients and communities, recognizing that we are guests in their .

life experience. It is only when we practice cultural humility—a recognition that our patients are the experts in defining what holds meaning in their lives, sharing this knowledge with the team, and integrating it into the plan of care—that we will truly advance health and value.

Care that is based on evidence-informed algorithms that speak to the mean response of the "average" patient is straightforward. When we place these algorithms against the backdrop of knowing our patients and understanding their unique lived experience, care becomes much more complex. Who is this average patient? None that I have ever met. I have been honored to serve patients who bring their rich, unique stories. By witnessing and listening to their stories, we understand the challenges that patients and communities face in implementing these algorithmic plans of care in the messy and wonderful real world. Do we have the courage and the creativity to blend the two perspectives, humanity and science? Absolutely! I witness this courage each and every day.

What does it take to sustain this courage and creativity? I believe there is much to learn from Watson's Theory of Caring Science. Our greatest assets in the healthcare system are not bricks and mortar. Our greatest assets are the people who serve. The challenge for leaders increasingly across disciplines is to care for those who care, including physicians, nurses, health professionals, frontline managers, and support staff. An engaged workforce is more critical now than ever to creating value. I go back to the reflective questions.

If staff and clinicians are the environment of care, how can leaders support them to be more present and loving to themselves, patients, families, communities, and one another?

Following Watson's principles of caring science, we advance staff engagement by sustaining humanistic values in complex environments. We create a congruity between organizational goals and the essence of why clinicians went into practice—to make a difference in the lives and health of their fellow human beings. We sustain loving kindness by creating systems that promote self-care practices that sustain and nourish the mind, body, and spirit of our staff. The alternative is for staff to shut down their hearts in the face of the human suffering and vulnerability that they witness every day. It is through authentic leadership that trusting, caring relationships are developed and sustained. It is through creating a culture of safety where all employees are expected to identify the strengths and opportunities in our systems. It is through empowering our teams at the point of care to creatively problem solve, serving as coaches and leaders who remove barriers while resisting the tendency to present our teams with solutions for them to implement. It is through infusing our organizations with caring science, advancing a culture that promotes healing, not just curing, for all those who entrust us with their lives and their health. Employee engagement and caring behaviors are truly the foundation of the value equation for those we are called to serve—patients, families, and communities—who want and need to feel known.

Chapter Key Point

- When patients feel known by their nurses they feel recognized as a unique human being; they feel safe; they feel a meaningful, personal, and mutual connection with their nurses; and they feel empowered to participate in their care.

References

American Nurses Association. (2015). *Code of ethics for nurses with interpretive statements.* Silver Spring, MD: Author.

Cathcart, E. B. (2008). The role of the chief nursing officer in leading the practice: Lessons from the Benner tradition. *Nursing Administrative Quarterly, 32*(2), 87–91.

Clifford, J. (1998). *Restructuring: The impact of hospital organizations on nursing leadership.* Chicago, IL: American Hospital Association.

Horvath, K., Secatore, J., & Reilly, P. (1990). Expert discussion groups: A strategy for clinical development, quality assurance and retention. In J. Clifford & K. Horvath (Eds.), *Advancing professional nursing practice* (pp. 256–71). New York, NY: Springer.

Jones, D. (2007). A synthesis of philosophical perspectives for knowledge development. In C. Roy & D. Jones (Eds.), *Nursing knowledge development and clinical practice.* (pp. 163–76). New York, NY: Springer.

Kunkle, C. (2016). *No time to care: A leadership game plan to ensure caregiver engagement.* Tampa, FL: Richter Publishing.

Minick, P. & Harvey, S. (2003). The early recognition of patient problems among medical-surgical nurses. *Med-Surg Nursing, 12*(5), 291–97.

Newman, M. (2008). *Transforming presence: The difference nursing makes.* Philadelphia, PA: F.A. Davis Company.

Radwin, L. E. & Alister, K. (2002). Individualized nursing care: An empirically generated definition. *International Nursing Review, 49(1)*, 54–63.

Somerville, J. (2009). *Development and psychometric evaluation of patients' perceptions of feeling known by their nurse's scale.* (Doctoral Dissertation). Retrieved from ProQuest LLC. UMI 3349962.

Tanner, C., Benner, P., Chesla, C., & Gordon, D. (1993). The phenomenology of knowing the patient. *Image: The Journal of Nursing Scholarship, 25*(4), 273–80.

Watson, J. (2008). *Nursing: The philosophy and science of caring* (Rev. ed.). Boulder, CO: University Press of Colorado.

Watson, J. (2017). Global advances in human caring literacy. In S. Lee, P. Palmieri, & J. Watson (Eds.), *Global advances in human caring literacy* (pp. 3–11). New York, NY: Springer.

Willis, D., Grace, P., & Roy, C. (2008). A central unifying focus for the discipline: Facilitating humanization, meaning, choice, quality of life and healing in living and dying. *Advances in Nursing Science, 31*(1), E28–E40. DOI: 10.1097/01. ANS.0000311534.04059.d9

Chapter 15

Integrative Nursing

Carolyn Hayes, PhD, RN, NEA-BC

To be 'in charge' is certainly not only to carry out the proper measures yourself but to see that everyone else does so too; to see that no one either willfully or ignorantly thwarts or prevents such measures. It is neither to do everything yourself nor to appoint a number of people to each duty, but to ensure that each does that duty to which he is appointed. This is the meaning which must be attached to the word by (above all) those 'in charge' of sick, whether of numbers or of individuals.

—Florence Nightingale (1992, p. 24)

This chapter challenges you to reflect upon and articulate what it is you are leading. Crucial questions for nurse leaders today include the following: Does it take a registered nurse to run operations? Does it require your education and experience to manage a workforce? In truth, unless you are leading the practice environment to facilitate nursing practice, then you are not necessary. You can, and arguably should, be replaced by alternately educated and probably lesser paid professionals. So how do you know that you are meeting the expectations of your role?

Every nurse is a leader expected to possess a certain moral comport-
ment while practicing evidence-based interventions embedded in
respectful and caring relationships with the recipients of those interventions and with colleagues. The social constructs of our profession
present a covenant with society that includes creating healing environments. Society, as recently as a 2016 Gallup poll, continues to rank
nurses as the most trusted profession in America (Gallup, n.d.). Our
discipline remains part art and part science. Formal nurse leaders are
expected to create and maintain healing environments that are relationship based and inclusive of self-care for staff, professional and para-
professional. To guide your reflection on what you are in charge of and
leading, this chapter presents the six principles of integrative nursing
woven into current leadership concepts about practice environments,
reflections from Nightingale, and questions and suggestions for leaders
in various roles.

Nursing is a privilege, granted by a society that has co-created a social
construct of nursing with us, members of a profession accountable
for self-regulation. Why do we so consistently rank as the number one
trusted profession? The American Nurses Association (ANA) *Social Policy
Statement* describes nursing as a "covenant," which is distinguishable
from and goes beyond a contract (Fowler, 2015). A covenant is defined as

> *an agreement or written promise between two or more parties that
> constitutes a pledge to do or refrain from doing something. Thus, an
> agreement that requires the performance of some act is termed an
> "affirmative covenant" while an agreement that restricts or refrains
> a person from performing something is called a "negative cove-
> nant." . . . The person making the pledge or promise is called the cove-
> nantor while the person to whom such promise is made is known as
> the covenantee.* ("Difference Between," 2015, para. 2)

In this definition you can see that the two parties do not have equal obligations and rights. Nurses are covenanters who have made promises to
perform some acts and refrain from others. If we had contracts with our
patients, we would have a very different relationship. A contract is

> *an oral or written promise that is enforceable by law. It is defined
> in law as a voluntary agreement between two or more parties, who
> intend to create legal obligations, in which there is a promise to do or*

*perform some work or service for a valuable consideration or benefit.
A contract is a common phenomenon. It is frequently used in deal-
ings between businesses, corporations, banks, owners of land, and
other transactions.* ("Difference Between," 2015, para. 4)

Nurses do not hold patients accountable for any reciprocal benefit. In
fact, we are most often employees of a third party with whom we do
have a contractual relationship, but our patients are cared for under our
professional obligations umbrella.

The specifics of these promises are the foundation of nursing ethics and
reside in the ANA *Code of Ethics, Social Policy Statement,* and professional
position statements. Limits to our practice exist in legal and regulatory
proclamations such as scopes of practice and state-based nurse-practice
acts. Further setting expectations for our professional practice are the
evidence-infused guidelines for practice environments, such as the
American Association of Critical-Care Nurses (2016) *Standards for
Establishing and Sustaining Healthy Work Environments* or the American
Nurses Credentialing Center's (n.d.) Magnet Recognition Program.
Leaders of a nursing workforce in the late 2010s should also be guided by
current leadership theories and an understanding of a multigenerational
workforce (Boychuk & Cowin, 2004).

While nursing has always espoused holism, other healthcare disciplines
have more recently incorporated this philosophy of care into their practice. Therefore, as medicine began to publish on integrative medicine,
there was a call for nursing to articulate itself. Drs. Mary Jo Kreitzer and
Mary Koithan (2014) took on that challenge and published results in a text
entitled *Integrative Nursing.* The six principles they forward (figure 15–1)
are a useful frame for leading the practice and practice environments as
described by the above documents and ideas. In addition, they can each
be reinforced by the writings of one of our founders, Nightingale.

The first principle is that "human beings are whole systems inseparable
from their environments" (Kreitzer & Koithan, 2014). This principle is
a call to be mindful of the environment that our patients, clients, and
communities exist in. In addition, it is a call to be mindful of the practice
environment for clinical staff. To reinforce this principle explicating the
interconnectedness of the people and environment, consider this quote
from Nightingale's writing:

People say the effect is only on the mind. It is no such thing. The effect is on the body, too. Little as we know about the way in which we are affected by form, by colour, and light, we do know this, that they have an actual physical effect. Variety of form and brilliancy of colour in the objects presented to patients are actual means of recovery. (Nightingale, 1992, p. 84)

Tending to the environment is a centuries-old concept in our practice and is essential for a leader to incorporate into their practice.

In this first principle we can also reflect on the ANA *Code of Ethics* (the Code), which places import on a respectful practice environment for patients but also calls to include colleagues and others as integral to a respectful approach to care. The Code states:

Respect for persons extends to all individuals with whom the nurse interacts. Nurses maintain professional, respectful, and caring relationships with colleagues and are committed to fair treatment, transparency, integrity, preserving compromise, and the best resolution of conflicts. (ANA, 2015, p. 4)

1. *Human beings are whole systems inseparable from their environments.*

2. *Human beings have the innate capacity for health and well-being.*

3. *Nature has healing and restorative properties that contribute to health and well-being.*

4. *Integrative nursing is person-centered and relationship-based.*

5. *Integrative nursing practice is informed by evidence and uses the full range of therapeutic modalities to support/augment the healing process, moving from least intensive/invasive to more, depending on need and context.*

6. *Integrative nursing focuses on the health and well-being of caregivers as well as those they serve.*

FIGURE 15–1. Integrative nursing principles

Is the environment you are leading a facilitator or barrier to these expectations? As a nurse director, do you encourage a collaborative practice environment, inclusive of all disciplines, that represents the best resolutions of conflicts? What unique role do you have in ensuring integrity-preserving compromise is the norm versus individuals experiencing being compromised by decisions made? Nurse directors are impactful in role modeling when actively engaged in interprofessional forums. A forum for ethical discussions is often a helpful way to ensure the collaborative environment is solid.

The second principle is that "human beings have the innate capacity for health and well-being" (Kreitzer & Koithan, 2014). To emphasize the importance of this principle Nightingale (1992) said:

> *It is often thought that medicine is a curative process. It is no such thing; medicine is the surgery of functions, as surgery proper is that of limbs and organs. Neither can do anything but remove obstructions; neither can cure; nature alone cures.* (p. 74)

She recognized that healing was in fact the work of the individual, not the interventionists. She implored the nurse to facilitate the patient's healing when stating:

> *A little needle-work, a little writing, a little cleaning, would be the greatest relief the sick could have, if they could do it; these are the greatest relief to you, though you do not know it. Reading, though it is often the only thing the sick can do, is not this relief.*
>
> *Bearing this in mind, bearing in mind that you have all these varieties of employment which the sick cannot have, bear also in mind to obtain for them all the varieties which they can enjoy.* (Nightingale, 1992, pp. 35–36)

As a nurse educator, when you introduce a new technological intervention, do you also role model including patient knowledge and preferences as essential to the patient's healing? Introducing patient-interfacing technology is an opportunity for you to engage the patient in the learning. Role model patient or family inclusion to reinforce to the learner that the relationship is a value and not just technical competence.

The third principle is that "nature has healing and restorative properties that contribute to health and well-being" (Kreitzer & Koithan, 2014). Our practice and our environments must be sensitive to creating ways to allow nature to interface with our patients, clients, and communities. Imagine a public-health nurse advocating to preserve green areas in a neighborhood or an acute care nurse helping a patient go outside for a breath of fresh air. Nightingale had a great deal to say about nature. For example, she noted, "No one who has watched the sick can doubt the fact, that some feel stimulus from looking at scarlet flowers, exhaustion from looking at deep blue" (Nightingale, 1992, pp. 35–36). To reinforce the direct impact nature had on healing she stated:

> While the nurse will leave the patient stewing in a corrupting atmo-sphere, the best ingredient of which is carbonic acid; she will deny him, on the plea of unhealthiness, a glass of cut-flowers, or a growing plant. Now, no one ever saw "overcrowding" by plants in a room or ward. And the carbonic acid they give off at night would not poison a fly. Nay, in overcrowded rooms, they actually absorb carbonic acid and give off oxygen. . . . It is true there are certain flowers, e.g. lilies, the smell of which is said to depress the nervous system. These are easily known by their smell and can be avoided. (Nightingale, 1992, p. 34)

As the director of the public health nurses, are you involved in the community politics, infusing this knowledge into decisions for the good of the community? As a nurse executive in acute care, are you advocating for nature when new patient care areas are being designed?

Nightingale further reflected on nature as healing by giving a great deal of thought and instruction on light. "It is a curious thing to observe how almost all patients lie with their faces to the light, exactly as plants always make their way towards the light" (Nightingale, 1992, p. 49). As modern-day scientists contemplate neuroplasticity and the effect light has on it, we can turn to Nightingale, who said:

> It is the unqualified result of all my experience with the sick, that second only to their need of fresh air is their need of light; that, after a close room, what hurts them most is a dark room, and it is not only light but direct sunlight that they want . . . People think the effect is on the spirits only. This is by no means the case. The sun is not only a painter, but a sculptor. (Nightingale, 1992, p. 37)

Without scans to prove her hypothesis, Nightingale had observed that light does not merely let us see what is there, but actually changes the form of what is the way a sculptor would. Do we as nurse leaders look for light in our environments? Does the acute care nurse director make it possible for clinical staff to take patients outside? Does the ambulatory nurse leader ensure patients have access to natural light in waiting areas or during treatments as possible? What about our employees?

The fourth principle is that "integrative nursing is person-centered and relationship-based" (Kreitzer & Koithan, 2014). Relationship-based care is a care delivery model that many choose today (Koloroutis, 2004). Do we as leaders ensure it is an attainable goal for clinical nurses to establish these relationships? Do nurse executives advocate that their respective organizations measure this as a key metric and determinant to patient outcomes? It is at the core of our patients' experiences. We are very attentive to the patient experience as one component of the Triple Aim, as articulated by the Institute for Healthcare Improvement (n.d.). Measurements of the patient experience are used as negotiation targets between providers and third-party payers.

For her part, Nightingale was clear that this was essential for nursing care and patient outcomes. She stated:

> *The effect in sickness of beautiful objects, of variety of objects, and especially brilliancy of colour is hardly at all appreciated. Such cravings are usually called the "fancies" of patients . . . their (so called) "fancies" are the most valuable indications of what is necessary for their recovery. And it would be well if nurses would watch these (so called) "fancies" closely.* (Nightingale, 1992, p. 40)

Nightingale reinforces in this quote the importance of knowing your patient and the patient's feeling known. She defines whatever is important to them as "necessary for their recovery" (1992, p. 40). Do your policies and procedures call for assessment of patient preferences?

The fifth principle is that "integrative nursing practice is informed by evidence and uses the full range of therapeutic modalities to support/ augment the healing process, moving from the least intensive/invasive to more, depending on need and context" (Kreitzer & Koithan, 2014). When members of the healthcare disciplines and many in the general public hear the term "integrative," they often think of integrative therapies, such as acupuncture or acupressure, therapeutic message, mindfulness, and others. In fact, this one principle of the *Integrative Nursing* frame highlights the use of these modalities as they are evidence based and, very often, less invasive than other options. However, these modalities are not new. Nightingale referenced many of them.

For example, presenting implementation of what we would now label as music therapy Nightingale stated:

> *The effect of music upon the sick has been scarcely at all noticed . . .
> I will only remark here, that wind instruments, including the human
> voice, and stringed instruments, capable of continuous sound, have
> generally a beneficent effect.* (Nightingale, 1992, p. 33)

With regard to what we would call pet therapy, she stated, "A small pet animal is often an excellent companion for the sick, for long chronic cases especially" (Nightingale, 1992, p. 58).

There has been increasing attention given to mindfulness practices for patients and nurses in recent literature. Nightingale was a proponent of this attention to the moment as well. She stated:

> *I have known a nurse in charge of a set of wards who not only
> carried in her head all the little varieties in the diets which
> each patient was allowed to fix for himself, but also exactly
> what each patient had taken during each day. I have known
> another nurse in charge of one single patient who took away
> his meals day after day all but untouched, and never knew
> if [sic]. If you cannot get the habit of observation one way or
> other, you had better give up the being a nurse, for it is not your
> calling, however kind and anxious you may be.* (Nightingale,
> 1992, p. 63)

It was so strongly held a belief that, for Nightingale, if a nurse could not be mindful, they should not be a nurse—it is that essential to practice. As a nurse in charge, do you make sure the clinical nurses are being mindful of their patients and completing tasks such as Nightingale's example of observing nutritional intake versus tray removal? Do you ask those questions when obtaining updates?

The sixth principle is that "integrative nursing focuses on the health and well-being of caregivers as well as those they serve" (Kreitzer & Koithan, 2014). This principle incorporates many current leadership concepts. For example, we speak of self-care when addressing relationship-based care (Koloroutis, 2004) and as a potential fourth aim to add to the Triple Aim mentioned previously (Bodenheimer & Sinsky, 2014). To give your best to your patients, clients, communities, or staff, you need to be at your highest and best, and that requires attention to care for the caretakers. As a leader, are you attentive to this principle? Does the nurse executive ensure institutional attention to employee wellness? Does the nurse director ensure breaks are happening and promote self-care at annual performance appraisals? It is easy to ask about self-care during meetings with our staff, and doing so reinforces the message that it is an expectation of the job. Do all nurse leaders role model self-care?

Nightingale had some strong beliefs about self-sacrifice versus balanced living. She said:

> The most devoted friend or nurse cannot be always there. Nor is it desirable that she should. And she may give up her health, all her other duties, and yet, for want of a little management, be not one-half so efficient as another who is not one-half so devoted, but who has this art of multiplying herself—that is to say, the patient of the first will not really be so well cared for, as the patient of the second . . . If you could but arrange that the thing should always be done whether you are there or not, he need never think at all about it. (Nightingale, pp. 20–21)

In this quote she not only advocates that a nurse should live their life in full versus sacrificing for the patient, but she also argues the patient is better served by a nurse in balance than by a self-sacrificing nurse.

Exemplars

There are acute and ambulatory settings that have put these principles into place and transformed practice. Boston Medical Center in Massachusetts adopted the burgeoning practice of taking a pause for the care team after an unsuccessful resuscitation. The pause acknowledges the humanity of the care team members who have just witnessed a traumatic event and the relationships some, if not all, of the members had with the now deceased. In April 2017, Sibley Memorial Hospital in Washington, DC, presented at the 2nd International Integrative Nursing Symposium: Creating Compassionate Healthcare Systems in Arizona. They presented on the influence of this thinking on designing new space and on practice changes they implemented, which had transformative value. Broward Health Imperial Point has implemented an adaptation of Watson's 10 Caritas Principles and developed a Pinky Promise for Quality Care (Gallison & Curtin, 2016). Many others have reported on implemented changes that have yielded improvements in patient experiences, retention, and other significant metrics.

What each reported effort has made clear is that there is a role leadership must play in the change. First, there is a need to be clear that relationships are expected to be a priority and self-care part of professional responsibility. Leaders also must eliminate barriers to independent practice regarding integrative therapies. Also pervasive in case reports is the identification of space for staff to take quiet time in the midst of their work. Being mindful of these principles is essential when facilitating projects and programs that center on the relationship of the nurse with the patient, client, or community. Of course, obtaining resources, time, and money as needed to support reflective practice and care of the caretaker is a common point of discussion and a great way to leverage your peers through consultation.

CASE STUDY

You are the nurse leader on a unit with a high turnover rate for staff. Your most senior staff are telling you that the turnover is because the nurses "can't do what they need for their patients with the staffing they have." Your patient-satisfaction scores are fair. Your executive leaders set targets for you to improve the scores with no additional resources. How could integrative nursing principles help you begin a change with seemingly incommensurate resource expectations?

Summary

Nursing is both art and science, and both aspects of practice require intentionality and mindfulness. While patient experience may be difficult to measure (Berkowitz, 2016), a highly engaged staff likely boosts patient experience, and patient-experience scores pertaining to interactions with nurses have the strongest association with a hospital's financial outcomes (Deloitte, 2016). This makes those interactions a priority for institutions. Nurse executives are accountable for the financial health of a hospital. Nurse leaders are also accountable for nursing practice as described in our foundational documents as covenantal. Examples in this chapter demonstrate that the two are not incommensurate goals but rather that focusing on relationship-based care as the underpinning of interactions is a time-honored approach articulated by nurse leaders starting with Nightingale.

Nurse leaders should develop habits of a reflective practice and understand, articulate, and role model the values embedded in our professional codes, the art of nursing, and relationship-based care. To lay claim to leading a clinical discipline, we must ensure that professional practice environments are healing for patients, clients, communities, and ourselves. We need to create practice expectations and environments that facilitate Nightingale's instruction that we ensure that each does that duty to which he is appointed. The six principles of integrative nursing, which include integrative therapies, can serve as a frame to create and sustain a healing environment. These ideas, while as old as nursing practice described by Florence Nightingale, impact the patient experience, which is an essential aspect of nursing's contribution to health.

Reflective Questions

- How would I describe the practice environment I am leading?

- Would the clinical nurses describe it the same way? Would non-RN colleagues? What is it that nurses want from their practice?

- What is it the patient, client, or community holds most valuable, and how do I know that?

- What would patients, clients, or community describe as key elements of their experience in the practice environment I lead?

- Do the patients, clients, or community members feel known? Do staff articulate self-care strategies?

- Do I role model respectful and caring relationships and self-care?

Chapter Key Points

- Leaders need to be clear that relationships are expected to be a priority and self-care part of professional responsibility

- Nursing is both art and science and both aspects of practice require intentionality and mindfulness.

- Relationship-based care should be the underpinning of interactions.

References

American Association of Critical-Care Nurses. (2016). *AACN standards for establishing and sustaining healthy work environments.* Aliso Viejo, CA: Author.

American Nurses Association. (2015). *Code of ethics for nurses with interpretive statements.* Silver Spring, MD: Author.

American Nurses Credentialing Center. (n.d.). *ANCC Magnet recognition program.* Retrieved from https://www.nursingworld.org/magnet

Berkowitz, B. (2016, January 31). The patient experience and patient satisfaction: Measurement of a complex dynamic. *Online Journal of Issues in Nursing, 21*(1).

Bodenheimer, T. & Sinsky, C. (2014). From Triple to Quadruple Aim: Care of the patient requires care of the provider. *Annals of Family Medicine, 12*(6), 573–76.

Boychuk D. J. & Cowin, L. (2004). Multigenerational nurses in the workplace. *The Journal of Nursing Administration, 34*(11), 493–501.

Difference between covenant and contract. (2015, March 29). Retrieved from https://www.differencebetween.com/difference-between-covenant-and-vs-contract

Deloitte. (2016). *The value of patient experience: Hospitals with better patient-reported experience perform better financially.* Retrieved from Deloitte: https://www2.deloitte.com/us/en/pages/life-sciences-and-health-care/articles/hospitals-patient-experience.html

Doidge, N. (2016). *The brain's way of healing.* New York, NY: Penguin Books.

Fowler, M. (2015) *Guide to nursing's social policy statement.* Silver Spring, MD: American Nurses Association.

Gallison, B. S. & Curtin, C. S. (2016). Creating a caring environment illuminates practice potential. *Beginnings, 36*(1), 20–24.

Gallup. (n.d.). *Honesty/ethics in professions.* Retrieved from https://news.gallup.com/poll/1654/honesty-ethics-professions.aspx

Institute for Healthcare Improvement. (n.d.). *IHI Triple Aim initiative.* Retrieved from http://www.ihi.org/Engage/Initiatives/TripleAim/Pages/default.aspx

Koloroutis, M. (Ed.). (2004). *Relationship-based care: A model for transforming practice.* Minneapolis, MN: Creative Health Management Inc.

Kreitzer, M. J. & Koithan, M. (2014). *Integrative nursing.* New York, NY: Oxford University Press.

LaVela, S. L. & Gallan, A. S. (2014). Evaluation and measurement of patient experience. *Patient Experience Journal, 1*(1). Available at https://pxjournal.org/cgi/viewcontent.cgi?referer=http://scholar.google.com/&httpsredir=1&article=1003&context=journal

Nightingale, F. (1992). *Notes on nursing: What it is, and what it is not* (Commemorative ed.). Philadelphia, PA: J.B. Lippincott Company.

Chapter 16

Leadership and Policy

Ashley Waddell, MS, RN, doctoral candidate

Patricia Noga, PhD, MBA, RN, NEA–BC, FAAN

Ideas are a medium of exchange and a mode of influence even more powerful than money and votes and guns. Shared meanings motivate people to action and meld individuals striving into collective action. Ideas are at the center of all political conflict. Policy making, in turn, is a constant struggle over the criteria for classification, the boundaries of categories, and the definition of ideas that guide the way people behave.

—Deborah Stone

All nurses can choose to be leaders; this is true in practice areas as well as in efforts to influence health policy. In fact, nurses can and should fulfill many critical roles in policy as part of the profession's commitment to improving the health of individuals, populations, and communities. According to Tyer-Viola et al. (2009): "As a human caring science, nursing has the expertise to advance society. As a profession, nursing also has the capacity to focus on the well-being of a society in advocating for social change" (p. 110). Society values the perspectives brought forward by nurses and respects the profession as a whole. Nurses' knowledge, training, and experience prepares them to participate in policy as honest translators or knowledge brokers, communicating the implications and results of health policies and the realities of healthcare delivery to public and policy decision-makers.

Nurse leaders must think about what members of the profession need, across academic and practice settings, to meet the needs of people. Long (2005) points out that public policy is a determinant of health and noted that a failure to influence policy-making results in policies originating from almost everywhere except the bedside. This impacts the well-being of patients and communities, both of which often suffer if policies do not successfully improve the quality, accessibility, and affordability of health-care services. Nurse scientists, whose focus is on developing knowledge, also have a large role in shaping policy and should commit to producing research with explicit policy implications. As policy impacts all facets of the profession, nurse leaders must identify opportunities across practice and research to effect change.

The nursing profession has been described as "a knowledge-based human resource capable of effecting major advances toward the goal of health equity among populations" (Duncan, Throne, & Rodney, 2015, p. 27). Participating in health policy is a logical intervention when nurses' assessments of client or community health problems specify a need for change (Gebbie, Wakefield, & Kerfoot, 2000), however, not all nurses have the skills or knowledge to do this (O'Grady, Mason, Hopkins Outlaw, & Gardner, 2016). As leaders, we must think about our role—and the role of our profession—in working toward a shared meaning of health equity in our society. What can we do to enhance nurses' contributions to health policy and ultimately improve the health of populations?

This chapter covers the need to prioritize health policy as a domain of nursing practice and the role of nurse leaders in creating space for health-policy efforts in practice and research settings. Nurse leaders must be deliberate in devoting time and efforts to inform discussions at all levels of policy.

Background: Prioritizing Health Policy in Practice and Research

Policy decisions are shaped by the way in which healthcare problems are defined and prioritized, and by the possible solutions (policies) and alternatives that are brought forward during the policy process. Nurses have knowledge of patient needs and have experienced the realities of healthcare delivery, including the implications of current policies and processes. When nurses' insights are not brought forward into the policy arena, policies fall short in adding value to the health-care system.

Researchers have worked to describe the skills needed by nurses to influence policy. Shariff (2015) describes links between nursing-leadership attributes and the attributes necessary for health-policy participation, noting political astuteness evolves with participation in legislative activities. Political skills such as social astuteness, interpersonal influence, networking ability, and apparent sincerity are described as essential for professional development and organizational leadership by Montalvo (2015), who further notes, "While the nursing profession has the ability to contribute to quality outcomes, decrease cost, and expand healthcare access, it needs to channel political knowledge and gain broader organizational influence" (p. 381). Cohen and Muench (2012) reviewed records of nurses' congressional testimony between the years 1993 and 2011, noting that over time nurses testified on issues that were clearly part of the nation's policy agenda. However, they identified a lack of testimony on important and consistent issues in healthcare such as quality and cost. Since that time, nurses and healthcare researchers from other disciplines have increasingly focused on quality outcomes and cost implications. Similarly, in the early 1990s, several scholars identified a variety of public policies that would have been different if the voices of nurses and women had been more influential in shaping them. Many of those policies are based in equity, with examples ranging from accessible family-planning and childcare services, a livable minimum wage, access to primary care, and substance abuse treatment; all are notable for their longevity in our nation's public-policy dialogue (Backer, Costello-Nikitas, Mason, McBride, & Vance, 1993).

As leaders, nurses must highlight the connections between population health problems that are evident in our patients, social determinants of health, community conditions, and public policy. Since nurses often limit their participation to procedure- and policy-making within their workplace or professional organization, their knowledge, experiences, and insights do not consistently make it to public policy–makers. Yet nurses' holistic, health-focused education enables us to provide a much-needed patient-centered perspective in policy discussions. Fyffe (2005) notes a lack of "apparent agreement and commitment within the nursing profession and professional organizations in the United Kingdom to devising a strategic approach to developing nursing's contribution to health policy"

(p. 5). We suggest that nursing leaders must devote resources, especially time, to strengthen the influence of nurses in health policy.

With approximately 4 million nurses in the United States, the profession makes up the largest sector of the healthcare workforce. Nurses are present in almost every setting and constituency where healthcare services are provided. They are integral members of the healthcare team and key coordinators of personalized care delivery. And as Tyer-Viola et al. (2009) state, "Because nurses represent the largest number of health care providers, the profession of nursing should claim leadership in social responsibility" (p. 110).

Recognizing the potential for collective impact, the Institute of Medicine (2011) report *The Future of Nursing: Leading Change, Advancing Health* called for the nursing profession to assume greater leadership roles in transforming the US healthcare system, a call reiterated in the follow-up report issued by the National Academies of Science, Engineering, and Medicine (2015). If more nurses were to make a concerted effort to contribute to policy, there would be the potential for great impact. Noting that policy issues surround nursing practice, Hahn (2010) underscores the need for nursing's impact on policy to be proportionate to the profession's size.

Engaging more nurses in policy couldn't be timelier. The United States is in a period of highly politicized and volatile debates about access to and cost of healthcare services. In 2015, healthcare expenditures rose 5.8% to $3.2 trillion, or nearly $10,000 per person (Centers for Medicare & Medicaid Services [CMS], 2017). Projections suggest that annual spending on healthcare services will be nearly 20% of the country's gross domestic product by 2025. These projections, based on the 2010 Patient Protection and Affordable Care Act's remaining in place, noted that the aging population and changes in economic conditions were largely fueling the 5.6% projected annual growth rate for healthcare spending (CMS, 2017).

Spending on healthcare services has been growing at an unsustainable pace, and people are questioning whether access to healthcare should be considered a human right. According to Lavizzo-Mourey (2014), "Health equity is connected to opportunity; and how we, as a nation, must balance the costs, benefits, and effectiveness of treatment and prevention to provide our people with care of the highest possible value" (p. 4). The nursing profession has the capacity to focus efforts on societal well-being and social change based on a commitment to the values of equity, access, and justice (Tyer-Viola et al., 2009). We can do this with a deliberate intention to influence policy.

Nursing is a professional discipline with arms addressing both science and practice (Donaldson & Crowley, 1978). Nurses are integral members of the healthcare team and are leaders in redesigning care delivery models. Fawcett (in press) explains the reciprocal relation between research and practice, noting that knowledge developed through research is applied in practice and that the results of the practice applications are used to refine knowledge through further scholarly inquiry. "Although practical problems may serve as a stimulus for scholarly inquiry, the starting point for the reciprocal relation between scholarly inquiry and practice always is scholarly inquiry" (Fawcett, in press). As the on-the-ground problem-solvers in healthcare, nurses are well informed to identify and define problems in need of policy change and also to generate ideas about pragmatic solutions to such problems.

Defining the Context of Policy Efforts Using the Nursing and Health Policy Conceptual Model

The policy-making process has been conceptualized as a set of six relatively predictable stages (Dye, 2013; Porche, 2010), which are described in table 16-1. Following this process, a problem gets identified and receives enough attention to get onto the agenda. Once it is on the agenda, various policy proposals are considered and then a solution is selected. The new policy or law is then implemented, and hopefully an evaluation of the policy is conducted after the law has been in place for some time.

While this linear conceptualization is useful to understand how policies come to be, it is overly simplistic and does not account for politics. As Ellenbecker and Edward (2016) state, "In actuality, policy development does not always occur in all these stages or in a linear fashion; stages may occur out of sequence, simultaneously, or be absent from the process" (p. 209). Stone (2002) describes politics as a "creative and valuable feature of social existence" (p. 8) that involves the preferences and priorities of policy decision-makers and stakeholders. Furthermore, power dynamics within the policy environment may bend otherwise rational or objective positions as individuals, interest groups, and decision-makers balance multiple and conflicting objectives and priorities (Hewison, 2008). Brehaut and Juzwishin (2005) explain that "the rightness or wrongness of a policy decision does not depend on whether appropriate evidence was used, but on whether the policy can be supported by the majority of citizens" (p. 4). When working to influence policy, one must consider both the policy context and process as well as the politics.

The Conceptual Model of Nursing and Health Policy (CMNHP; Russell & Fawcett, 2005) was developed to address the intersection of nursing and health policy, and it "provides a framework for analysis and evaluation of public, organizational and professional policies influencing the quality, cost and access to nursing and other health care services, as well as for any nursing-discipline specific and health services research" (p. 319). The CMNHP includes three sources of policies: the public, organizations, and professional associations. The three policy components include personnel, services, and expenditures; health policies address any or all of those components. Finally, the CMNHP has four levels, each with a focus and outcome ranging from efficacy, effectiveness, and efficiency of nursing practices within local healthcare delivery systems (levels 1 and 2); to access to healthcare systems and services within geopolitical communities, states, and nations (level 3); to global social justice (level 4).

The CMNHP model is useful for identifying the context or environments in which nurses engage in health-policy activities as well as the potential outcomes of policy-focused efforts. Reflecting on the context of health-policy efforts and activities is useful for both nurses in practice and researchers because policy stakeholders, decision-makers, and policy processes vary by institution and community. For example, hospitals have different processes for updating patient care policies; there may be a combination of committees, task forces, and subject-matter experts that contribute to the process. Similarly, each state of the United States has control over its policy process. Each state has a House of Representatives and a Senate, but within that structure, states have a lot of control over how they make decisions. In some states, members of the legislature hold other jobs, while in others, being a member of the legislature is a full-time job. There is even variation in the length of time that the House and Senate are in session.

Health policies determine who gets care, where they get it, when, from whom, and at what cost (O'Grady, Mason, Hopkins Outlaw, & Gardner,

2016). In order to participate in policy, nurses must be able to anticipate when and where policy topics will be discussed. Identifying opportunities using the levels discussed in the CMNHP is useful for discerning when and where policy decisions are made. Although the people involved in policy discussion will vary, if nurses know the time, place, and process for deliberation and decision-making, they will be better able to inform policy decisions. The nursing and health-policy outcomes associated with each level of this model can also guide health-policy goals and bring focus to policy recommendations generated by nurse scientists.

TABLE 16–1. Policy process

Steps	Description
Problem Identification	Problems suited for a policy solution are identified by individuals or groups
Agenda Setting	Garnering the attention of policy-makers, stakeholders, and the public to bring attention to a problem so that it becomes part of the policy agenda
Policy Formulation	The development and proposal of possible policy solutions by policy-makers, interest groups, experts, and other stakeholders
Policy Legitimation	Enacting policy through the legislative process, court decisions, or other authoritative decision-making processes within policy-making institutions
Policy Implementation	Executing or operationalizing the new policy or law. Often involves regulatory processes within government departments such as developing regulations, setting a compliance timeline, and defining enforcement mechanisms
Policy Evaluation	Exploring the extent to which policies solve the problems they were developed to solve. Evaluations can be conducted by a wide range of entities including governmental agencies, researchers, the media, and nonprofit organizations and should account for intended and unintended results of the new policy

Adapted from Dye (2013, p. 16).

Policy Leadership in Practice Settings

Nurses have the opportunity to engage in multiple levels of policy discussions, ranging from within organizations to across geopolitical communities (citywide, statewide, nationally, or globally). The focus of policy efforts varies widely from population health issues to professional practice regulations. This section focuses on efforts at a local level because opportunities to influence policy within one's organization, town, city, or state are often more accessible than efforts to shape federal or global policy. Opportunities to participate in policy are numerous and may include involvement in advisory groups, task forces, committees, coalitions, and board appointments. The provided examples highlight such opportunities and illustrate the collaborative nature of policy efforts.

Population Health Example: A Task Force to Combat Substance Use Disorders

Approximately 91 Americans die every day from an opioid overdose; and since 1999, prescription overdose deaths have quadrupled (Centers for Disease Control and Prevention, 2017). In one northeastern state, a nurse executive from a state hospital association partnered with a hospital CEO to form a task force to reduce opioid prescribing and slow the rise of substance use disorders. Approximately 10 nurses from hospitals, various community settings, and professional organizations across the state joined physicians, pharmacists, psychologists, social workers, and consumers in the effort and contributed to the work of the task force. Collectively, the group developed emergency department (ED), hospital, and physician practice guidelines, care management tools, and patient and provider fact sheets.

Hospital leaders in the state endorsed the guidelines and signed commitment letters to voluntarily implement the guidelines across the care settings. A website was developed that made publicly available the guidelines, education, tools, and fact sheets. Working in partnership and in parallel with key stakeholders—the state government, lobbyists, and the state's congressional delegation—nurses influenced passage of state legislation. They did this by sharing the ED guidelines, convening key stakeholders to converse, and imparting lessons from grant-funded activities along with experiences from their own community coalitions.

The nurse executive and colleagues have been sharing the impact of the task force through presentations and webinars available to healthcare organizations in various states and through the American Hospital Association. The nurse executive continues to oversee and guide the evolving work of task force members through expanding initiatives and coalitions in the three years since the task force's inception. Although the opioid-related deaths continue to rise, they now do so at a slower rate, and the number of prescriptions written for opioids decreased by 28% from the first quarter of 2015 to the second quarter of 2017 (Massachusetts Department of Public Health, 2017a, 2017b).

Questions for Consideration

The magnitude of this epidemic has put this issue squarely on the policy agenda. Now policy ideas are being debated, selected, implemented, and potentially evaluated.

1. As a nurse leader, to what extent are you involved in any collaborative policy efforts to address this epidemic?

2. If you are not currently participating, are you aware of efforts within your organization of employment, professional organization, school, or local community?

3. Who are the people leading and engaged in policy efforts to address the opioid addiction epidemic? Do you know of other nurses engaged in these efforts? If not, to what extent could the work be strengthened by adding a nursing perspective?

4. In what ways could you, or your colleagues contribute:

   a. In your workplace?

   b. Within your community? And with family and friends?

   c. Within professional societies and organizations?

   d. With elected officials and legislators in your community and state?

Keep in mind that health policies determine who gets care, where they get it, when, from whom, and at what cost.

5. What policy ideas are being discussed to address the opioid addiction crisis? Based on your perspective as a nurse, do the policy ideas make sense and address important aspects of the problem?

6. To what extent will the policy ideas improve access to treatment, efficacy of treatment, or cost of treatment? Do they address the training of healthcare personnel or changing how services are provided?

Professional Practice Example: Workplace Violence

In addition to patient safety in healthcare settings, worker safety has been of increasing focus. Along with federal rules and requirements, there are national hospital-accreditation standards, state laws, and state regulations addressing violence prevention in the healthcare workplace. Nurse leaders are leading conversations about how to ensure safe and healthy work environments for their patients and colleagues. In one state, proposed legislation and increasing episodes of violence in the healthcare workplace led to both a multipronged strategy to prevent workplace violence and an intensified partnership between professional organizations.

Nurse leaders from a regional nursing-leadership organization and a state hospital association formed a collaborative coalition to act on the issue, provide best practices and resources, and build an expanding forum of interested parties.

Preventing workplace violence became a key priority for nurse leaders and the board of the nursing-leadership organization. Its government-affairs committee focused on the topic, examined proposed legislation, supported and aligned itself with national resources, and developed and issued a position statement. Preventing workplace violence also became a strategic priority for the state hospital association. Spearheaded by a nurse leader, a workplace safety team was established, a successful workplace-safety summit for hospital teams was presented, legislation was drafted and introduced to improve on problematic areas in previously filed legislation, and a patient safety officer forum was developed. Moving forward, the goal of the nurse-led collaborative coalition is to continue to strive toward ensuring workplace safety by expanding the diverse workgroup committed to this issue, and further developing tools and resources, and educational forum ideas.

Questions for Consideration

1. In what ways is workplace violence impacting:

   a. You?

   b. Your ability to practice?

    c. Your colleagues?

    d. Your work environment?

    e. Your patients?

2. To what extent is the topic of improving workplace safety prioritized in your organization of employment? And in your local community? Are you aware of policy proposals to address workplace safety within your organization of employment or at the local, state, or national level?

3. How can you get involved to advocate for workplace safety? Can you identify committees, task forces, or councils focusing on this topic?

    a. Are these groups multidisciplinary and interprofessional? If not, should they be?

    b. How can you get involved with efforts to address these topics in professional societies or organizations? Is there an opportunity to foster interorganizational collaboration or coalition building?

    c. Have you held or attended forums with community leaders? How can you identify when and where these forums occur?

Professional Practice Example: Removing Scope-of-Practice Barriers for Advanced Practice Nurses

As a professional discipline, nursing operates within a social contract not only to develop and disseminate knowledge, but also to use that knowledge to care for people communities, and society (Donaldson & Crowley, 1978). The practice of nursing is regulated by the states. While nurses must pass one national licensure exam to be eligible for a license, each state has its own act that delineates the boundaries of nursing practice. Porter-O'Grady (2016) asserts that professions are held accountable to society based on a social mandate, noting that every profession has a social and legal right to "own and fully control the components of [its] practice separate from any institutional control by any entities or persons outside of its regulatory and professional agency" (p. 527). But he also notes that such rights have not been provided for the professional practice of nursing.

Mobilized by *The Future of Nursing* report (Institute of Medicine, 2011) and the Campaign for Action (2017) to advance and implement the report's recommendations, nurses in several states brought attention to the restrictive practice regulations governing advanced practice nurses (APRNs). *The Future of Nursing* report's recommendation to remove scope-of-practice barriers stimulated myriad nurse leaders to form an APRN workgroup.

While the quality of care and value of services provided by APRNs is well established, the politics around full practice authority and independent practice for APRNs are complex in some states. APRNs and nurse leaders from varied practice settings coalesced to engage with leaders of various professional nursing organizations, legislators, state regulators, and the public in order to inform and advance this discussion. One of the achievements of the APRN workgroup was a state-of-the-state report that shared the status of APRNs in their state for the four areas of advanced practice nursing (nurse practitioners, nurse anesthetists, nurse midwives, and psychiatric advanced practice nurses).

Subsequently, about one year later, a statewide APRN task force cochaired by a nurse and a physician was convened. All APRN specialties were represented along with relevant physician specialties and key stakeholders including those in anesthesia, OB/GYN, primary care, and psychiatry. Other group members represented the perspectives of patients, large private practices, home health, health insurers, attorneys, and policy-makers as they related to the scope of APRN practice. Frank discussion, differing positions and perspectives, and passionate, occasionally opposing viewpoints were offered by those on the task force when they were asked to comment on removing restrictive regulations. Although they weren't fully achieved, there were attempts to develop a consensus position for each of the APRN primary clinical practice areas. And where a consensus position was not fully achieved, the task force still made valuable contributions to the public-policy discussion. It did so by highlighting the various issues and perspectives involved in each practice area and attempting to narrow the differences among competing positions.

Nurse leaders participated in the task force in varying roles—as a cochair, as members, and as support staff. The varied roles of these nurse leaders and their established professional relationships allowed them to frankly express their viewpoints, confer with each other during and in between meetings, and leverage their respective task force roles to influence the outcome and recommendations.

This work has cumulatively raised awareness (problem identification and agenda setting) on the quality and cost of care and on the impact of APRNs on patient access. Evidence of an advanced policy discussion can be found in recommended healthcare-reform proposals (state Medicaid reform), improved traction for proposed APRN legislation, and testimony from multiple organizations. Both the report and the workgroup have been a source of reference and conversation by healthcare providers, lobbyists, legislators, and key stakeholders.

This example highlights how a focused priority—to address restrictive practice regulations for APRNs—was set at the national level and operationalized in one state. Progress was made incrementally and over time.

Questions for Consideration

1. Are you aware of the APRN scope-of-practice laws in your state?

    a. For nurse practitioners, clinical nurse specialists, nurse anesthetists, and nurse midwives?

2. Do APRNs in your state have full practice authority or restricted practice? How about within your organization of employment?

3. If APRNs do not have full practice authority, who is working toward such changes? Could such efforts be strengthened by increasing the number and diversity of the stakeholders involved?

4. To what extent do APRNs contribute to improved access to healthcare services? How do they compare to other providers when it comes to the quality and cost of services provided? How is this type of information collected? To how and to whom is it disseminated?

Professional Practice Example: Within Healthcare Organizations

Nurse leaders participate in policy within organizations in many ways. Regarding hospital board governance, evidence suggests that between 4% and 6% of hospitals have a nurse as a voting member of the board of trustees (Knowlton, 2014; Sundean, Polifroni, Libal, & McGrath, 2017). This startling statistic stimulated the formation of the Nurses on Boards Coalition in 2014 (Nurses on Boards Coalition, 2017). Additionally, where nurses do serve on the board of trustees, their potential contributions may be limited. Hughes (2010) describes traditional hierarchical structures and the dominance of the medical profession's authority leaving nurse board members feeling limited in their ability to contribute to decisions. Work remains at all levels of hospital and organizational governance as even chief nursing officers must continue to pursue parity with other hospital executives. "Without an equal voice in the boardroom, nurses cannot fulfill their professional obligation to society" (Sundean et al., 2017, p. 361).

Struggles of power within organizations have implications for institution-level policy that governs the delivery of healthcare services (Hughes, Carryer, & White, 2015). Richter et al. (2013) reports that nurses who participated in their study, Nurses Engagement in AIDS Policy Development, expressed a desire to be involved in policy work but lacked the opportunity to participate and engage in the process. They note that nurses are often asked to implement policies without having provided input into the policies' development, regardless of the source, which may be institutional, local, state, federal, or global.

While there remains a need for nurse leaders to address inequities in the governance of their employing organization, they should also consider developing strategies to encourage and support nurses' interactions with policy-makers. Waddell, Audette, DeLong, and Brostoff (2016) describe a collaboration between the nursing department and the office of government relations at an urban pediatric hospital. This mutually beneficial collaboration helped the government-relations staff better understand, and articulate to external audiences, how policy proposals align with the day-to-day needs and experiences of direct care providers. It also helped the participating nurses understand the value of engaging in the legislative process. From the government-relations staff, nurses learned essential policy skills such as how to prepare and deliver testimony, participate in legislative visits with state and federal elected officials, write and vet policy position statements with internal stakeholders, and develop and vet grassroots advocacy efforts within the hospital environment (Waddell et al., 2016).

Questions for Consideration

1. How do you contribute to and influence health-policy development and implementation? Do you do this through a formal role or through committee membership?

2. Are there opportunities for you, or your colleagues, to become more involved in policy decisions:

    a. Within your organization?

    b. Within your local community?

    c. At the state level?

    d. At the national level?

    e. On the global level?

3. At each of these levels of policy, what changes could be made to ensure a nursing perspective is represented?

Engaging more nurses in policy activities, for all levels of health policy, will require leaders to value and appreciate the contributions nurses make to such efforts. Leaders must prioritize policy-related activities for themselves and their staff so that contributions are not dependent on nurses finding free time to participate. This is challenging given the operational pressures described by nursing leaders in practice but should be a priority given the ideas being suggested to address challenges with the cost, quality, and access to healthcare services. Looking forward, leaders should consider whether some professional roles may need to be adjusted to create space for policy-related work.

Our experience in a multitude of policy situations, some of which are described in this chapter, has stimulated our thinking about what is needed by nurse leaders to increase nurses' contributions to policy. After watching attorneys engage in clinical practice issues and making recommendations to shape clinical practice, we must ask, "Where are our colleagues?" Leaders are aware that such decisions are being made, but they prioritize other efforts to the detriment of policy participation. Improvements are noted where deliberate efforts to engage nurses have occurred, but deepening and broadening participation cannot rely on the intentional efforts of a few (Thomas, Seifert, & Joyner, 2016). Improving population health through policy will require focused efforts by many leaders.

One may quantify exemplary nursing leadership in practice settings by accounting for the extent to which nurses—and nurse leaders—in an organization engage in policy-advocacy activities. "Although heads of medical and nursing departments have obvious leadership roles, the need for leadership by clinicians deeper in the organization—usually without any formal title, authority, or leadership job description— is increasingly recognized" (Bohmer, 2013, p. 1468). The role of the nurse leader must be to elevate the input of direct care nurses, both in organization-level governance and with external policy decision-makers (such as professional organizations and geopolitical communities). Leaders must work to foster collaborative relationships that will advance the dialogue related to important policy topics. Ultimately, exemplary nursing leadership must advance how members of the profession prioritize health-policy participation while building collaborations that facilitate policy participation.

Nurses Leaders in Health-Policy Research

Conducting timely and relevant research with health-policy implications is important as the United States explores options to improve health and healthcare delivery. When policy-makers ask policy questions, they often need answers in a shorter timeframe than what is normal for rigorous academic research projects. Martin, Currie, and Lockett (2011) describe "divergence between how research was valued by the institutions and actors of academia and those of government utilization" (p. 215). This draws attention to a value conflict between the desire to produce academically rigorous research that is suitable for publication in a reputable peer-reviewed journal and the more-applied research approaches that prioritize timeliness and insight to inform current policy proposals.

Ellenbecker and Edward (2016) explain that health-policy research addresses "current or future health problems and [informs] local, state, and national health policy solutions" (p. 211). They further note that methods of research will vary but that research is stronger when conducted by teams with disciplines such as nursing, economics, sociology, anthropology, political science, public health, and epidemiology represented. Research can target a specific step in the policy process (such as step 1, problem identification), and there are many examples of nursing research doing this. Ellenbecker and Edward (2016) provide examples of research addressing each step of the policy process. Nurse scientists should consider how explicitly they outline the policy implications of their research.

While publication of research findings is considered the ultimate dissemination among scholars, there can be a significant lag in the amount of time for research findings to make their way into policy discussions. Hewison (2008) cautions against a "reliance on evidence as the sole means of informing the policy process from a nursing perspective" (p. 295), as it can result in overemphasis of quantitative findings, it may not account for patient and provider preferences, and it may not inform steps toward incremental progress or system transformation. In addressing the challenges with traditional presentation of research findings, Crego and Islam (2016) state that "facts can speak for themselves but they frequently speak to themselves" (para. 36). Additionally, the specific and focused nature of many research findings make it difficult for policy-makers to interpret how easily the findings can be generalized or implemented broadly. Ideally, direct interactions between researchers and policy decision-makers benefit both parties, who will gain expanded insights and appreciation for each other's perspectives.

South and Cattan (2014) address the concept of knowledge transfer, defined as "a dynamic and iterative process that includes the synthesis, dissemination, exchange and ethically sound application of knowledge to improve the health of [people], provide more effective health services and products and strengthen the health care system" (Canadian Institutes of Health Research, 2012, para. 5). Knowledge transfer goes beyond a focus on dissemination and addresses a more intentional approach to bringing evidence into relevant forums. Knowledge translation may require a different skill set or research planning process from what is traditionally associated with academic research. For example, with emphasis on partnership, nurse scientists should engage with policy-makers if at all possible. If not, leaders should seek a member of the scholarly team to work as a "knowledge broker" (Martin, Currie, & Lockett, 2011, p. 215) to facilitate a direct interaction between the producers and users of research. Nurse scientists who are less inclined to interact directly with policy-makers may want to consider using social media platforms or blog posts to interpret, share, and promote research findings.

Exemplary nursing leadership in the area of policy research should involve deliberate efforts to delineate specific policy implications. The logistics of bringing into line the needs of policy-makers with the needs of the producers of research is challenging, but this work is well aligned with the role of nurse leaders as translators of policy-relevant information.

Nurse scientists may want to consider describing the stage of the policy process and the level of health policy most relevant to their research findings. Such efforts will simplify advocating the research findings and will help those without explicit health or research expertise. Ultimately, such efforts may increase the inclusion of nursing research in health-policy discussions. As the nursing profession works to increase influence in policy, journal editors may want to consider the extent to which they require policy implications to be discussed in manuscripts.

Similarly, nurse leaders must consider how they value and support dissemination of research findings to policy decision-makers and stakeholders. This involves examining the extent to which participation in policy activities is supported and appreciated as part of the academic role for tenured or tenure-track faculty. Director-level positions at academic institutions should be considered as a way to structurally address nursing's service to community and population health. Individuals or teams of researchers should be encouraged to produce policy positions that are easily understood by those who are not trained scientists, and researchers may want to consider disseminating research findings and policy recommendations over social media or through other media outlets. Leaders of professional nursing organizations may also want to evaluate how their organizations promote and share policy positions.

Nurse leaders may also want to consider how much they work to build interprofessional and diverse research teams. South and Cattan (2014) describe a framework for the co-construction of knowledge throughout the stages of study design, delivery, and dissemination. Deliberate efforts could enhance the evidence for community-based health-promotion interventions or policy-oriented research. In their efforts to describe or address current policy problems, leaders should think broadly about ways to expand collaborations designed to provide complementary knowledge, skills, or expertise. Leaders may find it useful to evaluate the extent to which academic and practice groups are working together—are there opportunities to strengthen collaborations in a way that would present a unified front or strengthened position on a policy topic?

Bringing It All Together

Today's challenge is to align nursing's strengths with problems on the policy agenda (at all levels) to elevate the contributions of nursing within a society that cares deeply about business interests and competition and is noncommittal when it comes to prioritizing health and care. Policy-making can be thought of as the evolving "criteria for classification, the boundaries of categories, and the definition of ideas that guide the way people behave" (Stone, 2002, p. 11). Nursing is about providing service to human beings within the context of society; accepting this makes the intersection of nursing work and policy more tangible. Individual nurses work through multiple structures to influence and govern nursing practice and contribute to decisions regarding the provision of healthcare services. And the profession as a whole must work to identify policy preferences and make them known to the public and to decision-makers in a timely fashion.

Nursing is both a practice-based and an academic discipline, which positions it well to influence policy discussions. Nurses make up the largest sector of the healthcare workforce and are present in nearly every setting in which healthcare services are delivered. Nurses can identify examples of policies that are not meeting the needs of clients, and such observations must make their way into policy discussions. When communicating policy ideas, nurses may find it useful to couple research findings or data describing a problem with real-word examples or stories, as the combination of qualitative and quantitative information is very powerful. Crego and Islam (2016) note that feelings are more likely than facts to influence thinking and behavior, an important point to note when working to shape policy. Nurse leaders should consider how to share their knowledge, expertise, and experiences in the most effective way to improve health policy and the health of populations.

If policy reflects the dominant belief of a culture, then efforts must continue to obtain power, as it is needed to influence and create change (MacDonnell, 2010). Given the range of proposed ideas to address access to healthcare services and the cost of such services, nurse leaders should be courageous and bold when messaging concerns or support about policy proposals. It is increasingly important for leaders to gain confidence in translating implications of current policies and proposed policy ideas. Nurse leaders need to be comfortable stating outrage if in fact a policy proposal is outrageous! We can do this with an honest yet tactful and professional message. The same is true for policy ideas that would advance the health of people and populations; we should not withhold support. The public, elected officials and their staff, and fellow nurses are looking to nurse leaders for reactions and interpretation of policy ideas.

Health-policy efforts are inherently interprofessional; diversity among collaborators is an asset and a source of power. Creating shared meanings and purpose motivates people and creates excitement, and nurse leaders should work to foster dynamic collaborations with the goal of improving population health through practice, research, and policy. Nurse leaders should consider collaboration broadly. For example, are professional organizations collaborating with each other to form consistent positions, recommendations, and messages on important policy topics? How about experts in academic and practice settings or colleges within a university? Patient advocates, community-based organizations, or other important stakeholders? Scanning the environment, or one's professional network, for answers to these questions will inform next steps.

Translation is a large part of the nurse leader's role in policy—translation of healthcare realities, translation of patient needs and experiences, and translation of research findings. The question is, Do nurses see that as part of their professional role? Do they prioritize policy efforts and protect time to engage with policy-makers or the public on policy topics? Nurse leaders must create opportunities for nurses to participate in such efforts. In addressing nursing's social responsibility, Tyer-Viola et al. (2009) highlight the values of equity, access, and justice, noting that participation in policy links the concept of caring to the welfare of society. With a social mandate to serve society, nurse leaders must think about what is needed for members of the profession—across academic and practice settings—to more completely fulfill that mandate.

Nurse leaders must design and operationalize models that facilitate participation in policy. Martin, Currie, and Lockett (2011) asked the question, "What can be done upstream to . . . assist the production of research knowledge that is more readily utilized by health care managers and other stakeholders downstream?" (p. 212). Nurse leaders conducting research should also consider this question and may want to engage with policy-makers to gain insight into this area. In colleges, universities, hospitals, and healthcare delivery organizations that have a commitment to public, population, or community health, nurse leaders should work to operationalize that aspect of the organization's mission into professional roles designed to influence policy. The need for quality- and patient-focused policy is as important now as ever, and nurses have a tremendous opportunity to contribute to such efforts.

Chapter Key Points

- The skill of translation is important in a nurse's role in influencing policy.

- Nursing is practice based and an academic discipline.

- Nurse leaders should focus on the question, What can be changed upstream?

References

Backer, Costello-Nikitas, Mason, McBride, & Vance (1993, summer). Legislative update power at the policy table when women and nurses are involved. *Revolution*, 68–75.

Bohmer, R. M. (2013). Leading clinicians and clinicians leading. *New England Journal of Medicine, 368*(16), 1468–70. DOI: 10.1056/NEJMp1301814.

Brehaut, J. D. & Juzwishin, D. (2005). *Bridging the gap: The use of research evidence in policy development.* Edmonton, Canada: Alberta Heritage Foundation for Medical Research.

Campaign for Action (2017). *State action coalitions.* Retrieved from http://campaignforaction.org/our-network/state-action-coalitions/

Canadian Institutes of Health Research. (2009). *About us.* Retrieved from http://www.cihr-irsc.gc.ca/e/29418.html

Centers for Disease Control and Prevention. (2017). *Understanding the epidemic.* Retrieved from https://www.cdc.gov/drugoverdose/epidemic/index.html.

Centers for Medicare & Medicaid Services. (2017). *NHE fact sheet.* Retrieved from https://www.cms.gov/research-statistics-data-and-systems/statistics-trends-and-reports/nationalhealthexpenddata/nhe-fact-sheet.html

Cohen, S. S. & Muench, U. (2012). Nursing testimony before congress, 1993-2011. *Policy, Politics & Nursing Practice, 13*(3), 170–78. DOI: 10.1177/1527154412471201

Crego, E. & Islam, F. (2016, December 6). 2016 presidential election analysis: The Trump cards. *The Huffington Post.* Retrieved from http://www.huffingtonpost.com/entry/2016-presidential-election-analysis-the-trump-cards_us_5845bdd3e4b0707e4c81715b

Donaldson, S. K. & Crowley, D. M. (1978). The discipline of nursing. *Nursing Outlook, 26*(2), 113–20.

Duncan, S., Throne, S., & Rodney, P. (2015). Evolving trends in nursing regulation: What are the policy impacts for nursing's social mandate? *Nursing Inquiry, 22*(1), 27–38. DOI: 10.1111/nin.12087

Dye, T. R. (2013). *Understanding public policy* (14th ed.). Englewood Cliffs, NJ: Pearson.

Ellenbecker, C. & Edward, J. (2017). Conducting nursing research to advance and inform health policy. *Policy, Politics & Nursing Practice, 17*(4), 208–17. DOI: 10.1177/1527154417700634

Fawcett, J. (in press). Transitions in nursology from pre-history to contemporary times and adapting to the current age of uncertainty, disquiet, and upheaval. *Japanese Journal of Nursing Research.*

Fyffe, T. (2005). *"The tipping point" Developing nursing's influence on policy & politics.* London, England: Florence Nightingale Foundation.

Gebbie, K., Wakefield, M., & Kerfoot, K. (2000). Nursing and health policy. *Journal of Nursing Scholarship, 32*(3), 307–15. DOI: 10.1111/j.1547-5069.2000.00307.x

Hahn, J. (2010). Integrating professionalism and political awareness into the curriculum. *Nurse Educator, 35*(3), 110–13. DOI: 10.1097/NNE.0b013e3181d95040

Hewison, A. (2008). Evidence-based policy. *Policy, Politics & Nursing Practice, 9*(4), 288–98. DOI: 10.1177/1527154408323242

Hughes, A. (2010). The challenge of contributing to policy making in primary care: The gendered experiences and strategies of nurses. *Sociology of Health & Illness, 32*(7), 977–92. DOI: 10.1111/j.1467-9566.2010.01258.x

Hughes, K. A., Carryer, J., & White, J. (2015). Structural positioning of nurse leaders and empowerment. *Journal of Clinical Nursing, 24*(15/16), 2125–32. DOI: 10.1111/jocn.12839

Institute of Medicine. (2010). *The future of nursing: Leading change, advancing health.* Washington, DC: National Academies Press.

Knowlton, D. L. (2014, October 9). Hospitals must recruit nurses to their leadership boards [blog post]. Retrieved from https://www.rwjf.org/en/culture-of-health/2014/10/hospitals_must_recru.html

Lavizzo-Mourey, R. (2014). *Building a culture of health: 2014 president's message.* Retrieved from Robert Wood Johnson Foundation: http://www.rwjf.org/content/dam/files/rwjf-web-files/Annual_Message/2014_RWJF_AnnualMessage_final.pdf

Long, R. (2005). From revelation to revolution: critical care nurses' emerging roles in public policy. Critical Care Nursing Clinics of North America, 17, 191–99.

MacDonnell, J. (2010). Policy talk: Gender and the regulation of nursing knowledges and practices. *Advances in Nursing Science, 33*(3), 219–33. DOI: 10.1097/ANS.0b013e3181eb4215

Martin, G., Currie, G., & Lockett, A. (2011). Prospects for knowledge exchange in health policy and management: Institutional and epistemic boundaries. *Journal of Health Services Research & Policy, 16*(4), 211–17. DOI: 10.1258/jhsrp.2011.010132

Massachusetts Department of Public Health. (2017a). *Data brief: Opioid-related overdose deaths among Massachusetts residents (August 2017).* Retrieved from https://www.mass.gov/files/documents/2017/08/31/data-brief-overdose-deaths-aug-2017.pdf

Massachusetts Department of Public Health. (2017b). *MA Prescription Monitoring Program county-level data measures (2017 quarter 2).* Retrieved from https://www.mass.gov/files/documents/2017/08/31/prescription-monitoring-program-data-aug-2017.pdf

Montalvo, W. (2015). Political skill and its relevance to nursing. *The Journal of Nursing Administration, 45*(7/8), 337–83.

National Academies of Science, Engineering, and Medicine. (2015). *Assessing progress on the Institute of Medicine report The Future of Nursing.* Washington, DC: National Academies Press.

Nurses on Boards Coalition (2017). *Our story.* Retrieved from https://www.nursesonboardscoalition.org/about/

O'Grady, E. T., Mason, D. J., Hopkins Outlaw, F., & Gardner, D. B. (2016). Frameworks for action in policy and politics. In D. J. Mason, D. B. Gardner, F. Hopkins Outlaw, & E. T. O'Grady (Eds.), *Policy & Politics in Nursing and Health Care* (7th ed., pp. 1–21). St. Louis, MO: Elsevier.

Porche, D. J. (2010). *Health policy: Application for nurses and other healthcare professionals.* Sudbury, MA: Jones & Bartlett.

Porter-O'Grady, T. (2016). Re: Joseph M., & Borgue, R. (2016). A theory-based approach to nursing shared governance. 64. Pp. 339 to 351 [letter to the editor]. *Nursing Outlook, 64*(6), 527–29. DOI: 10.1016/j.outlook.2016.09.001

Richter, M.S., Mill, J., Muller, C. E., Kahwa, E., Etowa, J., Dawkins, P., & Hepburn, C. (2013). Nurses' engagement in AIDS policy development. *International Nursing Review, 60*(1), 52–58. DOI: 10.1111/j.1466-7657.2012.01010.x

Russell, G. & Fawcett, J. (2005). The conceptual model for nursing and health policy revisited. *Policy, Politics & Nursing Practice, 6*(4), 319–26. DOI: 10.1177/1527154405283304

Shariff, N. (2015). A Delphi survey of leadership attributes necessary for national nurse leaders' participation in health policy development: An East African perspective. *BMC Nursing, 14*(13), 1–8. DOI: 10.1186/s12912-015-0063-0

South, J. & Cattan, M. (2014). Developing evidence for public health policy and practice: The implementation of a knowledge translation approach in a staged, multi-methods study in England, 2007–09. *Evidence and Policy: A Journal of Research, Debate and Practice, 10*(3), 379–96. DOI: 10.1332/174426414X13920508946082

Stone, D. (2002). *Policy Paradox: The art of political decision making* (revised ed.) New York, NY: Norton & Company.

Sundean, L., Polifroni, E. C., Libal, K., & McGrath, J. M. (2017). Nurses on health care governing boards: An integrative review. *Nursing Outlook, 65*(4), 361–71. DOI: 10.1016/j.outlook.2017.01.009

Thomas, T.W., Seifert, P.C., & Joyner, J.C. (2016). Registered nruses leading innovative changes. *Online Journal in Nursing, 21*(3).

Tyer-Viola, L., Nicholas, P. K., Corless, I. B., Barry, D. M., Hoyt, P., Fitzpatrick, J. J., & Davis, S. M. (2009). Social responsibility of nursing: A global perspective. *Policy, Politics & Nursing Practice, 10*(2), 110–18. DOI: 10.1177/1527154409339528

Waddell, A., Audette, K., DeLong, A., & Brostoff, M. (2016). A hospital-based interdisciplinary model for increasing nurses' engagement in legislative advocacy. *Policy, Politics & Nursing Practice, 17*(1), 15–23. DOI: 10.1177/1527154416630638

Afterword

Consilience Spiraling Upward: MILE TWO

Jeffrey M. Adams, PhD, RN, NEA-BC, FAAN
Jennifer Mensik, PhD, RN, NEA-BC, FAAN
Patricia Reid Ponte, DNSc, RN, NEA-BC, FAAN
Jacqueline Somerville, PhD, RN, FAAN

\Con*sil"i*ence\, n. [con- + salire to leap.] Act of concurring; coincidence; concurrence. The consilience of inductions takes place when one class of facts coincides with an induction obtained from another different class.

("Consilience," n.d.)

Throughout this book we've shared exemplars of strategies to quantifiably influence the advancement of leadership practice, research, education, policy, practice, theory, media and industry. This endeavor was written to embrace the breadth and depth of existing nursing-leadership knowledge while supporting a need and opportunity for assimilation of new knowledge. This assimilation brings an ever-increasing clarity, professional unity, articulation, and integration to the care of individuals, groups, and communities and also to the care for those who lead and provide this care. The application of consilience within the framework of nursing and nursing's relationship with other disciplines can help bring new clarity to the dialogue.

The concept of consilience was discussed by philosophers of science for more than 100 years, but it was not until Edward O. Wilson's book *Consilience: The Unity of Knowledge* was published that the concept became much more a part of the scientific vernacular. Wilson's (1998) concept of consilience suggests that knowledge should not be explained through a separation and isolation of common themes. Rather, consilience of knowledge can only be achieved by unifying these themes. This is appropriate for our approach to articulate quantifiable "good" leadership.

Consilience in Nursing

Jacobs (2001) suggested that consilience in nursing could best be explained by identifying common themes in nursing literature (nursing, science, art, holism, knowledge, truth, and ethics) as concepts under which nursing knowledge and practice is specialized and classified. This approach builds on the notion that in nursing's early stages, it was developed with multiple, seemingly disconnected theories to describe the discipline (Smith, 1999). Jacobs also suggested that nursing knowledge and practice are inconsistent and often dichotomous as applied within roles of specialization. This construct of role or content in specialty nursing currently spans education, policy, practice, research, and theory. It is melded into the bucket of "nursing knowledge."

Our intent of this book being to span and unite the approach to understanding nursing leadership, we have purposefully included evidence from emergent thinking to work more mature in its development. Similar to Benner's novice-to-expert competency model (Benner, 2001), each reader of this book has their own unique combination of competencies, experiences, and values that have influenced their own development in these areas.

Traditionally, knowledge is developed and utilized in silos where many dissertations, capstones, and theses are shelved as "learning experiences" of the student and not integrated effectively into advancing knowledge of the whole. Tenure for academics rewards the publish-or-perish mindset over the optimized research methods or innovative approaches necessary. Practice scholars struggle to find buy-out time and are often faced with the realization of the need to do more with less.

Nurses work with and lead others to address the complexity of humans while being constantly influenced and forever responding and changing. Admittedly with 4 million nurses in the United States alone, and 19+ million globally, nursing is perhaps the most complex of disciplines because of our expansive depth and breadth of roles, reach, and impact. Melding basic science with social science, having multiple educational preparations, and having an expansive array of roles across specializations is just the tip of the iceberg.

It is important to identify the way we know—empirically, personally, aesthetically, ethically (Carper, 1978), sociopolitically (White, 1995), or emancipatory (Chinn & Kramer, 2011)—with proper language (Reid Ponte, Somerville, & Adams, 2016) in order to frame, describe, and influence others based on what we know and contribute. It is the totality of these ways of knowing that provide an individual and a discipline with a focused perspective on knowledge and a structured mechanism for describing the work and value the discipline brings.

It was our development of this book and bringing together what many see as the seemingly differing "silos" that led us to conceptualize the graphic Model of Influential Leadership Enhancements—Toward Wellness Outcomes (MILE TWO), depicted in figure A-1.

The MILE TWO represents a "spiraling upward" (Havens, 2008) toward optimized leadership, both in the global knowledge and the individual. As each piece or siloed area of knowledge is attained, it contributes to the greater whole and becomes part of the readily accessible pool informing others and incrementally growing knowledge toward a unified goal. In the scenarios contained within this book, the MILE TWO represents an ever-growing endeavor to optimize and unify leadership across a variety of topics to enhance the wellness of patient populations, the workforce, and organizations.

I did then what I knew how to do.
Now that I know better, I do better.

—Maya Angelou

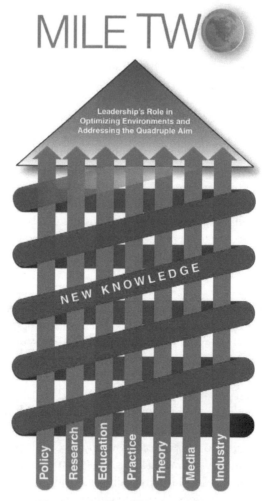

Model of Influential Leadership Enhancements –
Toward Wellness Outcomes (MILE TWO)

FIGURE A–1.   MILE TWO (©Jeff Adams, LLC)

As the American Nurses Association (n.d.) states, all nurses are leaders. It's not just those in formal leadership positions, but also bedside nurses, nursing students, all nurses. Although we tend to think that all leaders are managers and all managers are leaders, this is not entirely true. The danger in this thinking is that those not in management believe they need a formal title to effect change and that those with a formal title are the ones that control change, allowing only certain change to occur. There is too much work in our profession, let alone in healthcare, for only a small group to be leaders. If we continue to perpetuate this thinking, then we will lose our power: the power of 4 million nurses who have the ability to change the health policy of this country through our influence, the trust placed in us, and our voices.

In leadership, there is a tendency to follow the leadership trend of the month. Usually a new book or set of research states that certain leadership traits, individually or organizationally, are the key to effective change. What we know, however, through experience and research is that there is not necessarily one right way but many potential ways to accomplish a goal. There are many ways to think about leadership and know that leaders do not silence others based on a lack of years of experience, degrees, or credentials or based on job title. Leaders recognize the inherit value of each person and invite them to the table. As you read this book, you can recognize that leadership is a complex concept composed of many different components. Each leader works to organize, optimize, and utilize these components differently to effectively and purposefully influence change.

A great leader knows when to use the right intervention at the right time, in the right dose, delivered to the right people, for the right reason. Be that leader.

References

American Nurses Association. (n.d.). *About ANA*. Retrieved August 20, 2018, from http://www.nursingworld.org/FunctionalMenuCategories/AboutANA

Benner, P. (2001). *From novice to expert: Excellence and power in clinical nursing practice* (2nd ed.). Upper Saddle River, NJ: Prentice Hall Press.

Carper, B. A. (1978). Fundamental patterns of knowing in nursing. *Advances in Nursing Science, 1*(1), 13–23.

Chinn, P. L., & Kramer, M. K. (2011). *Integrated theory and knowledge development in nursing* (8th ed.). St. Louis, MO: Mosby.

Consilience. (n.d.). In *Online Etymology Dictionary*. Retrieved June 4, 2016, from http://dictionary.reference.com/browse/consilience

Havens, D.S. (2008). *Spiraling upward for nurse retention and quality care*. Department of Health and Human Services, Health Resources and Services Administration—Nurse Education, Practice, and Retention Grants Program, HRSA-D11HP09752-01-01. July 2008–June 2013.

Jacobs, B. B. (2001). Respect for human dignity: A central phenomenon to philosophically unite nursing theory and practice through consilience of knowledge. *Advances in Nursing Science, 24*(1), 17–35.

Reid Ponte, P., Somerville, J., & Adams J. M. (2016) Assuring the capture of standardized nursing data: A call to action for chief nursing officers. *International Journal of Nursing Knowledge, 27*(3), 48–55.

Smith, M. C. (1999). Caring and the science of unitary human beings. *Advances in Nursing Science, 21*(4), 14–28.

Wilson, E. O. (1998). *Consilience: The unity of knowledge*. New York, NY: Random House.

White, J. (1995). Patterns of knowing: Review, critique and update. *Advances in Nursing Science, 17*(4), 73–86.

Index